T0306115

# Emergency Department Leadership and Management

## Best Principles and Practice

# Emergency Department Leadership and Management

## Best Principles and Practice

Editor-in-Chief

### Stephanie Kayden MD, MPH

Chief,
Division of International Emergency Medicine and Humanitarian Programs,
Department of Emergency Medicine, Brigham and Women's Hospital
and Harvard Medical School, Boston, MA, USA

Editors

### Philip D. Anderson MD, MPH

Associate Director of Quality Assurance,
Department of Emergency Medicine, Beth Israel Deaconess Medical Center, Harvard Medical School,
Boston, MA, USA

### Robert Freitas MHA

Executive Director,
Emergency Medicine Consulting Division, Harvard Medical Faculty Physicians at Beth Israel
Deaconess Medical Center, Boston, MA, USA

### Elke Platz MD, MS

Director of Emergency Ultrasound Research,
Department of Emergency Medicine, Brigham and Women's Hospital and Harvard Medical School,
Boston, MA, USA

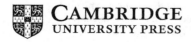

CAMBRIDGE
UNIVERSITY PRESS

# CAMBRIDGE
## UNIVERSITY PRESS

University Printing House, Cambridge CB2 8BS, United Kingdom

One Liberty Plaza, 20th Floor, New York, NY 10006, USA

477 Williamstown Road, Port Melbourne, VIC 3207, Australia

4843/24, 2nd Floor, Ansari Road, Daryaganj, Delhi - 110002, India

79 Anson Road, #06-04/06, Singapore 079906

Cambridge University Press is part of the University of Cambridge.

It furthers the University's mission by disseminating knowledge in the pursuit of education, learning and research at the highest international levels of excellence.

www.cambridge.org
Information on this title: www.cambridge.org/9781107007390

© Cambridge University Press 2015

First published 2015

*A catalogue record for this publication is available from the British Library*

*Library of Congress Cataloging in Publication data*
Emergency department leadership and management : best
principles and practice / editor-in-chief, Stephanie Kayden ;
editors, Philip D. Anderson, Robert Freitas, Elke Platz.
        p. ; cm.
Includes bibliographical references and index.
ISBN 978-1-107-00739-0 (Hardback)
I.  Kayden, Stephanie, editor of compilation.    II.  Anderson, PhilipD.
(Philip Dean), editor of compilation.    III.  Freitas, Robert, editor of
compilation.    IV.  Platz, Elke, editor of compilation.
[DNLM: 1.  Emergency Service, Hospital–organization &
administration. 2.  Leadership.  WX 215]
RA971
362.11068–dc23        2013050334

ISBN  978-1-107-00739-0  Hardback

For my family
S.K.

To Sophie and Kate
P.A.

With thanks to my family for their support
R.F.

To my parents
E.P.

# Contents

## Section 4 – Special topics

# Contributors

**Venkataraman Anantharaman MBBS, FRCP (Edin), FRCS Ed (A&E), FAMS**
Department of Emergency Medicine, Singapore General Hospital, Singapore

**Philip D. Anderson MD**
Department of Emergency Medicine, Beth Israel Deaconess Medical Center, Boston, MA, USA

**Christopher W. Baugh MD MBA**
Department of Emergency Medicine, Brigham and Women's Hospital, Boston, MA, USA

**J. Stephen Bohan MD MS FACP FACEP**
Department of Emergency Medicine, Brigham and Women's Hospital, Boston, MA, USA

**Kirsten Boyd RN MHA**
Department of Emergency Medicine, Beth Israel Deaconess Medical Center, Boston, MA, USA

**Matthias Brachmann PhD**
Bredehorst Clinic, Medical Management GmbH, Düsseldorf, Germany

**Peter R. Brown**
Chief of Staff, Office of the CEO, Partners HealthCare, Boston, MA, USA

**Shelley Calder MSN RN**
Department of Emergency Medicine, Beth Israel Deaconess Medical Center, Boston, MA, USA

**David Callaway MD**
Department of Emergency Medicine, Carolinas Medical Center, Charlotte, NC, USA

**Peter Cameron MBBS MD FACEM FIFEM**
Department of Emergency Medicine, Hamad Medical Corporation, Doha, Qatar

**Jody Crane MD**
Fredericksburg Emergency, Medical Alliance Inc., Mary Washington Hospital Emergency, Fredericksburg, VA, USA

**Meaghan Cussen MA**
Department of Emergency Medicine, Beth Israel Deaconess Medical Center, Boston, MA, USA

**Christina Dempsey BSN MBA CNOR**
Chief Nursing Officer, Press Ganey Associates, South Bend, IN, USA

**Jonathan A. Edlow MD FACEP**
Department of Emergency Medicine, Beth Israel Deaconess Medical Center, Boston, MA, USA

**Thomas Fleischmann MD FCEM FESEM MHBA**
Department of Emergency Medicine, Salzgitter Hospital, Salzgitter, Germany

**Robert L. Freitas MHA**
Harvard Medical Faculty Physicians at Beth Israel Deaconess Medical Center, Boston, MA, USA

**John D. Halamka MD MS**
Department of Emergency Medicine, Beth Israel Deaconess Medical Center, Boston, MA

**Manuel Hernandez MD MBA FACEP**
CannonDesign, Chicago, IL, USA; Department of Emergency Medicine, University of Florida College of Medicine at Jacksonville, Jacksonville, FL, USA

**Cherri Hobgood MD**
Department of Emergency Medicine, Indiana University, School of Medicine, Indianapolis, IN, USA

**Jock Hoffman MA MD**
Division of Emergency Medicine, David Geffen
School of Medicine, UCLA Emergency Medical
Centre, Los Angeles, CA, USA

**Steven Horng MD**
Department of Emergency Medicine, Beth Israel
Deaconess Medical Center, Boston, MA, USA

**Kirk B. Jensen MD MBA FACEP**
Chief Medical Officer, BestPractices Inc., Raleigh,
NC, USA; Executive Vice President, EmCare, Dallas,
TX, USA

**Jennifer R. Johnson BS**
Independent Project Manager, Eugene, OR, USA

**Stephanie Kayden MD MPH**
Department of Emergency Medicine,
Brigham and Women's Hospital, Boston,
MA, USA

**Tasnim Khan MD MHCM**
Medical Director Level III, Executive Health
Resources, United Health Care Group, Newtown
Square, PA, USA

**Daniel G. Kirkpatrick MHA FACHE**
Founder and Managing Partner, Partners in
Improvement, Rocky Mount, NC, USA

**James Lennon AIA ACHA**
Lennon Associates Inc., Del Mar, CA, USA

**Mary Leupold MA**
Director, Human Resources Operations, Harvard
Medical Faculty Physicians at Beth Israel Deaconess
Medical Center, Boston, MA, USA

**Thom Mayer MD FACEP FAAP**
Founder and CEO, BestPractices Inc., Fairfax, VA,
USA

**J. Lawrence Mottley MD**
Department of Emergency Medicine, Beth Israel
Deaconess Medical Center, Boston, MA, USA

**Scott B. Murray MD**
Chief, Emergency Department, Nashoba Valley
Medical Center, Ayer, MA, USA

**Deirdre Mylod PhD**
Vice President of Hospital Services, Press Ganey
Associates, South Bend, IN, USA

**Larry A. Nathanson MD**
Department of Emergency Medicine,
Beth Israel Deaconess Medical Center, Boston,
MA, USA

**Michael P. Pietrzak MD**
Director of Strategic Initiatives, MedStar Institute for
Innovation (MI2), Washington, DC, USA

**Elke Platz MD MS**
Department of Emergency Medicine, Brigham and
Women's Hospital, Boston, MA, USA

**Nadeem Qureshi MD**
Department of Emergency Medicine, King Faisal
Specialist Hospital and Research Center, Riyadh,
Saudi Arabia

**Matthew M. Rice MD JD FACEP**
Department of Emergency Medicine,
Summit Pacific Community Hospital,
Madigan Army Medical Center, Gig Harbor,
WA, USA

**Andrew Schenkel MBA DIC PhD**
Assistant Professor, Stockholm School of Economics,
Stockholm, Sweden

**Chet Schrader MD FACEP**
Department of Emergency Medicine, John Peter
Smith Hospital, Fort Worth, TX, USA

**Puneet Seth MD**
Department of Emergency Medicine, Singapore
General Hospital, Singapore

**Richard B. Siegrist, Jr. MBA MS**
Department of Health Policy and Management,
Harvard School of Public Health, Boston, MA, USA

**David Smith MD**
Department of Emergency Medicine, King Faisal
Specialist Hospital and Research Center, Riyadh,
Saudi Arabia

**Robert E. Suter DO MHA FACEP FAAEM
FACOEP-D FIFEM**
Division of Emergency Medicine, University of Texas
Southwestern, Dallas, TX, USA

**Carrie Tibbles MD**
Department of Emergency Medicine,
Beth Israel Deaconess Medical Center,
Boston, MA, USA

**Sebastian N. Walker BSc (Eng) Aero**
Global Program Manager, Thomas Reuters

**Lee A. Wallis MBChB MD FRCSEd FCEM FCEM(SA)**
Head of Medicine, University of Cape Town, Cape Town, South Africa

**Julie Welch MD**
Department of Emergency Medicine, Indiana University, School of Medicine, Indianapolis, IN, USA

**Leana S. Wen MD MSc**
Director of Patient-Centered Care Research, Department of Emergency Medicine, George Washington University, Washington, DC, USA

# Foreword

In the *Chicago Sun-Times*, Ashley Montagu once said that "no history of art can be more dramatic than that of medicine, for there is hardly an aspect of life and society upon which it does not touch." When he wrote those words, emergency medicine (EM) was not born, but in my opinion it is more appropriate to emergency medicine than to any other specialty.

The history of emergency medicine takes us back to Charak, an Indian physician of 300 BC, and to Iwty of Egypt, from the Nineteenth Dynasty. Whilst they both practiced what is now known as emergency medicine, however, there is no evidence to suggest that either of them could be thought of as providing pioneering leadership to modern emergency medicine.

I do not wish either to interpret the past or to forecast the future, because leaders, like historians, often get many things wrong when they interpret the past – and most things wrong when they forecast the future. However, there is now some evidence of what I said in the first George Podgorny lecture (ICEM 2002), that "the twenty-first century will be the century for and of emergency medicine."

The twentieth century saw the development of a number of new disciplines and subspecialties in medicine. The first ever professional organization created for emergency medicine (then known as casualty medicine and surgery, or accident and emergency medicine) was the Casualty Surgeons' Association in the UK, established in 1967, which staged the first International Conference on Emergency Medicine in London in 1986. I was fortunate to be one of the organizers. This subsequently led to the formation of the International Federation for Emergency Medicine (IFEM) in 1991, the foundation of which was due to the foresight shown by the leadership of the four founding members of IFEM, the Casualty Surgeons' Association (now the College of Emergency Medicine in the UK), the American College of Emergency Physicians, the Australasian College for Emergency Medicine, and the Canadian Association of Emergency Physicians. It is believed that this initiative changed the perception of emergency medicine and the provision of emergency care worldwide. The founders acted on the principle of Mark Twain that if you do what you did, you get what you got.

Further progress by IFEM made it clear that for anything that needs progression, the leaders must provide leadership with sincerity and dedication, competency to manage, clear purpose, and reputable status. They require attending to all details and, if required, recreating a modern organization with some autonomy. This applies to any organizational and management aspects. For effective leadership, a leader needs to guide colleagues by persuasion, by appropriate and positive actions or opinions, because a leader holds a dominant or a superior position in the field and is able to exercise a high degree of control or influence over others.

There are two types of leaders. One is the type described by Confucius, easy to serve but difficult to please. Another is General Patton's type: "Lead me, follow me, or get out of my way." I suggest that the ideal is a mixture of the two, a leader who is easy to follow and also easy to help. In my opinion there are six principles of an effective leader: passion, art of presentation (communication), policies and actions, skills to deliver, ability to meet challenges, and clear goals for the future. As leaders, we need to remember not to associate with people we would not trust our lives to or give our lives for. A leader needs to identify the tasks, the teams, and the individuals for these teams. For effective leadership, one needs to have Gandhi's humanity and humility, Mandela's warmth and integrity, and Churchill's vision and toughness. Because vision without action is a dream, and action without vision is passing time, but vision with action changes the world. Leadership is all about creating a vision to which others can aspire, and energizing them to work towards that vision.

In the modern world we need to appreciate that whilst we deal with the sick and injured, for further development and wider acceptance of the specialty there is a need for us to understand that we are influenced by local governments and politics. Cooperation from law makers will enhance our cause. There is a need to appreciate the usefulness of wider participation in international agencies such as the WHO and regional emergency medicine organizations. Understand that the politics, the usefulness of wider participation, and the uniqueness of our specialty make a distinguished triad. A leader cannot ignore the fact that there are different systems of delivering care, along with geographical and cultural variations, in the global society.

There are six **C**'s of success. Leadership needs to demonstrate a clear **C**onception, to have strong **C**onfidence, to have focused **C**oncentration on what is being done, and to do that with **C**onsistency. Character and emotional **C**ommitment of leadership will bring success.

In the culture of an ever-changing world, we need to remember that if it isn't broken, don't mend it. A leader is responsible for the success, as well as the failure, of a group. As Confucius once said, our greatest glory is not in never falling but in rising every time we fall.

This book is the first of its kind, totally focused on all aspects of leadership in emergency medicine. Very many distinguished leaders in the field have contributed to a detailed discussion of the principles of leadership, management, and organization in emergency medicine. The special topics are of particular interest. And I am confident that the book as a whole will provide material for all grades of emergency physicians, from specialist trainees to established leaders. Let us hope that the development of effective leadership in emergency medicine worldwide goes a long way towards the provision of high-quality emergency medical care for our patients.

I feel very honored and privileged to have been asked to write this foreword. I wish you and this book a great success.

*Gautam G. Bodiwala, CBE, DL, JP, DSc (Hon), MS, FRCS, FRCP, FCEM, FIFEM*
*Former President, International Federation for Emergency Medicine*

# Leadership in emergency medicine

Robert L. Freitas

## Key learning points

- Understand the difference between leadership and management, and recognize competencies that make a good emergency department leader.
- Studies of leadership have produced little evidence to explain what works, but more recent studies of emotional intelligence can be used to develop or improve leadership skills.
- Good leaders are risk takers who use occasional failures to learn to become better leaders.

## Introduction

Healthcare organizations (HCOs) and emergency departments (EDs) will usually have many managers but few true leaders, even though in today's ED leadership is more important than ever. The ED leader of today deals with constant change, rising expectations of payers and patients, fewer resources with which to treat more patients, tough competition for talented clinicians and managers, mountains of information and data to sort out, and increasing acuity of patients. Some ED leaders also face chronic staff or equipment shortages, pandemics and disasters, and a variety of other challenges every day. These challenges force us to be creative, to build teams and harness their collective power, and often to change the way patient care is provided in radical ways.

Many of the studies written about leadership have focused on for-profit organizations. *Stodgill's Handbook of Leadership* makes references to thousands of scholarly studies of leadership.[1] Unfortunately, few academic works address leadership in health care, and almost none deals with emergency medicine. This lack of science is complicated by the fact that much of the

world's health care is provided by public agencies, which adds a political component to the ED leader's job. While it can be argued that leadership is different within public and private entities, modern healthcare systems are starting to operate more like private businesses, with a focus on providing cost-conscious, efficient, and high-quality services. Public healthcare leaders need to be just as innovative, entrepreneurial, and motivated as their private-sector counterparts.

Nevertheless, leaders in a public healthcare system must use power in a somewhat unique way. First, these leaders must understand the politicians who often set policy, allocate resources, and determine time frames for action. Second, they must take into account citizens, patients, and patients' rights groups. Finally, they must translate all of this into meaningful action understood by clinical staff members who often resist change wrought by the "political good."

## Leadership versus management

There is much debate about the differences between managers and leaders. It is usually said that the four key activities of managers are budgeting, controlling, planning, and organizing. Thus, the line between leader and manager can be blurred by the activities of the individual.[2] Some who think they are leaders are in fact managers because of the way they approach work; some managers are leaders by virtue of how they get the job done. Title alone does not separate the manager from the leader.

The goal of managers is to provide stability, deal with organizational complexity, and implement decisions. Managers put out fires and typically work in a top-down fashion. Managerial roles often arise out of necessity rather than desire. Managers deal with the many details of the staff. In the ED, among

*Emergency Department Leadership and Management*, ed. Stephanie Kayden, *et al.* Published by Cambridge University Press.
© Cambridge University Press 2015.

**Table 1.1** Differences between leadership and management

| Leadership | Management |
|---|---|
| Changes status quo | Is part of status quo |
| Proactive | Reactive |
| Provides vision to believe in | Establishes structure |
| Changes rules | Enforces rules |
| Looks to the future | Deals with "here and now" |
| Takes risks | Manages risks |
| Energizes followers | Directs subordinates |
| Is empathetic | Is sympathetic |
| Shares authority | Shares responsibility |
| Thrives on chaos | Thrives on order |

many other tasks, managers make the work schedule, hire a nurse for the night shift, handle the daily disagreements between nurses and physicians, develop and enforce rules or policies, and ask for more funds from the hospital leadership. In stable times strong management may be enough to keep the ED running smoothly, but in turbulent times leadership is a necessity.

Leadership is different than management: it is a mindset, an approach to the job. It is often said that managers do things right, whereas leaders do the right things. There can be many leaders in the ED, not just the person who holds the top position. Dawson states that "leadership exists when someone exercises influence over others in their group ... and emphasises values that are espoused, directions in which future developments are guided, and the manner in which everyday tasks are accomplished."[3] In the ED, leaders might decide that the current work schedule does not take into account the work–life balance of the doctors and nurses, allowing for critical gaps in coverage that impact patient care. They therefore assemble a team to design a new, more flexible work schedule; or decide after analysis of patient flow that two nurses are needed at night but with different starting times; or develop a team-building program to minimize interdepartmental conflict. An ED leader might go to the hospital to ask for more funds based on innovative new strategies that make it possible to see more patients or provide new services that improve

patient care. Whereas managers put out fires, leaders ignite fires with new ideas and innovations, creative thinking for problem solving, and building teams to harness the power of the staff (Table 1.1).

Leaders promote change and question the status quo by promoting new ideas and challenging old ideas, whereas managers are more interested in keeping the status quo. Managers like stability in an organization. They like work to be orderly and uncomplicated, and they make rules and policies to keep things running smoothly. Leaders argue that emergency physicians (EPs) can intubate, that an EP can manage an ED without other specialty services, or that a well-trained nurse can order an x-ray without a physician seeing the patient first – all in order to provide faster, more efficient patient care. Leaders understand there is a sense of urgency to change. Participants from all over the world in the International Emergency Department Leadership Institute (IEDLI) say that they feel an urgency to do things, whether it be to create a new model of emergency medicine in their countries, or to solve a horrible overcrowding situation in their departments. But urgency should not be confused with activity. Rushing around from meeting to meeting is not urgency but frenetic activity. Urgent behavior does not need to be driven by the belief that everything is in a terrible condition, but more by a sense of what is important and "*the determination to move, and win, now.*"[4] This sense of urgency leads to positive behaviors in which people are proactive and alert, constantly scanning the internal and external environment for opportunities and threats that help determine ultimate success and survival.

Leaders understand the importance of *context*, how a particular event fits into the larger environment and how it is shaped by current or past events. There is a widespread tendency to portray leaders as people who shape events rather than are shaped by them. The multiple challenges facing the ED every day do not lend themselves to being shaped – one cannot shape the arrival of 50 trauma patients from a train crash. Instead, the ED leader is shaped by the reality of patients streaming through the door, and he or she determines a plan of action in response. Think back to our earlier example of the ED schedule. The leader who comes up with a new, innovative work schedule that makes the staff happier and provides better care to patients was shaped by the need reflected from patients and staff, not the other way around. Good leaders sense the context of situations. They want to know what is going on and why, what happened before in previous similar challenges, and then use adaptive capacity to achieve success. Adaptive capacity includes such skills as the ability to make sense of a given situation, see how it fits into a bigger picture, and then adapt a plan to deal with it. It also means being able to recognize and seize opportunities. Further, adaptive capacity is the ability to see all of the alternatives to a given situation before weighing the most apparent solution to a problem. Constantly thinking through problems in the same way every time means that new, creative options will often be overlooked for the tried and true path. The issues confronting the ED of today are not simple to resolve; they will take creative thinking. Einstein is often quoted as saying, "We cannot solve problems by the same kind of thinking that created them."[5] When all you have is a hammer, everything starts to look like a nail.

---

**Case study 1.1**

Dr. Karen Kornet has been the ED chief at her hospital for over two years. Overall the doctors and nurses are very happy. She has instituted some evidence-based protocols, has improved their chronically overcrowded waiting room with changes in triage, and has built a great working relationship between the doctors, nurses, and other ED staff members by using team training. But as more of the doctors are getting older, they are starting to talk about a desire for a better quality of life. They don't want to work nights and weekends forever. Unfortunately she just doesn't have the budget to add additional staff, even though she has asked hospital leadership for additional positions. She has already made changes in the schedule that were well received: by making the evening shift one hour shorter and having the night doctor start two hours earlier, she now has an extra doctor on duty from 21:00 to 23:00. By making the night shift a bit longer, she has lessened the load on the evening-shift doctor, decreasing door-to-doctor time during those busy hours but also allowing the evening-shift doctor to feel less fatigued and stressed at the end of the shift. The impact on the night-shift doctor was minimal, because usually things started to slow down after 01:30, and the night doctor could sleep for a couple of hours.

One thing Dr. Kornet has learned is that it is important to know not only what is going on in her hospital, but also what is going on in neighboring hospitals. This allows her to get great ideas from other ED leaders, some more experienced than she.

She was talking with a colleague from another hospital whose ED was overstaffed. The hospital leadership had been talking about firing some doctors, even though they were very competent. Knowing there were no funds from her own hospital to hire additional doctors, but still wanting to help her staff have a better work–life balance, Dr. Kornet developed a proposal to get coverage for night shifts by using the doctors from the other hospital on a part-time basis. In fact, one of the other doctors who was to be fired, Dr. Hassan, preferred to work only nights because she had young children at home. Dr. Kornet's hospital was receptive to the idea of paying the other hospital for the night-shift physicians, because it allowed Kornet's hospital to add additional staff without the expense of insurance, retirement, or other benefit costs. Because both were regional hospitals, the employer for both was the same, and the exchange was easy. Dr. Hassan's hospital was able to save her job by reducing its overall expense. All the staff doctors were happy with Dr. Kornet because there were two fewer night shifts per week to work.

By demonstrating adaptive capacity to the situation of staffing and coming up with a novel approach, Dr. Kornet again showed her ability to come up with a win–win solution for all.

---

Overcrowding is a problem that is often at the top of an ED leader's list of dilemmas. Many studies describe overcrowding's effect on patient care, and it takes real leadership to solve this worldwide problem.[6-8] Some hospital senior staff now recognize that it is not just an ED problem; overcrowding has to do with hospital capacity. As more hospitals shut inpatient beds, many try to manage inpatients with fewer staff, or run shortages of ancillary hospital services like laboratory or x-ray. One study in Ireland describes ED overcrowding as due to discharged ED patients waiting to find services in the community to receive further care.[9]

What does this have to do with leadership? A necessary component of leadership involves building networks and being connected in multidisciplinary, intradisciplinary, and even extradisciplinary groups. For example, trying to solve overcrowding by convening all your ED staff to get ideas will usually not solve the problem by itself. You also may need to reach out to primary care doctors to increase their hours of coverage; to inpatient physicians, senior leaders, and nursing leaders to discharge inpatients faster; and to the community to understand how community health is impacting the ED. You may need to network with ED leaders locally, regionally, and worldwide to find out how they are solving the problem. The leader of the ED must be connected to professional medical groups both inside and outside of his or her own hospital, civic groups on the local and regional level, and – if the hospital is government-operated – local politicians so they may advocate for the ED's causes. If there is not an organized group of emergency physicians or nurses in your area, consider starting one.

Leaders use these networks to build collaborations and find new ways to solve old problems. The founder of the Mayo Clinic in Rochester, Minnesota, Dr. William W. Mayo, was first approached with the idea of building a hospital after the local Franciscan Sisters were called on to help during a deadly tornado in 1883.[10] When the emergency was over, the head of the convent, Mother Alfred, asked Dr. Mayo if he and his two sons, Dr. William J. Mayo and Dr. Charles Mayo, would staff a hospital the nuns were considering building. Dr. Mayo originally declined. Hospitals during the nineteenth century were viewed as places people went to die, not to be healed. Also, he thought Rochester was too small to support a hospital. Despite Dr. Mayo's objections, Mother Alfred persisted, and the hospital opened as a 28-bed facility in 1888. Today, St. Mary's Hospital has 1265 beds and is one of the flagship hospitals of the Mayo Clinic. And it all started with a collaboration over 130 years ago.

Leaders are proactive, whereas managers are reactive. Many ED chiefs say that all they do is put out fires all day. These are reactive tasks. An ED chief who is putting out fires all day rarely has time to lead. The role of a leader is to set the agenda. Rushing from one crisis to another means that others are setting the agenda. For some ED chiefs, putting out fires all day is very rewarding because they can use it like a shield to avoid the harder work of planning, innovating, and thinking about change. Moreover, not all fires that are brought to the ED chief are important. Triage is as important for the leader as it is for the clinician. Working on a small finger laceration when another patient is having a myocardial infarction would be horrible patient care, but this is no different from spending all your time dealing with minor problems when quality is low in the ED. People soon learn that the only way to get your attention is by bringing larger and larger problems to you every day, reinforcing your role as firefighter. The ED leader soon finds that

a lot of energy is being spent to accomplish very little. It usually makes more sense to empower people to solve their own problems, allowing ED leaders time to create vision and innovations such as new ways to treat patients, to deal with strategic issues such as building a new department, or to re-engineer the model of emergency medicine practiced in the department.

## Theories of leadership

It would be easy to tell the ED leader, "Do the following things and you will be successful in your new job" – but, like medicine, leadership is both art and science. While it would be folly to expect a physician or nurse to work in the ED without basic courses in chemistry and biology, it is also ridiculous to talk about leadership without a brief discussion of leadership's history and theory. Until the twentieth century, most countries and companies were governed by the ruling classes. This gave credence to the *great man* theory of leadership, also called the *trait* theory, which held that people were born into the leader's role and therefore possessed the personal traits necessary to lead from birth.[11] One of the interesting parts of this theory, and its name, was that it excluded women from leadership positions. Much research was conducted on this theory to try to understand what gave these "great men" their superiority. The great man theory persisted until the early 1920s, when studies indicated that there was no universal set of leadership characteristics and that leaders did not possess a superior level of intelligence. Over time, it became more apparent that ordinary men and women could learn leadership skills.

The next leadership theory to emerge was the *style* theory, also called the *behavioral* theory of leadership. Researchers determined that leadership behavior was essentially composed of two types of behaviors: task behaviors and relationship behaviors. The task style of leader was focused on achieving objectives, while the relationship-oriented leader was focused on helping followers feel comfortable with themselves, about the job, and with each other. This led to the belief that leaders had one dominant style used in almost all situations, with another style that could be used when the first was not successful. This theory's major shortcoming was that it only described observed behaviors, instead of telling leaders how they might behave to become better leaders.

Because of the failures of earlier theories to adequately explain or predict good leadership, research continued. The *contingency* theory, also called the *situational* theory, asserts that no single way of behaving will work all the time, and that leadership style depends on the situation.[12] Research suggested that a leader's behavior was based on understanding of the effort of subordinates, their ability to do their jobs, the clarity of their job responsibilities, the organization of the work, and the cooperation and cohesiveness of the work group. After leaders assess the above variables, they then pick a leadership style that is most appropriate. If, for example, employees are competent and have the expertise to perform their work, then an employee-oriented leadership style might be appropriate. If the employees do not possess the skills and competency, a more production-oriented style is suggested, composed of more direction, rules, and policies. This theory had promise because it forced leaders to understand culture and have a handle on what was going on in the workplace by spending time with employees. Each employee was to be treated differently according to his or her unique needs, and the way the leader treated each employee might change from the beginning of the subordinate's career to later in that career as the employee understood the job better. This theory seems on the surface to have lots of promise, but there were very few research studies done to validate it. It also failed to explain why some leaders with particular styles were more effective in some situations than in others, and also what organizations should do when there is a not a good match between the leader and the situation.

All of these earlier theories of leadership are considered *transactional*. The goal of transactional leadership styles is to get other people to do things for something in return: money, prestige, or other rewards. Contemporary theories of leadership are different. The first contemporary leadership style, studied considerably since the 1980s, was called *transformational* leadership. Transformational leadership focuses on intrinsic motivation.[13] This style of leadership is concerned with values, standards, and ethical behavior and focuses more on long-term rather than short-term goals. Transformational leaders treat followers not as mere workers, but as human beings with issues, motivations, and needs. People are actually changed after exposure to the leader. The connection between leaders and followers becomes almost moral in nature, and raises the conduct and aspirations of both.[2]

It is in writing about transformational leadership that we start to see mention of vision in leadership. Vision provides a map of where the organization is going and gives everyone a sense of purpose and identity. This style of leader is considered a change agent. Most transformational leaders have lots of charisma. Gandhi, John F. Kennedy, Winston Churchill, and Mother Theresa are prime examples, but some transformational leaders have led their followers astray, such as Adolf Hitler. Leaders like Hitler begin to act independent of their followers, or put their own interests ahead of the interests of their followers. One argument against the theory of transformational leadership is that this charismatic, visionary style may be nothing more than a personality trait.[14] However, the theory is beneficial in that it partly explains what leaders can do to motivate followers, and that how they do it counts.

## Emotional intelligence

Leadership is difficult. Everyone knows people that should have been superstars as leaders; they were intelligent, creative, and brave. Some of them failed miserably and were never heard from again. Just as incompetent clinicians can harm patients, incompetent leaders can damage or destroy organizations. Leadership can be lonely when the things the leader must do are unpopular or when subordinates do not share the leader's vision. But the leader must press on. In the 1995 book *Emotional Intelligence*, psychologist Daniel Goleman explored emotions and how some people were able to better manage them than others.[15] Using neurobiological data, he studied why some people with lower intelligence quotients (IQ) were successful while those with higher IQs were often unsuccessful. These successful people were not at the top of their class, and yet they went on to do great things, leading innovative companies that were employee-centric and known for great products. In fact, Gardner reports that 80% of the success factors he studied had nothing to do with an individual's IQ.[16] Goleman set out to study this 80%, in particular those characteristics that are defined as emotional intelligence: the ability to persist in spite of setbacks, to premeditate, to delay gratification, to regulate emotions in the daily grind of life, and to empathize and have hope.

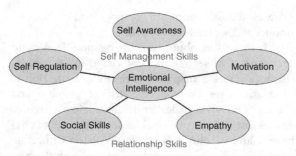

**Figure 1.1** Components of emotional intelligence, after Goleman 1995, 1998.[15,17]

Later work by Goleman translated his earlier studies into how emotional intelligence effects leadership ability.[17] Goleman sought to understand how people could change their behavior to become better leaders. He broke down his theory into five major competencies: self-awareness, self-regulation, motivation, empathy, and social skills (Fig. 1.1). He calls self-awareness, self-regulation, and motivation "self management skills," and empathy and social skills "relationship skills." Each of these is further broken down into sub-competencies.

## Self-awareness

Self-awareness comprises emotional awareness, accurate self-assessment, and self-confidence. People who have emotional awareness know how they are feeling and why, and are unafraid to let other people know. They understand what they think, do, and perceive, as well as how their emotions effect everyone around them, including patients, colleagues, and subordinates. As an emotionally aware leader, you know when you come to work that all your subordinates are aware of your moods and can tell when you are happy, tired, or emotionally drained. To have these emotions is understandable for everyone, but the leader must know when his emotions are in play in order to gauge how a particular emotion affects performance. For example, ED work is stressful; being the physician or nurse leader is stressful as well. If you see patients in addition to your administrative duties, the stresses of one part of your job can overflow into the other part. If you have just worked a stressful shift with many sick patients, it might not be the best time to conduct a subordinate's performance evaluation.

Having emotional awareness also means understanding your values and goals. It has been said that "the most important thing in life is to know what is

important."[18] Any career decision should always be measured against your core values. If your goal is to really make a difference in emergency medicine and in the lives of your patients, then taking a job solely based on salary or prestige, even though the hospital's leadership has no interest in moving emergency medicine forward, will usually lead to an unhappy experience. At the same time, if one of your core values is that the patient always comes first, many decisions as a leader become easier: dealing with outside consultants who do not want to come in after hours, or with recalcitrant hospital administrators who do not want to fund an essential piece of equipment.

A good leader should be able to make an accurate self-assessment and be aware of her strengths and weaknesses. Leaders often have blind spots that can put their careers at risk. According to Kaplan, some of the most common blind spots are blind ambition or the goal of winning at all costs; relentless striving at the expense of other important things in life such as family and friends; pushing others too hard; the insatiable need for recognition; or the need to seem perfect all the time.[19] Blind spots cause leaders to make mistakes. The ED nursing director who feels the need to work harder than everyone else in the department (especially those he or she considers lazy) is a perfect example of this. Most workplace competencies are behaviors learned over time, and with effort the negative behaviors can be changed. Someone who is impolite and interrupts subordinates can learn to do better, through coaching, by accepting feedback from those surrounding them, or by learning new behaviors. The leader should also know her strengths. This means knowing whether you are the right person for a particular task or should instead defer to others who are stronger in that area. A good example would be an ED chief who takes the lead on the development of an ED information system because of her strength with computers while delegating the project of building a new ED to the associate chief because of his past experience with two similar building projects. Self-assessment also means seeking feedback from peers, colleagues, superiors, and subordinates. There are many tools that can be used for this, including 360-degree feedback, performance evaluations, and behavioral surveys.

Self-confidence makes up the last sub-competency of self-awareness. People who have self-confidence are able to take on big challenges and master new jobs or skills without difficulty. They feel that they compare favorably to others of their level but are not afraid of constructive criticism. The self-confident have charisma, which can inspire confidence in subordinates. One must have self-confidence to go to the chiefs of other services to advocate for emergency medicine, or to go to a community meeting to understand the local community's displeasure with an event that occurred in the ED. Decisiveness is a key component of self-confidence. There are many decisions that must be made in leadership positions: hiring and firing decisions, resource allocations, and new program implementation. After you have gathered information about a problem, assembled a team to deal with it, set up a schedule, it will then be time to act. Do so with confidence, so that your subordinates can see that you are serious about the problem and dedicated to the solution.

As a leader, you must also be able to speak out with confidence when a core value of yours or the organization has been threatened. Standing up for your values demonstrates to the ED team that you are able to represent them. For example, allowing doctors from other specialties to intimidate or berate the ED staff without your intervention will demonstrate to the staff that you do not have the confidence to stand up for them.

## Self-regulation

Self-regulation is another emotional competency that makes up emotional intelligence. Self-control is an important part of self-regulation. The good leader will regulate emotional upsets as well as those feelings that could cause distress. Stress is cumulative and will build up whether the source is from home or from work. The ED is an emotional place: our staff are high-energy people who do not always agree with us, many patients are very sick, and family members can be demanding. As mentioned above, it is important to have and show our feelings, but lashing out at staff members, or sulking when things do not go as planned, is counterproductive. You will have many trying moments as a leader – senior hospital administrators may not be convinced of your compelling idea, or a child may die in the ED, causing grief among your staff – but it is important to be seen as a composed role model who maintains a positive attitude. On occasion, just being the calming voice or opinion in a stressful situation is all that is needed. Even time management is considered self-regulation. As more

and more demands are placed on leaders, the ability to stay focused and keep a personal schedule becomes more important. If subordinates see the leader always being late it sets the tone for the rest of the department; consequently meetings never start on time, staff members show up late for work, and important meetings can be missed.

Another part of self-regulation is being trustworthy and conscientious. Leaders must act ethically and should not put themselves in a position where their ethics can be questioned. The practice of taking gifts from ED suppliers – forbidden in many countries – can be construed as unethical even if it is common in your region. Unethical behavior by others also must not be tolerated, even if a ban on these practices is unpopular. If the ED chief knows that staff members occasionally take small supplies like bandages home for personal use and does not act decisively to stop it early, it will be harder to stop in the future when the practice becomes commonplace and excessive. Being popular is not the goal of the ED leader; following one's principles should be.

Everyone makes mistakes from time to time. Part of being a good leader is to occasionally take risks, some of which may have unsuccessful outcomes. The leader with emotional intelligence admits his mistakes, thus demonstrating trustworthiness. Trust in their leader is something that subordinates must have. If the leader promises to do something, he or she must follow through, or at least explain why the promise cannot be met.

Having self-control also means being adaptable and open to new ideas. The good leader seeks out new ideas not only to run the department but also to treat patients in a more efficient manner. New ways of doing things can come from journals, conferences, meetings of business executives, and even the local café. Seek ideas for longstanding problems from within the staff, as they are usually closest to the problem. The innovative leader does not always need to be the source of the next big idea. Instead, you should foster an environment in which staff feel empowered to offer suggestions.

### Case study 1.2

In 2000 the US Institute of Medicine published a report called *To Err is Human: Building a Safer Health System*.[20] Among many things cited in the report was the cost of medication errors in hospitals. Medication errors caused 7000 preventable deaths, caused harm to 1.5 million people, and had an annual cost to the health system of US$3.5 billion. Instead of trying to solve this from the top of the organization, Kaiser Permanente Health Systems' leaders took the innovative approach of going to the nurses, physicians, and pharmacists, and even patients, to enlist their support and ideas on how to prevent the problem in their hospitals. The hospital system had already studied the fact that interruptions and distractions while preparing and dispensing medicines were the biggest cause of medication errors in their hospitals.[21] They assembled a two-day focus group with over 70 people to come up with ideas to minimize distractions. The group produced over 400 ideas, many of which are still used today, including having nurses who are preparing medications wear a bright yellow sash that signifies they are not to be disturbed and a painted zone around the medication dispensing zones indicating that those within the zone are not to be disturbed. By the leaders being innovative and allowing their subordinates to use their own innovations to solve a problem, the hospital system is saving over US$900 000 annually.

## Motivation

Good leaders are highly motivated to achieve, have commitment to a personal and organizational vision, and take initiative. The leader who is not interested in achieving excellence will usually end up as a manager, solely interested in keeping things as they are. Leaders strive to achieve excellence, both in patient care and in ED efficiency. They foster cordial relations between staff and patients, thus creating a good place to work or to get emergency treatment. The good ED leader wants to achieve quality targets and takes them seriously. An interest in achievement should belong not only to the leader but to the entire staff as well. Allowing subordinates to attend educational conferences, to take professional courses, and to try new things contributes to their personal satisfaction and a fulfilling work experience.

Leaders must have vision. Having vision means seeing the ideal future direction while realistically taking into account internal and external forces.[22] The leader meshes her personal vision with the vision of the organization and, if the two visions are at odds, works to meld them. Leaders then must have the communication skills necessary to articulate the vision to followers in a clear and concise way. Leaders should embody the vision in their values and actions each day. This vision keeps the leader going when things are difficult and acts as fuel for tired staff at the end of a long shift. Having a vision about the design of the new ED you are hoping to build and communicating it regularly to the staff can often keep them optimistic about working in an old, outdated facility. Articulating the vision is best done in person, in one-to-one or group meetings. Communicating the vision via email or text message will not work, though these methods can be used to reinforce a vision. ED workers are rarely the type to blindly follow someone without knowing where they are going; communicating your vision allows the ED staff to trust you to lead.

The motivated leader must also be optimistic. Optimism is key to vision, innovation, and risk taking. In Italy, where a residency program in emergency medicine was established in 2009, the dean of the medical school in Florence, a champion of the program, remained optimistic throughout longstanding, arduous political battles with government officials and doctors from other specialties who argued against the need for such a program (G. Gensini, personal interview, February 7, 2012). Today this residency has spread to 25 of the 26 regions of the country and first-year classes continue to grow. Optimism is the order of the day for those in emergency medicine. You must believe that the things you do benefit patients, the leadership skills you bring will make your department a good place to work, and the initiatives you begin will end in success. Your subordinates will sense your optimism and may be more optimistic because of it. Without optimism, you will give up on yourself, your causes and, ultimately, your patients and subordinates.

## Empathy

Goleman describes the next two competencies of emotional intelligence as "relationship skills" because they involve working with others. Using emotional intelligence to become a better leader means having strong social skills. Building teams, empowering staff to make decisions, and knowing what is going on with your staff are important components of successful leadership that involve managing many relationships. Leaders sometimes feel "lonely at the top." Inesi and Galinsky cite many reasons for this, all related to trust. The main reason is that leaders sometimes believe that the only reason subordinates are nice to them or do the things they ask is because of the leader's power.[23] Many brilliant leaders are in fact loners. Research indicates that when loners become leaders they have a tendency to retreat into solitude, trying to solve vexing problems by themselves, trusting their intuition and decision-making processes rather than seeking counsel from others.[24] The successful leader will instead build networks that allow her to take advantage of many ideas. Empathy, the ability to sense how others are feeling, is a key leadership skill. People rarely tell us in words how they are feeling; rather, it is through their facial expressions, hand gestures, and posture that they signal their emotions. Freud said, "mortals can keep no secrets; if their lips are silent they gossip with their fingertips."[25] Goleman calls this "social radar," and notes that sensing emotion is not enough; the leader must also respond appropriately to the sensed emotions.[17]

How does this relate to the business of leading an ED? We expect our subordinates to come to work every day and do their best; yet sometimes they do not. A leader who can sense that something is wrong can help the employee perform better. For example, the doctor who is normally very good, but now seems preoccupied or short-tempered may have problems at home: a sick child or spouse, financial difficulties, and so on. Some leaders might be tempted to say, "All we care about here is performance, not what is going on in someone's personal life." But the leader who recognizes the staff's personal problems and offers appropriate assistance will engender loyalty and commitment in all employees. The leader who communicates with employees solely through voicemail and email will not be able to determine how those employees feel. Regardless of how busy the ED nursing director or ED chief might be, it is still important to spend face-to-face time with subordinates. Most employees and colleagues also are good at picking up on non-verbal signals from their leaders, so it is important not only to say empathetic words but also to demonstrate our empathy with non-verbal signals. Being empathetic should be viewed not as a weakness but as a strength.

Empathizing with people does not mean agreeing with them. Disagreements are less likely to develop into full-blown battles if the leader attempts to understand the other's position, even if it is contrary to her own. Another thing that leaders are called on to do is arbitrate between two or more differing opinions between subordinates. When arbitrating, it is important to understand the emotional positions of all sides and to be seen to do what is best for the department rather than to take sides in the dispute.

In practical terms, being empathetic also means helping employees develop themselves. The good leader should have a sense of where subordinates want to go with their careers, not only through performance evaluations but also through direct observation of what part of the job gives the subordinates joy. Does a particular nurse who might not always have a good attitude seem to take substantial gratification in taking care of children, or does one doctor always seem to like taking on technical tasks? Caring enough about our employee's success to want to mentor them pays off in many ways. According to Orpen, mentoring employees allows them to perform at higher levels, increases their level of job satisfaction, improves loyalty to the organization, and lowers turnover rates.[26]

Of course the good leader knows how to respect employees' privacy and should also know when not to intrude in employees' personal lives, but in the end, to be an empathetic leader means that people should know you are a caring, compassionate person who attempts to understand the feelings of those around you. A note of caution: be wary of using false empathy, or giving the appearance of understanding people's emotions without really feeling empathy towards them. People will know by your actions where you really stand. Machiavelli said, "It is unnecessary for a prince to have all the good qualities I have enumerated, but it is necessary to appear to have them."[27] Empathy is a quality that cannot be faked.

## Social skills

The last of the five key components of emotional intelligence is having social skills. Having social skills means more than being friends with the staff, or telling jokes at a party. According to psychologist David McClelland, people have three important needs: the need for achievement, the need for power, and the need for affiliation.[28] They possess these needs in varying degrees. Those with a high need for affiliation wish to be part of groups, to have good relations with those around them, and to avoid conflicts. Often those with high affiliation needs perform poorly compared to others. Leaders are often faced with difficult decisions, and those decisions may lead to conflict. Consequently, leaders with high affiliation needs may find themselves frustrated with colleagues or subordinates after unpopular decisions they must make. It is sometimes said that it is better to be friendly with everyone than to be everyone's friend.

To lead successfully there must be group interactions between the leader and followers. The good leader gets people to willingly follow her, rather than relying solely on administrative fiat. Social skills can be further broken down into influence, communication, conflict management, and change catalyst. Those with emotional intelligence know how to influence those around them. Connecting emotionally to an audience, whether you are discussing patients at shift change, trying to sell a new policy to the staff, or convincing the CEO of the hospital to let you build a new ED, is an important part of being an influential leader. It is important to notice whether people are listening to you speak, reading your emails, or accepting your ideas. Being a leader is about making things happen in your organization. If you notice that you often fail to get buy-in, have a negative impact on things, or are being ignored, look at how you attempt to influence people. Are you open to their ideas, or are you stubborn and resistant? Do you rely on a familiar strategy to get things done, even if you know it is not always successful? Influencing people requires a positive outlook, strong communication skills, a willingness to listen, and empathy towards the audience, not a Machiavellian approach bent on winning at all costs.

Communicating openly with staff is another strong social skill that is part of the emotionally intelligent leader. It is difficult to influence people without listening first to what they have to say. Everyone knows someone who dominates the conversation, cutting the speaker off mid-sentence and ignoring the speaker's verbal or physical messages. It is always better to try to come to a mutual understanding when communicating and to make others feel free to offer suggestions. Ask good questions to show you are listening and do not shut yourself up in the office. Most ED communication is informal, so being where the workers are is necessary if you want to know what is going on in your department. Many ED leaders

today work at least a few shifts per month, including off hours, to stay in touch with their ED staff.

The ED leader must sometimes deliver bad news: hospital or department financial problems, impending lay-offs, or the death or serious illness of an employee. The leader's emotional self-control will help him deal with his own feelings about the situation. A study of more than 100 executives and managers found that their colleagues preferred leaders who best handled their own emotions during difficult circumstances.[29]

The ED is often filled with conflict between nurses and physicians, staff and patients, ED staff and the staff of other departments, and between colleagues of equal rank. Conflict resolution is therefore a key skill for the ED leader. The best way to deal with conflict is to stop it before it starts. Often simply understanding the perspectives of all parties can lead to a mutually beneficial solution. Always strive for a win–win resolution, even though it might take longer to reach. Using tact during conflict is a sign of a good leader. Some problems, such as a disruptive physician, are difficult, and there may be no win–win solution. In such a case the leader must decide what is best for the department as a whole. A person who consistently generates conflict with other staff should not be tolerated and will often need to be replaced. Avoid resolving a conflict by simply passing an edict on the case. This often will drive the conflict underground only to surface again in the future. If no resolution can be reached between two parties, consider allowing them to "agree to disagree."

Finally, the leader with emotional intelligence needs to be a change catalyst. While some of the problems in health care today are definitely related to the poor global economy, health systems in many countries were already in crisis, and the foundering economy only exacerbated the problem. Those developing countries with improving economies have the problem of trying to provide higher-quality health care as standards of living improve and their citizens become more demanding. Heifetz, Grashow, and Linsky write in their *Harvard Business Review* article that with an improved economy, things are not likely to return to normal. They call this "leadership in a permanent crisis," and go on to say that the leader of today must be able to foster adaptation.[30] Today's leaders must develop not only best practices but also "next practices" to lead into the future. They advise embracing a state of "disequilibrium" to keep people

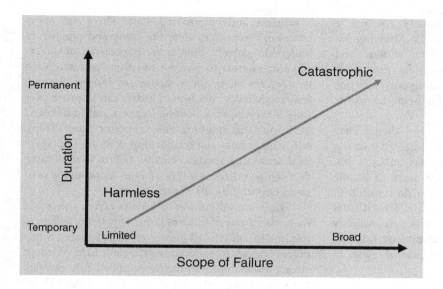

**Figure 1.2** Organizational impact of failure, after Henry 2011.[32]

just uncomfortable enough to allow them to accept change. However, there is always a risk that people will begin to suffer from "change fatigue," as cited by Kotter, and those affected may eventually leave the ED. Kotter states that for change to move throughout an organization, at least 75% of those involved must accept the change.[4]

Revolutionary change is difficult in medicine where changes often evolve over time, especially in government-operated systems. By creating a staff of people with leadership skills, this 'evolutionary' change will often happen faster. Leaders can hasten such change by giving staff authority to make decisions and allowing them to take calculated risks (under leadership supervision to ensure no risk to patients). Later in this text there is more on dealing with and implementing change, but leaders especially must embrace change and allow as many staff members as possible to assist with change efforts.

## Dealing with failure

Good leaders occasionally fail, and all leaders should be prepared for failure at some point in their careers. Emotional intelligence can help minimize failures if leaders use intuition to know when a course of action might be problematic. Leaders must be self-aware and understand their environment if they want to reduce the chance of major failure, but often our self-confidence gets the better of us. Walshe and Shortell studied major failures in the healthcare

systems of the United States, the United Kingdom, New Zealand, Australia, the Netherlands, and Canada.[31] They found that some leaders believe that not every patient can be successfully treated. They see these failures of treatment as part of the normal course of business and therefore do not view them as potential drivers of change. This author believes this notion of accepting failure as a course of business cannot be tolerated. Change agents must be willing to risk failure, even in the ED, as long as the failure does not negatively affect patient care. Unfortunately, most catastrophic leadership failures do affect patients.

Good leaders learn from their mistakes in ways that allow for personal and professional growth. Henry states that short-term failures with little fallout are easily tolerated in an organization, whereas more long-term, wider-reaching failures may be catastrophic (Fig. 1.2).[32] This also applies to the ED. A small, short-term schedule problem resulting from an innovative schedule change that disrupts the ED for a couple of days has less impact than does the failure to account for future volume growth when designing a new ED.

Emotional intelligence can help the leader deal effectively with failure. After a failure, the leader must have the self-confidence to go on with the job. Failures of the head, based on inadequate or faulty information, can be remedied by a commitment to learning new skills and doing things better in the future. Failures of the heart, such as a leader lacking the motivation to adequately research a problem, can be more difficult to fix. Studying his motivations, seeking feedback from others, and recognizing his lack of self-awareness can allow a leader to turn a failure into an opportunity for personal growth. Failure also can help the leader learn empathy for others.

Strong leaders put failures behind them. They accept their poor decisions, examine what went wrong and move on. Their self-esteem may suffer a bit, and they may decide to learn new ways to handle the problem that led to the failure or do research to ensure the failure does not happen again. They discuss the failure freely with the staff and take responsibility for it, but in the end they should understand that, like all humans, they are prone to occasional failure.

## Conclusion

There is no perfect recipe for success in leadership. Each country or hospital will have certain nuances that inform the development of a personal leadership strategy to create an ED that provides high-quality care by a satisfied and empowered staff. There are many common things that unite the study and practice of leadership globally. First is the importance of understanding context to analyze situations and accepting that we are all in for a lifetime of change. Second, leaders are made, not born. Leaders can improve over time if they become lifelong learners and understand the impact that emotions have on performance. Third, self-management and relationship skills are important in determining success. Finally, failure is something that can be tolerated if it is small in scope and is used as an opportunity for improvement.

There are millions of ED visits across the world each year. Some of these millions of patients will go to minimally staffed and poorly equipped places, while others will go to modern, world-class EDs. Without strong leadership even highly equipped EDs can fail, but with strong leadership even the most basic ED can provide excellent care. The challenges of leadership are many, but anyone can become a better ED leader through perseverance, the desire to be a lifelong learner, and a commitment to providing the best care to patients with the resources at hand.

## References

1. Bass B, Bass M. *Stogdill's Handbook of Leadership Theory, Research and Managerial Applications*. New York, NY: Free Press, 1990.

2. Goodwin N. *Leadership in Healthcare: a European Perspective*. London: Routledge, 2006.

3. Dawson S. *Analysing Organisations*, 3rd edn. Basingstoke: Palgrave Macmillan, 1996.

4. Kotter JP. *A Sense of Urgency*. Boston, MA: Harvard Business School, 2008.

5. Gunderman RB. *Leadership in Healthcare*. London: Springer-Verlag, 2009.

6. Coughlan M, Corry M. The experiences of patients and relatives/significant others of crowding in accident and emergency in Ireland: A qualitative descriptive study. *Accident and Emergency Nursing* 2007; **15**: 201–9.

7. Weiss SJ, Derlet R, Arndahl J, *et al*. Estimating the degree of emergency department crowding in academic medical centers: results of the National ED crowding study (NEDOCS). *Academic Emergency Medicine* 2004; **11**: 38–50.

8. Cameron PA. Hospital crowding: a threat to public safety? Managing access blocks involves reducing hospital demand and optimizing bed capacity. *Medical Journal of Australia* 2006; **184**: 203–4.

9. Jayapresh N, O'Sullivan R, Bey T, *et al*. Crowding and delivery of healthcare in emergency departments: the European perspective. *Western Journal of Emergency Medicine* 2009; **10**: 233–9.

10. Berry LL, Seltman KD. *Management Lessons from the Mayo Clinic*. New York, NY: McGraw-Hill, 2008.

11. Bass BM, Bass R. *The Bass Handbook of Leadership: Theory, Research, and Managerial Applications*, 4th edn. New York, NY: Free Press, 2008.

12. Gordon JR. *A Diagnostic Approach to Organizational Behavior*. Boston, MA: Allen and Bacon, 1983.

13. Bass BM, Riggio RE. *Transformational Leadership*, 2nd edn. Mahwah, NJ: Lawrence Earlbaum Associates, 2006.

14. Bass BM. *Leadership and Performance Beyond Expectations*. New York, NY: Free Press, 1985.

15. Goleman D. *Emotional Intelligence: Why it can Matter More than IQ*. New York, NY: Bantam Dell, 1995.

16. Gardner H. *Intelligence Reframed: Multiple Intelligences for the 21st Century.* New York, NY: Basic Books,1999.

17. Goleman D. *Working with Emotional Intelligence.* New York, NY: Bantam, 1998.

18. Blanchard K, O'Connor M. *Managing by Values: How to Put Your Values into Action for Extraordinary Results.* San Francisco, CA: Berrett Koehler, 2003.

19. Kaplan RE, Drath WH, Kofodimos JR. *Beyond Ambition: Driven Managers Can Lead Better and Live Better.* Ann Arbor, MI: Jossey Bass, 1991.

20. Institute of Medicine. *To Err is Human: Building a Safer Health System.* Washington, DC, National Academies Press, 2000.

21. Cleary N. Kaiser Permanente's innovation on the front lines. *Harvard Business Review* September 2010: 92–7.

22. Dym B, Egmont S, Watkins L. *Misson, Vision, and Effective Nonprofit Leadership.* Upper Saddle River, NJ: FT Press, 2011.

23. Inesi ME, Galinsky AD. Five Reasons Why it's Lonely at the Top. *Wall Street Journal* March 25, 2012.

24. George B, McLean B, Craig N. *Finding Your True North.* San Francisco, CA: Jossey-Bass, 2008.

25. Gray P. *Freud: a Life In Our Time.* New York, NY: WW Norton & Company, 1998.

26. Orpen C. The effect of mentoring on employee's career success. *Journal of Social Psychology,* **135**: 1995.

27. Machiavelli N. *The Prince.* New York, NY: Signet Classics, 2008.

28. McClelland D. *Human Motivation.* Cambridge: Cambridge University Press, 1987.

29. Walter V. *Clarke Associates. Self Regulation and Communication.* Pittsburgh, PA: Clarke Associates, 1997.

30. Heifetz R, Grashow A, Linsky M. Leadership in a permanent crisis. *Harvard Business Review* July–August 2009: 62–9.

31. K. Walshe, S. Shortell. When things go wrong: how healthcare organizations deal with major failure. *Health Affairs,* **23** (3): 103–11.

32. Henry A. *Storage for the Internet Presentation.* Web 2.0 Summit. San Francisco, CA, October 18, 2011.

# Identifying and resolving conflict in the workplace

Robert E. Suter and Jennifer R. Johnson

## Key learning points

- Recognize conflict within the workplace.
- Employ proven theories and strategies to resolve the conflict.
- Turn the conflict into positive, productive gain.

## Introduction

It is inevitable that conflict will occur in any workplace, including the hectic environment of the emergency department (ED). The reasons for conflict are varied and often quite complex. In addition, there are significant cultural differences in the level of acceptance of open conflict. Tolerance for conflict can even vary between regions or groups of people within the same country.

Regardless of the culture, if it is not addressed, true conflict can do serious damage to a workplace. Low morale and discontent can lead to loss of experienced employees, resulting in higher expenses and staffing costs. Conflict also affects productivity, as attention that is paid to conflict detracts from job duties, and may lower efficiency and productivity. Leadership should have some training on conflict resolution that includes identifying it, addressing it with proven strategies, and finally following up to ensure that the conflict has been resolved. Doing so improves financial success and employee health, and in the healthcare setting can have a positive impact on the quality of patient care. Minimizing conflict in the ED should therefore be viewed as an ethical imperative.

The cost to replace an employee is typically double the annual salary of the position. With that knowledge in mind, many organizations are implementing employee retention measures – not only to help offset this cost drain but also as a measure to increase the number of satisfied employees. Employers understand that keeping valuable employees happy increases productivity and efficiency for their organization, which contributes to their overall financial and quality outcomes success. Lack of efficiency increases the cost to operate the facility or department as job duties are not completed in a timely manner, much less in an effective one.

ED leaders can minimize conflict in the workplace by identifying it before it escalates, and then employing proven strategies to resolve the situation, hopefully to the satisfaction of all involved. By doing so, leaders can cultivate a happy and productive work environment.

## Identifying and recognizing conflict within the workplace

Conflict has been defined as a "state of disharmony between incompatible or antithetical persons, ideas, or interests; a clash."[1] Perceptions, emotions, and behavior form an interactive system. Interestingly, it has been asserted that for true conflict to exist, it must also be perceived by the involved parties, although this premise could be challenged.

Many people try to ignore conflict, either because of discomfort rooted in past negative experiences or simply because of an aversion related to their personality. This may be especially true of doctors, nurses, and other workers who gravitated to health care because of their desire to be in a compassionate, nurturing environment. Others may respond to conflict in a manner that increases the severity of the situation instead of defusing it.

*Emergency Department Leadership and Management*, ed. Stephanie Kayden, *et al.* Published by Cambridge University Press.
© Cambridge University Press 2015.

Human beings have defense mechanisms that must be overcome when addressing conflict. The typical initial response is to perceive the conflict as an attack, and to go on the defensive. If conflict is handled with that perception in mind, it can end up spiraling down into a counterproductive exacerbation of the conflict.

## Sources of conflict in the emergency department

The ED is a complex environment that can lead to a number of sources of dissatisfaction and resultant conflict. Overcrowding, lack of on-call specialists, scheduling issues, salary discrepancies, difficult patients and family, problems with staff, consultants, and administrators or supervisors are all potential generators of conflict.

Conflict in the ED can result from sudden immediate circumstances or can build over time as the result of longstanding issues in the department.

Before discussing strategies and communication styles that are proven tactics in resolving conflict, it is important to understand the types of behavior associated with conflict situations.

## Behaviors associated with conflict

People tend to demonstrate five different behaviors when conflict arises (Table 2.1).[2]

(1) **Competing**. This behavior is very aggressive in that the ultimate objective is to win in the situation regardless of the consequences or impact on the other individual or individuals involved. It is rooted in power, and the person employs any and all tools necessary to accomplish the win. The motivation behind this tactic is a strong belief that they are right in their opinion or perspective. This behavior is rationalized by the individual as defending the right course of action. Individuals

**Table 2.1** Behaviors associated with conflict

| |
|---|
| Competing |
| Accommodating |
| Avoidance |
| Collaboration |
| Compromise |

exhibiting competing behavior do not demonstrate any willingness to cooperate, as it would offset the desired outcome. It's a "my way is the only way" concept.

(2) **Accommodating**. This is the direct opposite of competing, meaning non-assertive but cooperative. Often this person will sacrifice communicating thoughts, ideas, solutions, or opinions in order to create harmony. The reason for this behavior is varied. For example, it might have roots in self-sacrifice, or yielding to a more dominant personality. The self-sacrifice concept is interesting, as this "selfless act" can create a sense of martyrdom (look at what was sacrificed for the good of all). This not an ideal way to resolve conflict, since not all avenues are examined.

(3) **Avoidance**. This behavior is neither assertive nor cooperative. Individuals who show this behavior are very conflict-adverse and do all in their power to eliminate the potential for being in a confrontational setting. In this regard, individuals might demonstrate actions to avoid situations that have issues which might become confrontational. They might leave in the middle of a discussion that appears to be escalating into conflict. Or they might not respond to written communication where conflict might arise. For example, an employee emails her manager two separate times requesting a meeting to discuss job duties that the employee is concerned might not be evenly distributed. The manager, being conflict-adverse, does not respond at all to either email communication, and when approached personally by the employee, tells her she will get back to her with a date and time. Of course, this does not happen. With avoidance behavior, conflict does not get resolved, and often the results are even more severe.

(4) **Collaboration**. This is the most time-consuming mode of behavior, but also the most effective and productive. It requires a much greater depth of effort from all parties involved. In this case, all parties express their thoughts, goals, concerns, and solutions. All are then examined, and as a cooperative and collaborative whole a decision is made on how to proceed. This is a very clear definition of a team concept, working towards a common goal as defined by these individuals. It is both cooperative and assertive, as agendas are

directed more towards finding a solution rather than towards achieving individual desires. It requires a heightened level of understanding and flexibility of thinking, as each individual has to be receptive to other perceptions and ideas.

(5) **Compromise**. This is mildly assertive and cooperative. This mode is generally most effective, and most often utilized, where a more immediate resolution is necessary. Compromising behavior falls in the middle between accommodating and competing behaviors, as it takes from each – though more from accommodating – in order to find a solution. The solution, as with most compromises, does not entirely satisfy but is accepted by all parties involved. As mentioned, this concept is good for an immediate correction – but with the notion that to achieve a more ideal outcome it could be followed up with a collaborative action. So, while the ideal is not achieved, it is still a correction of the conflict.

Exploring and understanding each of these behaviors will assist when choosing the most effective method for resolving the conflict, and will lead to its more effective resolution.

The identification of conflict can come from many sources. Feedback about issues can come from physicians, employees, and patients quite readily. Should leadership be present and visible in the department, as recommended earlier, conflict can often be identified and contained before it escalates. Once the conflict type is identified, a strategy should be chosen. One example might be peer-to-peer conflict that is becoming visible to patients, which means it has to be handled immediately. Or perhaps conflict exists such that patient throughput is very slow, in whch case an action committee might be formed to identify inefficiencies and implement corrective actions. When conflict is quickly identified, a strategy is chosen, and actions are taken, this should result in productive gains in employee/patient satisfaction, more efficient work processes which increase productivity, and a healthier, happier workplace.

---

**Case study 2.1.  Peer-to-peer conflict**

Melissa and Tiffany worked at a front desk as administrative assistants. Near the end of one work day, Melissa was very busy trying to check patients out so asked Tiffany is she would assist her. Tiffany told Melissa no, stating that she was doing medical records right then for mail-out the next day. The patient who was at check-out with Melissa was unhappy with this exchange, and two days later reported it to the manager. Prior to this, however, Melissa had asked to speak privately with Tiffany the next day, mentioning how she felt when she asked for help and was turned down. Tiffany said that she felt pressure to get those medical records out since the supervisor earlier that day had spoken to her about it being a priority. What Tiffany had forgotten was that patient care comes first, as management had stated multiple times. They both agreed to be more mindful of each other's job duties and to make an effort to be better team players.

---

# Employ proven theories and strategies to resolve the conflict

Conflict management follows the principle that not all conflicts can necessarily be resolved, but learning how to manage conflicts can decrease the odds of non-productive escalation. Conflict management involves acquiring skills related to conflict resolution, building self-awareness about conflict modes, developing conflict communication skills, and establishing a structure for management of conflict in your environment.[3]

Managing conflict in the workplace should be of paramount interest. In an ideal work environment, while conflict may be inevitable, it should be managed relatively easily. Training, coaching, mentoring, and role playing all demonstrate a certain level of aptitude towards resolving conflict. As with anything, practice makes proficiency. Continuous communication and education is also quite helpful. Explaining and demonstrating proper communication is important, as it is crucial for resolution of conflict. At some point, crucial conversations, those with a high likelihood of containing conflict, will take place. Understanding that these "high-risk" conversations exist and recognizing when they occur allows for healthy conversations.[4]

A healthy conversation is one where appropriate, effective communication takes place. For example, a co-worker is irritated with a peer because he or she is not working as hard as others or is doing things in a way that causes more work for others. A healthy conversation would be to discuss it with that person directly, utilizing professional, appropriate, and courteous communication.

Concerns should be addressed in a way that is not threatening or aggressive. A good opening phrase may be something along the lines of "Can you help me out? When one of us disappears from our workplace for an extended length of time, it causes backup with our patients. I know that we have to have lunch and breaks, but what do you think we can do to better help each other?"

Working and communicating together to find solutions is effective. Often people demonstrate actions that promote unhealthy approaches to resolving the conflict. Realistically speaking, most people find conflict difficult or uncomfortable, so it is easier to take alternative routes that bypass but worsen the conflict. These approaches include saying negative comments behind a person's back, or using passive aggressive behaviors such as doing the same things that a low-performing employee does as retaliation. These actions do nothing to resolve the conflict but only encourage low morale and result in substandard productivity. All detract from the overall objectives of the organization. Therefore, mastering crucial conversations can increase any leader's effectiveness and success in all areas of life.

The roots of conflict resolution are in mediation and arbitration, but more far-reaching actions need to be incorporated in order to effectively address the conflict. It is very difficult to be neutral in conflict, as our instinctive and very natural ojective is to achieve our own personal agendas, and acting as a completely neutral party is not possible.[5]

Finding a way to achieve consistent fairness is a more realistic approach to resolving conflict situations. Being actively engaged in every step of the conflict is important. It is important to understand conflict so it can be effectively contained and resolved. The best solution to a problem results from identifying all factors involved and addressing them accordingly. To do this requires strong knowledge of the issue in its entirety. Keep the desired outcome in mind, and hold the same standard for all parties involved. The overall goal should be to thoroughly and effectively find a workable solution to a problem which results in a better work environment with more effective work operations. Worry less about individual wants and needs and more about the overall good of the entire team and organization.

Communication is always a challenge, no matter what the situation. In areas of conflict it is even more challenging. With the advent of email and cellphones, our face-to-face communications have substantially decreased. This not only allows for conflict to manifest more readily but also allows for conflict to be more easily ignored. Understanding how the new technologies impact workplaces should encourage leadership to implement measures that promote appropriate and timely resolution of conflict.

While email is a comfortable and easy way for most people to communicate, it is still important to develop and maintain personal interactions. These interactions allow for more efficient and effective communication without increasing the risk of misinterpretation or confusion that can stem from written formats. Further, personal interactions should reflect and demonstrate that communications are professional, appropriate, and courteous. Attention to these traits will help minimize confrontational situations, especially if there is disagreement over the content of the discussion.

Conflict resolution in a workplace should be a priority for all team members, not just for leadership. Every individual should be committed to making the workplace a happy and productive environment. This attitude extends beyond the workplace and becomes an additional benefit to clients, patients, and customers. An understanding of strategies to resolve conflict, and the willingness to practice these strategies, will allow an individual to resolve issues instead of contributing to them.

When confronted with conflict it is important to overcome the initial defensive response by taking a step back, taking a deep breath, and then identifying what is truly the issue at hand. Extrapolating from the emotions to the root cause of the conflict should be an initial step. Is it a personality conflict with a fellow employee or patient? Is it a frustration with a current work process that is not allowing for a smooth workflow? Is the lack of a good working relationship with a supervisor contributing to some of the conflict? For leadership to have a true understanding of what conflict is occurring in the department, leaders need to be visible and accessible. Ways to achieve a better understanding can be varied, such as working a couple of shifts per month, spending time in the department interacting with employees and patients, or, at the minimum, having an open-door policy. An open-door policy is not necessarily the most efficient, since it moves away from scheduled time such as doing a shift and moves into allowing for casual walk-in appointments, often causing difficulty with time management.

Once identified, the next steps are very specific, depending on the type of conflict. Some situations require an immediate response, with the understanding that it is only a temporary fix until time can be allocated to resolving the conflict more thoroughly. Other situations are more time-consuming and involved. One example might involve identifying process improvement projects in order to overhaul an unpopular operational system change, such as going from a paper medical record to an electronic medical record.

Another example is a lack of satisfaction with leadership. This is one of the more difficult and most ignored types of conflict. Often the employee will not mention this discontent for fear of retribution. Organizations should encourage employees to voice their thoughts, ideas, and challenges, and remove the stigma of retaliation.

Unfortunately, when concern is expressed about leadership, leaders can and do retaliate – which leaves little or no form of recourse for the employee. This risk of increased conflict in an already uncomfortable situation only emphasizes to the employee that addressing the situation is not a benefit, and in fact can have more of a negative impact on that person's work life should he/she proceed with the issue or complaint. If, on the other hand, the root of the conflict is identified, and the individuals involved are willing, they can then proceed with correcting the situation with proven strategies, a few examples of which are given below.

---

**Case study 2.2. Employee-to-supervisor conflict**

Janet was employed as a manager of a large medical practice, responsible for 50 employees. Her director, Randall, made it clear that she was accountable for all that occurred in the practice. One of the concerns Janet had was with her assistant director, Brigid, who consistently made unilateral decisions regarding process changes and hiring of new staff without Janet's knowledge. This caused much strain on Janet as she routinely tried to manage the impact of this lack of positive and appropriate communication. It clearly conveyed to the employees that there was a distinct break in the relationship between Janet and Brigid. This cultivated an environment of distrust, discomfort, and strain which then permeated the entire practice. Janet asked for a face-to-face meeting to address her concerns with Brigid. When Janet mentioned her concerns, Brigid's response was that

she did not have to let Janet know in advance of decisions made, as it was her call. Upon further contemplation, Janet decided to take it up another level, where her director resolved the conflict through reinforcement of the expectations on Janet, but also through relationship and communication-building exercises to help develop a more positive and productive working relationship.

---

## How to turn the conflict into positive, productive gain

Conflict management is the use of strategies and tactics to move all parties toward containment or resolution of the dispute in a manner that avoids escalation or the destruction of relationships.

Once conflict is identified, one of the key components in resolving the situation should be finding the solution to include a productive gain. For example, in a medical practice, employees are experiencing frustration with processes that are in place on how the patients are brought back to see the doctor. This conflict is leading to lower morale and a higher rate of patient and physician complaints. The manager puts together a collaborative team that addresses the key areas that appear to cause the problem. This team then comes up with a solution of redistributing job duties for a more effective flow process. The next step is to take the solution to the rest of the employees and implement. Once implemented, they follow up in one week, in one month, and in two months to receive feedback on the new process. Slight modifications to the process are likely necessary. What they find is an overall benefit to the patients, the employees, and the physicians. Job duties are accomplished in a timely manner that is much smoother and more efficient. This more efficient flow allows employees to spend time identifying other problem areas and creating solutions for better outcomes. This enhanced productivity results in many gains. Productivity from a financial standpoint and employee productivity working in a happy and healthy environment, added to patient satisfaction, creates a highly effective organization.

Note that the above example includes team members helping to come up with a solution, which is a highly regarded technique in accomplishing employee happiness. Unilateral decision making by management has been proven over time to be a less effective way of making changes. Getting the employee to "buy in" on the solution or concept is very important in the implementation process if it is to be effective. The best way to achieve that end is to have their input. Furthermore, many times conflict between employee and leadership arises from management's opinion that they know more about an employee's job than the employee does. Given that employees do the job day in and day out, their opinions and thoughts should have high relevance.

---

**Case study 2.3.  Team member conflict with customer/client/patient**

Kendra was a front-desk supervisor at a large medical oncology practice. One day a patient came in for an appointment, but it was the wrong day. The patient actually was supposed to have an appointment for a scan that morning in the diagnostic center, but had got confused. The patient was very insistent that her appointment was at the practice. Kendra kept arguing with her until one of her staff called the manager. When the manager, Jackie, arrived, Kendra was upset and had an elevated tone of voice. The patient was in tears and her husband was visibly angry at Kendra. The manager, speaking in a very calm, quiet manner, asked the patient to explain what had happened. When Kendra tried to interrupt, Jackie said that she wanted to hear the patient's viewpoint. After hearing the story, Jackie offered some coffee or tea to the patient and then stated that she was going to ask the doctor if he could fit this patient into his schedule. Jackie made it clear that there was no guarantee and that there might be a little wait. The patient was very happy, even with an additional 30-minute wait to see the doctor, who fit her in his schedule. Kendra, however, was pulled into Jackie's office for some coaching and mentoring on how to handle conflict situations like this, especially with patients.

---

## Cultural differences in conflict resolution

Today's world is increasingly a global society, with team members from a variety of backgrounds. In this setting, it is important to understand different customs and values that an employee brings to an organization. For example, the appropriate physical distance between individuals who are talking to each other varies greatly. The Spanish consider being within half an arm's length acceptable, whereas in the United States this distance is considered intrusive.

Realizing differences, being respectful, and behaving accordingly greatly enhances the ability to either avoid conflict or achieve a positive outcome. Cultural differences are not just between countries but can be regional or ethnic as well. In the United States, religion is not discussed in the workplace in the Northeast. In the Southeastern United States, however, this type of discussion is much more accepted. Ignoring or failing to learn cultural differences can result in very uncomfortable situations.

## Conclusion

It is important to understand that conflict is inevitable in any workplace. Many variables contribute to conflict, and the ability to identify them will be critical in successful resolution. Technology such as cellular phones and email has resulted in an increase in the number of avenues available for the avoidance of conflict resolution. In addition, these same technologies have detracted from developing good interpersonal traits, as interactions no longer routinely include face-to-face communication. This degree of separation reduces the ability to form a positive working bond with others involved and lends to an increased risk for misinterpretation.

How leadership manages conflict will translate to how employees handle conflict. It should be the responsibility of all employees to take an active role in addressing conflict appropriately in order to promote a healthy, happy, and productive work environment. To achieve this goal, strong organizations give leadership and employees training in productive ways to address conflict, and also tools to enhance communication. Communication truly is the root of successful conflict resolution. However, without understanding behaviors associated with conflict (why people do and say what they do) and the strategies that effectively resolve the conflict, communication will not be enough. Further, it is very important, even crucial, to eliminate the initial desire to achieve a personal agenda in order to create a solution for the good of the whole. It should be standard practice to think very carefully about an action before actually taking it, as impulse actions tend to increase conflict. A heightened awareness and concentration when involved with a "crucial conversation" are key components to achieving a good outcome. And finally, finding a way to get a productive gain with the solution is ideal. All parties are then happy with the results, which in turn often have farther-reaching impact such as patient satisfaction and financial gain.

Finally, it should be mentioned that becoming proficient at conflict resolution is not immediate. It can take years and many experiences to achieve a strategy that works. Each individual should utilize a basic concept, then adapt it to suit his or her own personality and abilities. This is a work in progress, meaning it should be understood that this is essentially a trial-and-error concept where mistakes or missteps will occur. Learning from those mistakes and doing better the next time is where success is found in resolving conflict.

## References

1.  American Heritage Dictionary of the English Language, 4th edn. Boston, MA: Houghton Mifflin, 2000.

2.  Killman T. *Conflict Mode Instrument*. Palo Alto, CA: Consulting Psychologists Press.

3.  Foundation Coalition. Understanding Conflict and Conflict Managment. http://www.foundationcoalition.org/publications/brochures/conflict.pdf (accessed January 2014).

4.  Patterson G, Grenny J, McMillian R. *Crucial Conversations: Tools for Talking when Stakes are High*. New York, NY: McGraw-Hill. 2002.

5.  Mayer B. *Beyond Neutrality: Confronting the Crisis in Conflict Resolution*. San Francisco, CA: Jossey-Bass; 2004.

## Further reading

Covey SR. *The 7 Habits of Highly Effective People*. New York, NY: Simon & Shuster, 1989, 2004. A great resource for information.

Covey SR. *The 8th Habit: from Effectiveness to Greatness*. New York, NY: Free Press, 2004. A continuation of the book listed above.

Mayer B. *Beyond Neutrality: Confronting the Crisis in Conflict Resolution*. San Francisco, CA: Jossey-Bass; 2004. Another great resource for handling and managing conflict.

The *Journal of Conflict Resolution*, online at http://jcr.sagepub.com, is a great resource. Focuses on the full range of human conflict and deals primarily on an international level but also addresses more specific forms of conflict.

Avoiding common ED communication pitfalls. *Emergency Physicians Monthly*, March 16, 2011.

Chapter

# 3

# Leading change: an overview of three dominant strategies for change

Andrew Schenkel

## Key learning points

- Understand three dominant strategies of change.
- Understand the managerial implications of the strategies.
- Know when to use the respective strategies.

## Introduction

Change is a constant rather than an exception in today's organization. This applies to both the private and the public sector, and emergency medicine (EM) is no exception. From an external perspective, forces in the external environment can consist of changes in technology, social trends, political or legal decisions, environmental or ethical changes. Internal forces for change can emanate from many specific parts of an organization not functioning efficiently or effectively, with the parts of an organization being vision, strategy, structure, culture, human relations management (HRM), and systems. Alternatively, another internal force for change could be a misalignment between the parts of an organization, meaning the individual parts are working fine independently but the parts are not aligned. EM in particular is experiencing numerous pressures promoting change. These include restructurings in which the focus is on whether facilities should be centralized or decentralized, the implementation of new protocols or work practices, and in addition trying to change the internal culture such that EM is an accepted discipline. For most managers, the ability to lead change remains an elusive challenge. Thus, the first question is, why is change so difficult?

Change is problematic for most organizations, and EM is no exception – but it has some unique features that pose additional challenges. On a general level, people react negatively to change for numerous reasons: change is threatening, people are satisfied with the status quo, a change results in increased work, people perceive that they are losing out from the change, the change consists of the wrong goal or an incorrect means to achieve the goal, change is viewed as doomed to fail, or people may be suffering from change fatigue from numerous change efforts and/or a lack of motivation to change. In addition, health care and by extension EM makes leading change more complex as well as challenging. Firstly, studies have shown that reactions to change vary according to occupational and professional groups, specialization, generation, educational background, and employment status, as well as the extent to which the person feels associated with the organization.[1] In addition, professional groups with a perceived higher status as well as professional identity have a greater openness to organizational change, and reduced levels of change-related uncertainty.[2] These studies suggest that change in EM has special features compared to change in other organizations, and that these features have the consequence that reactions to change are more heterogeneous. At the same time, the challenges as well as conditions facing EM vary from organization to organization. In turn, leading the change requires a broad palette of strategies that need to be suited to the change effort, organization, and conditions in order to obtain the desired results.

This chapter reviews three strategies of change, with each strategy having a set of distinct assumptions, with the purpose of broadening the palette of options available in understanding and leading change. Assumptions are important, since they underlie our thoughts, interpretations, and behavior toward change. Thus, to formulate a strategy for

*Emergency Department Leadership and Management*, ed. Stephanie Kayden, *et al.* Published by Cambridge University Press.
© Cambridge University Press 2015.

change as well as its subsequent execution requires that we focus on the underlying assumptions. It is likely that no one change strategy will work for all organizations all the time. Hence, three strategies with very different underlying assumptions will be discussed. The first strategy is based on the concept of *programmed change*. The second outlines change from a *political* perspective. The third perspective is change from an *organizational development* perspective. The final section of the chapter sums up key points of the three strategies and proposes a framework to guide the EM practitioner, with the purpose of understanding when to use each change strategy.

## Programmed perspective of change

### Case study 3.1

Liz works in a small hospital that is establishing EM and a corresponding emergency department (ED). To accomplish this, parts of existing departments at the hospital will have to be merged. Everyone is excited about this change, because a specially designed facility with state-of-the-art equipment has been purposely built. For years the large majority of administrators, doctors from different professions, nurses, and technicians have supported the idea of a new multiprofessional facility. Unfortunately, funds were not present to build it. Now that tax revenues have increased, politicians have allocated funds to build the facility and it is becoming a reality. People involved in the project recognize that it is urgent to open the facility because more capacity for patient treatment is required. The ED facility now stands finished and people from other departments have merged into one department called simply ED. New routines and procedures have to be designed for this new department to work as a dedicated ED.

Liz has read Kotter, and implements his eight-step model of change. This means forming a powerful guiding coalition with the vision of establishing a world-class ED, and bringing in operational as well as functional department heads to form the vision. Thereafter, a strategy is developed by the guiding coalition. Part of the strategy is to open the facility on a limited trial basis, and once this has succeeded to completely open up the facility. The first patients are treated successfully, and they are surprised. Part of the operational plan is to spread the news of this success in order to encourage people involved in the change. Spreading the news is achieved through an internal magazine as well as through a celebration in which cake is served to the people who work in the department. The next stage of the plan is to fully open the ED, and this meets with more success.

Liz understood the power of programmed change and drew upon the widely used framework of Philip Kotter's eight-step model.[4] Kotter's model is based upon numerous rational and bureaucratic assumptions. The rational assumptions are that organizations exist to achieve established goals and work best when rationality prevails over personal preferences and external pressures. The bureaucratic assumption is that the organization is hierarchical, and that labor is specialized and governed by explicit and impartial rules that are impersonally applied by professionals.[3] Further, these rules are followed. The following section draws widely on the work of Kotter and describes his framework.[4]

The first step of Kotter's model is to create a sense of urgency. As a leader this means creating a state such that the organization recognizes that a change has to take place. This particular step does not consider what the change will be, and rather describes a psychological state of readiness in which people are prepared to make a change. This can be seen as one of the most critical steps in his model, as without this psychological state change cannot proceed. Kotter describes numerous ways in which this can be accomplished, for example through comparison with another organization in the form of a rivalry or benchmarking, or through bringing in an expert to create a gap that leads to a crisis.

The second step is to build a powerful guiding coalition. Kotter does not describe in great detail what a powerful coalition is, and instead points out its attributes. Specifically, he says that its members should have the same vision and a similar attitude toward creating a common vision or goal, and the means of achieving this goal. Further, the powerful guiding coalition should be trustworthy and have the requisite resources to carry out the change.

The third step is to create and operationalize a vision. Operationalization refers to concrete actions in terms of who is doing what and when these actions should be done. It is in principle a plan that outlines how the vision should be obtained.

The fourth step is closely linked with the third step in that it consists of communicating the vision. According to Kotter there are three components to this: What is the vision? Why this vision? How are you going to achieve the goal? He points out that the vision should be communicated simply and through multiple media, and that when communicating the vision, it is key that the guiding coalition walks the talk, as this decreases skepticism and builds credibility.

Once the vision is communicated, the fifth step consists of empowering people to act. This means giving people the formal capacity to act, including necessary skills as well as required resources. For the change leader this means assessing that these requisites are in place – and, if they are not, ensuring that they are put in place.

The sixth step is to plan for and create short-term wins. The wins need not be large, as change projects often consist of many small steps of interdependent actions. Short-term wins act as a means to keep the bandwagon rolling and to gain support along the way, as well as a mechanism for skeptics to lose ground. In the process of creating supporters, skeptics are won over, and become the minority as critical mass is created.

The seventh step is that of consolidating improvements with the purpose of generating more changes. It consists of building more short-term wins such that the change seems inevitable. It can be seen as constructing a larger whole out of small components. The purpose of this step is to maintain and build the momentum, culminating in realization of the initial goal.

The eighth step consists of anchoring as well as institutionalizing the new approaches. This step focuses on making the change stick through making it part of the organization's routines and procedures as well as its culture. These changes represent the cumulative learning of the organization,[5] and as they become a part of everyday organizational life they constitute the culture of the organization.[6] However, altering the path is difficult – and thus making the change stick is key.

Kotter's model of change is widely used and attractive because it becomes a question of following the steps as outlined above. Having said that, these eight steps – as previously mentioned – build upon the following two assumptions: (1) organizations exist to achieve established goals, and (2) rationality prevails over personal preferences such that decisions

lead to action. Thus, provided that these assumptions hold, and as long as resources are not scarce, the coalition is powerful, and a sense of urgency exists, change is in fact possible.

# Political perspective of change

**Case study 3.2**

Sarah was embarking on a change to shorten the waiting times at the ED. As the project leader and MD her goal was to reduce the waiting time on weekends from the current 3 hours on the average to 1.5 hours. She thought she had found a solution to the problem. Specifically, she was aware that the hospital had many fractures and other orthopedic injuries on weekends. Under the current system, patients with orthopedic injuries were the responsibility of the ED, but the ED did not control the resources to treat them. Instead, these patients had to be transferred to another wing of the hospital to be examined and treated by the orthopedic department. Her solution involved transferring some of the physicians from the orthopedics department and making them part of the ED. This way the ED could work as an integrative team and shorten the waiting times.

While everyone agreed that it was beneficial to shorten the waiting time, Sarah had a challenge with her proposal. In particular, while everyone agreed on Sarah's strategy on how to achieve the goal, shifting manpower from the orthopedics department to the ED met with a high degree of resistance from the orthopedics department. They simply did not want to give up resources to the ED. They thought that a better solution would be to maintain the status quo, as that was the way things had always been done. Immediately, a case of conflict occurred as a result of the different solutions.

Sarah's challenge was to achieve the goal of reduced waiting times. From her perspective, this was the overarching issue. She saw that a rational dialogue, describing why the change should be made, just did not work. Instead of improving matters, dialogue only inflamed the issue. She quickly realized that the best argument does not always win and said, "So much for rationality. We have different goals, scarce resources, different strategies for solving problems, and the only result of this situation is conflict." She knew that if there had been more resources the problem would be solved, as she would not have to rely on the orthopedics department. However, this was a zero sum game in that there would be winners and losers. Upon reflecting on the situation, she said to a colleague in the department, "Our organization is like a jungle and I need to think like the king of a jungle and act like the lion. That is the only thing that the orthopedics department understands. For the change to be implemented, I need to show them I am king and that I have more power then they do. Once I have more power the change will occur." She mapped out the power that she had, as well as the power of the orthopedics department. She found that she had power as an expert, since she was a leading authority on EM and on how to organize EDs in the country. However, the head of the orthopedics department, the person she was discussing the issue with, had formal power and access to resources in the form of the physicians in his department. In this case, his power was greater then her power, and both partners found the issue important. Quite simply, Sarah required more power in order to obtain her goal.

What Sarah did was to engage in politics through building an alliance with the hospital administrators and local politicians. This would have the effect of increasing her power enough to obtain her goal, in that she would have more power than the head of the orthopedics department. Sarah thus contacted the hospital administrator and a local politician and asked for a joint meeting. On the agenda, which she set, was only one issue: How do we shorten waiting times? During this meeting she explained what she wanted to do in order to decrease the waiting times. They fully understood her argument, since she was a leading expert on the matter. At the end of the meeting the hospital administrator and leading local politician said, "Let us think about what you have said." Shortly thereafter she received a telephone call from the hospital administrator, who stated that she had received the support of the local politician as well as the administrator of the hospital in order to carry out the change. However, the hospital administrator pointed out that he would rather the issue of transferring resources were handled between Sarah and the head of the orthopedics department, since the hospital had a decentralized decision-making system. Sarah consulted the head of the orthopedics department and told him that she had the hospital administrator and local politicians on her side in terms of the proposed change. She said, "The choice is yours: you can provide me with the extra resources that I need or we can bring it to the hospital board to make a decision." The head of the orthopedics department saw that Sarah had

gained more power then he had and that he had essentially lost. He could have brought the matter to the board, but at this point the cards seemed stacked against him. Simply put, he said, "I am not going to win this one, and bringing it to the board will mean that I lose face. Further, they will think that I am resource-hungry." Thus he acquiesced to the change and orthopedic specialists moved to the EM department. Once in place, the result of this change was that waiting times on weekends were substantially reduced. Sarah had succeeded in navigating in the jungle and becoming the king.

In the above example, Sarah understands the politics of change. She sees that organizations are not always rational, and do not always have the same goals. Further, she quickly realizes that scarce resources, combined with different goals as well as different means of achieving those goals, only leads to conflict. She quickly comes to the conclusion that organizations are more like a jungle, and to win you have to become the king of the jungle – the lion. The following section discusses change from a political perspective, beginning by outlining the assumptions of this perspective toward change.

The political perspective is based on a series of assumptions that are quite different than those presented above, in the discussion of programmed change. The first assumption underlying the political perspective is that conflict or the perceived incongruency between two or more parties is a natural part of an organization. The second assumption is that the person or group who has the most power obtains the desired goal. In this respect power is the adjudicator of who gets what. These assumptions act as the foundation of a political strategy toward change. The following paragraphs begin by outlining a strategy for change from a political perspective, drawing on Pfeffer.[7]

The first step is to analyze whether the conditions for conflict are present. There are several causes of differences in organizations that in turn lead to conflict, with one of the most fundamental causes being that of scarce resources.[7] This is evident in Sarah's example, as if resources were abundant there would not have been a conflict with the orthopedics department. There are different resources, and examples include financial and physical capital, knowledge, goodwill, reputation, brand, intellectual property and culture.[8] The challenge is that to carry out change

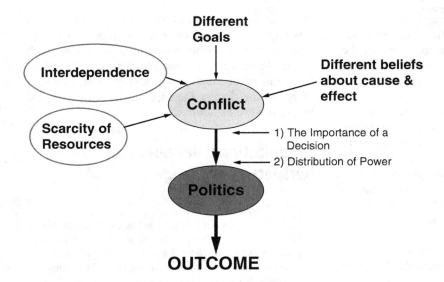

**Figure 3.1** Differentiation between conflict and politics.

often involves scarce resources, or the actual change alters the balance of resources. The next cause of differences that can lead to conflict is the extent to which people or groups affected directly share the same goal. When goals are not homogeneous, conflict can occur. The final cause of conflict is the extent to which actors agree on cause and effect.[7] When actors do not agree on cause and effect this can lead to conflict. From a change perspective, understanding cause and effect encompasses identifying what is the problem and how to address it. Thus, if actors do not agree on the means for change, conflict occurs. This is the case in Sarah's example, in which she has one belief about how to solve the problem and the head of the orthopedics department another. Nevertheless, they share the same goal – but other reasons for conflict, as cited about, lead to conflict.

The second step is to identify the extent to which the conditions for politics exist. For conflict to lead to politics, or the active gathering and use of power, the issue at hand must be perceived as of high importance by both participants.[7] In our example, both Sarah and the head of the orthopedics department perceive the issue as important, and hence politics takes place. Figure 3.1 illustrates a framework for conflict and politics.

When the importance of the issue at hand is high, actors will jostle to gain more power such that one actor has an excess of power compared to the other, because outcomes are determined by who has the most power.[7] Thus, the first activity for the change

leader in this context is to assess who has what type of power, as well as how much power they have. There are numerous types of power, with some of the main sources of power as follows:[9]

- formal power (power that comes with the formal position)
- bureaucratic power (the ability to control rules, regulations, and procedures)
- information and expertise
- control of rewards
- coercive power, in the form of the ability to constrain or punish
- control of or access to resources
- alliances and networks
- agenda setting
- personal power (charisma, political skills, or verbal facility)
- culture

Power can be assessed in numerous ways; for example, power can be manifested in terms of symbols such as parking spaces or the corner offices. Additionally, power is embedded in structures, and thus one can identify who sits on formal committees or in formal posts. This was the case of the head of the orthopedics department in the example described above. Finally, perceptions are real, because people act on them. Thus, asking people about who is viewed as powerful provides a good indicator of the power that they have.

Ascertaining the political landscape only provides actors with an indication of who has what power and how much they have. Based upon this analysis, they can ascertain whether they have enough power to obtain the goal or if they should engage in politics in order to gain more power.

In the event that the actor leading the change has more power as a result of analyzing the power landscape, this analysis suggests that it is likely that the change will be accomplished. In the event that the leading actor does not have more power than the other actors involved, and views the issue at hand as important, she has two options. The first is to avoid conflict. The second is to engage in politics with the purpose of increasing her power.

There are numerous means to reduce conflict, and they can be seen as focused on reducing the conditions for conflict. The conditions for conflict are dependency upon scarce resources, different goals, and heterogeneous beliefs in terms of cause and effect,[7] and thus, to reduce conflict, the change leader has the following options available at hand:

- increase resources
- decrease dependency
- align goals
- establish similar views of cause and effect

In the case of Sarah, changing the conditions that led to conflict did not seem to be possible. In this situation, an actor can use the different sources of power:

- use formal authority
- control knowledge and information
- build alliances and networks
- manage culture (meanings and symbols)
- build reputation as an expert
- foster others' identification such that personal power is increased
- increase perceived dependence on resources
- use information to persuade
- use resources to obtain compliance (push and pull)

This section has outlined change from a political perspective, and discussed the ensuing strategies. Politics is important from a change perspective, since one of the most common mistakes in implementing change is the lack of a thorough understanding of the conditions for conflict and politics. This entails mapping out the differences leading to conflict and

the conditions for politics. With respect to the latter, it is important to map out the landscape of power in terms of who has what power as well as how much power. As pointed out, when the change leader establishes that he or she does not have adequate power to carry out the change, then appropriate strategies and tactics need to be adopted.

## Organizational development perspective of change

### Case study 3.3

Michelle was recently appointed as the head of the ED. She saw there was a need to improve service to patients as well as to increase the quality of health care delivered. She thought about how she would accomplish this. Michelle felt like she had seen it all in terms of carrying out change. When thinking back over why change programs did not work, she cited two reasons. First, was there was almost always active resistance against the proposed changes and ensuing organizational politics. Second, there was a high degree of passivity among people involved in the actual change. The passivity mainly emanated from disillusionment with the change process, as the ED as well as the hospital had gone through numerous change programs.

Michelle thought about this and came to the conclusion that she had three options. The first was to actively engage in politics in order to overcome any resistance to the change effort. She thought carefully about this option and decided against it, as resorting to politics was against her values as well as detrimental to the organization. Further, she had seen numerous heads of other departments try a political perspective, but the desired change had not been achieved. The second option was that of programmed change. She argued against this approach for the reason that often using this strategy starts and ends with the same Powerpoint presentation. In other words, little happens except for a Powerpoint presentation that is later archived in a desk drawer. Upon reflecting on the third option, she asked herself, "What are my values and what is my management style?" She came to the conclusion that she had a strong belief in people and their ability to accomplish goals if given the right conditions. She felt that her role was like a gardener, and that she had to arrange for a rich and fertile soil for the seeds and give the seedlings water in order for them to flourish. Therefore, her change strategy consisted of actively involving people in the change effort as well as empowering them to make changes. Thus, they were no longer recipients of change, but creators. At the same time, she still was the gardener and responsible for deciding what plants to plant as well as where they should be located. In other words, she was responsible for the vision as the leader.

In terms of carrying out the change, this meant that the first thing Michelle did was to gather her top management team in the ED and formulate a vision as well as a strategy. Thereafter, a task force was established to understand what obstacles had to be removed in order to achieve the desired vision. This group consisted of respected people in the organization, some of whom were deemed critical to carrying out the change. The task force set about understanding barriers to change through interviewing people in the organization on this particular question. The task force compiled the answers to the questions and reported back to Michelle and her top management team.

Michelle and the group were told that several hinderances prevented them from attaining their goals. Specifically, the following obstacles were cited: (1) a bureaucratic structure, (2) poor coordination across functions, (3) closed vertical communication, and (4) low motivation because of the first three issues. Michelle and her top management team said they would discuss what the group had said and report back to the group. After discussion, Michelle and her team accepted the recommendations of the group and said they would take actions to address the issues that had been highlighted. Thus, layers were removed in the structure in order to make it flatter, and designated liaisons between departments and functions (a person working in two different entities) were appointed to improve coordination and communication. Further, the question of how people coordinated and communicated their activities in the ED became part of the annual employee evaluation. Michelle said to her management team, "What you measure matters." She saw that evaluating communication was a means to make better communication and coordination part of the organizational culture.

With these changes in hand, the people involved in the change effort felt that the change was obtainable, with the necessary preconditions to carry out the change in place. Flattening the organization and ensuring delegation of responsibility resulted in a change of attitude in people in the organization, from one of being watched upon to one in which they were trusted and empowered. At the same time,

the desired goal required more communication between functions as well as departments. Thus, appointing liaisons between departments and functions assisted in providing the necessary underlying conditions for change to occur. The organizational changes were made, and thereafter the initial strategy was carried out. The result of providing the conditions for the change, as well as carrying out the change, resulted in the achievement of the articulated goals of improving services to patients as well as increasing the quality of health care.

People are an important part of making change happen in organizations. The role of the leader, as Michelle illustrates, is to believe in people and create the "right" conditions so they are motivated and can develop. Michelle uses this principle to achieve change, and sees that a win–win situation is created as people carrying out the change become satisfied and the organization achieves its goals. The mutual beneficial and dependent relationship between people and organizations underlies the organizational development (OD) perspective of change – the focus of this section. Further, without people, Michelle could not make the changes or get work done. Similarly, people in the organization also need to work. When organizational performance is at the desired level a so-called "fit" is achieved. Conversely, when there is a performance gap – that is to say, desired performance is not achieved – this is an indication of a misfit between people and organization. To address this "gap" the organization has to improve employee conditions such that they provide motivation for people and their needs are met. Motivation is considered as the forces acting on or within an organism to initiate and direct behavior.[10] As a change leader, Michelle clearly works on satisfying the needs of people in her department, and she sees this as a means of facilitating change as well as a necessary prerequisite for change.

In this section we consider two of the most widely cited scholars discussing the issue of needs in the OD area: Maslow[11] and Herzberg.[12] These theories are institutionalized,[13] and thus they influence both an employee's expectations as well as an employer's way of designing work. According to Maslow, needs exist in a pyramid. At the top of this pyramid, and at the highest level of needs, is self-actualization.[11] In declining importance are the following needs: esteem, love/belonging, safety/security, and physical needs at the bottom of the pyramid.[11] Herzberg built upon Maslow's work, and outlined the following needs as motivating people: achievement, recognition, work itself, responsibility, promotion, and growth.[12] Unlike Maslow, he stated that there are factors at work which create dissatisfaction, which he called hygiene factors. Several of the hygiene factors that he mentioned are pay/benefits, company policy, relationships with co-workers, supervisions, job security, status, responsibility, and working conditions.[12] What is important to point out is that a minimum level of hygiene factors is required, but increasing them above a certain level does not lead to an increase in motivation.

The main role of the leader in the change process, according to the OD perspective, is to create the conditions such that people's needs are fulfilled. In turn, people will be motivated to fulfill their needs. Thus, underperformance in an organization requires that motivation be increased, since there is an inherent mismatch between the organization's needs and the people who work there. In the case of Michelle, improving motivation and putting the necessary conditions were important in terms of her achieving the change. However, this was not enough in and of itself, as changes in structure had to be made as well as attempts at having a culture that would support the strategy. Knowing what to do is important, but it is not the same as getting the change done. For the latter, it is necessary to generate a state of readiness for the change to occur, in the form of dissatisfaction with the current state. This is done through having people become part of the change process. The advantage that this approach has is that resistance and passivity – two reasons why change projects fail to achieve the intended goals – are overcome. Thus, people involved in the change process become co-creators of change through a so called "honest conversation" in which the barriers that stand in the way of achieving the change are discussed in an open way.[14] This is exactly what Michelle did when she asked for feedback from the task force in terms of identifying the barriers preventing the organization achieving its goals. In turn, it is suggested that this process leads to dissatisfaction, self-designed models, internal commitment, and actions that provide the motivation and the means for change, as well as the process that overcomes any resistance that may be present.[14] Overall, to achieve change, the dissatisfaction with the current state that is generated has to be greater than the potential loss emanating from the change.[15]

## Summary

This chapter has reviewed three strategies of change: programmed, political, and organizational development perspectives of change. There is no one change perspective that works for all organizations all of the time, since the context varies and organizations are not all the same. Often managers continue to use the change theory that they previously used. However, effective change is not necessarily accomplished by attacking old problems with what we already know or have done. This is especially the case when change has not been previously implemented in a successful way. When it comes to change strategy, there is a strong tendency to choose the programmed approach, as this is how we would like organizations to work. As suggested, one of the disadvantages of the programmed change perspective is that the issues of power and conflict are largely not considered. Having said that, a purely political approach can be seen as being too cynical – but at the same time it likely mirrors the heterogeneity of EM.

The OD approach builds very much on a participative bottom-up approach that in turn leads to a high degree of commitment. The OD change process is based upon building capabilities or the underlying processes through which goods and services are directly or indirectly produced or delivered through the transformation of resources.[14] Research suggests that there is a positive linkage between the quality of capabilities and financial performance.[16,17] While the OD approach is attractive, it is criticized for being naïve.

Each of the outlined change strategies is associated with different metaphors to describe the leader, different tasks, and a distinct set of leadership processes. Table 3.1 summarizes these, for both effective and ineffective change leadership.

While Table 3.1 provides insight into the different types of change management strategies, what it does not do is point out which strategy should be used when. Effective change leadership requires matching the critical aspects of change with the strategy of change. These aspects are associated with the five questions that are listed in Table 3.2.

This chapter has outlined three change strategies, with the purpose of describing three dominant approaches, and at the same time it is hoped that the discussion will assist in providing the leader with a range of tool kits to choose from.

**Table 3.1** Effective and ineffective change leadership

| Change strategy | Effective change leader | | | Ineffective change leader | |
| | Leader | Task | Leadership Process | Leader | Leadership Process |
|---|---|---|---|---|---|
| Programmed change | Analyst City planner | Align structures and systems Plan the change Follow the plan | Analysis planning | Petty tyrant | Management by Excel, or a person who looks at numbers and charts |
| Organizational development | Coach | Align organizational and human needs Believe in people Empower people Increase participation | Supporting, empowering | Lightweight, or a person who cannot carry out the actions and is not well respected | Creating conditions |
| Political | Maneuverer Networker Negotiator Politician | Assess conditions for conflict Assess power distribution Engage in politics | Assessing the landscape | Con artist thug or a bully | Manipulation Fraud |

Inspired by Bolman and Deal (2003).[9]

**Table 3.2** Choosing a change strategy

| Critical question | Change strategy if answer is yes | Change strategy if answer is no |
|---|---|---|
| Are individual commitment and motivation essential for the success of the change? | Organization development | Programmed Political |
| Is the quality of the change process important? | Organization development | Programmed Political |
| Are there high levels of ambiguity and uncertainty? | Organization development Political | Programmed |
| Are conditions for conflict present? | Political | Programmed Organization development |
| Are you working from the bottom up? | Organization development | Programmed Political |

Inspired by Bolman and Deal (2003).[9]

# References

1. Fitzgerald A, Teal G. (2003). Health reform, professional identity and occupational sub-cultures: the changing interprofessional relations between doctors and nurses. *Contemporary Nurse* 2003; **16** (1–2): 9–19.

2. Callan VJ, Gallois C, Mayhew MG, *et al.* Restructuring the multi-professional organization: professional identity and adjustment to change in a public hospital. *Journal of Health and Human Services Adminstration* 2007; **29**: 448–77.

3. Weber M. *The Theory of Social and Economic Organization.* Translated by AM Henderson & Talcott Parsons. New York, NY: Free Press, 1947.

4. Kotter JP. *Leading Change.* Boston, MA: Harvard Business School Press, 1996.

5.  Nelson RR, Winter SG. *An Evolutionary Theory of Economic Change*. Cambridge, MA: Belknap Press, 1982.

6.  Schein E. *Organizational Culture and Leadership*. San Francisco, CA: Jossey-Bass, 1985.

7.  Pfeffer J. *Power in Organizations*. Marshfield, MA: Pitman, 1981.

8.  Grant RM. *Contemporary Strategy Analysis*. Oxford: Blackwell, 2008.

9.  Bolman L, Deal T. *Reframing Organizations: Artistry, Choice and Leadership*, 3rd edn. San Francisco, CA: Jossey-Bass, 2003.

10. Petri H, Govern J. *Motivation: Theory, Research, and Applications*. Belmont, CA: Wadsworth, 2003.

11. Maslow A. *Motivation and Personality*. New York, NY: Harper & Row, 1954.

12. Herzberg F. One more time. How do you motivate employees? *Harvard Business Review* 1968; **46** (1): 53–62.

13. Miner J. *Organizational Behavior I: Essential Theories of Motivation and Leadership*. Armonk: ME Sharpe, 2005.

14. Beer M, Nohria N. *Breaking the Code of Change*. Boston, MA: HBS Press, 2000.

15. Beckhard R, Harris RT. *Organizational Transitions: Managing Complex Change*. Reading, MA: Addison-Wesley, 1987.

16. Hahn W, Powers TL. Strategic plan quality, implementation capability and firm performance. *Academy of Strategic Management Journal* 2010; **9** (1).

17. Tang EC, Liou FM. Does firm performance reveal its own causes? The role of Bayesian inference. *Strategic Management Journal* 2010; **31** (1): 37–51.

**Chapter**

# 4

# Building the leadership team

Peter Cameron

## Key learning points

- Understand the essentials of team building, and the key roles in a successful emergency department (ED) leadership team.
- Know how to appoint the right people, how to mentor junior team members, how to manage underperformance.
- Understand succession planning and the importance of achieving an appropriate work–life balance.

An ED depends on a team culture and environment. A dysfunctional team will result in an unpleasant work environment and poor patient outcomes.

## Building the leadership team

To build an effective leadership team, there are a few essential characteristics, as outlined in the following sections.

## Authenticity

A leadership team requires a leader that other members of the team can respect and trust. The leader must believe in what he or she is doing and be enthusiastic and passionate about the outcomes. Although many managers will go through the motions of conveying a mission statement and strategic vision for their organization, this becomes pointless unless they are able to make the organizational members believe in the desired outcomes. If you can't articulate what it is that the organization stands for – and believe it yourself – then you will not succeed as a leader. In colloquial language, this means being able to "walk the talk."

## Ethics

Although none of us is perfect, if a leader wants a team to be ethical in its approach, then the leader has to model the behavior. Showing respect and being polite to patients and other team members (even those at the "bottom of the food chain") is an important starting point. Being punctual, being meticulous about claiming expenses and taking leave, and doing your share of the less popular shifts and duties suggests that you are serious about modeling good behavior. Clearly, as a director, you will have less time to do many tasks, but at least offering shows intent to shoulder the load.

## Communication
### To staff

For a team to function effectively, there must be good communication channels. There are formal and informal methods of communication. Generally each department will have some formal meetings such as a weekly leadership meeting. There may also be a weekly newsletter or email listing major news or changes for the department. Websites are also useful for posting important items such as events, policies, and meetings. Unfortunately, despite formal channels, most staff, most of the time, somehow do not seem to get the key messages that you want to relate. This is where informal channels are important. For key people in the organization (such as the nurse manager), it is worth having a coffee/drink regularly. An open-door policy is very helpful in allowing staff to bring up problems or issues early – before they result in discontentment and poor morale. Clearly there will be times when the office door needs to be closed, but this should be limited and is generally respected by staff. A few minutes each day passing

*Emergency Department Leadership and Management*, ed. Stephanie Kayden, *et al.* Published by Cambridge University Press.
© Cambridge University Press 2015.

through the work area (especially around handover time) shows that you care and are willing to listen to the small issues that staff may feel embarrassed bringing up in a formal meeting.

### To managers and superiors

The way you interact with your superiors is very important in determining your relationship with your own team. The team must know that you are an effective advocate for them and that you have credibility and respect from your seniors. Make sure that when you do have "wins" they are relayed to team members so that they understand that you are working for them. In much the same way, your superiors need to know that you are working for the whole organization. When budgets, throughput, and other numbers are improving, this should be relayed in clear concise language that is accessible to all. It is worth devoting some time to clear, rapid, and effective communication of the achievements of your department throughout the organization. A good website, short emails, newsletters, presentations, and media stories are all useful conduits.

## Meetings

It is possible to fill every day with meetings and not get anything done. Every meeting commitment should be assessed for its value to your department. Where there is no value then time should not be wasted. Regular meetings on a particular area (e.g., psychiatry liaison) can often be replaced by ad hoc meetings that are scheduled only when there is an issue. Meetings outside the department should be delegated to other senior staff where appropriate, to free up your time.

Meeting etiquette dictates that every meeting should start on time and finish on time. In general, business meetings longer than one hour are wasting time. Those attending the meeting should be focused and not reading emails and texts. Minutes are essential for useful business meetings (remember, whoever is taking the minutes determines the agenda, so make sure your allies are taking the minutes).

As a general rule, all business should be sorted before the meeting. A meeting that you chair in which there are surprise disagreements implies poor preparation. A quick call to participants before the meeting will ensure that major issues are sorted beforehand. If key points are sorted in a confrontational way during the meeting, there will be a winner – but more importantly a loser, who will not be happy. This person will work against you in the future. An intelligent discussion before the meeting will normally allow everyone to be a winner and ensure that there is total support for the proposal.

## Collaboration

An effective unit or department requires help from outside. The ED is very much a part of an integrated hospital or larger institutional/organizational group. With any major project or undertaking, always consult those affected and make them a part of the process. Ownership of the outcome is important in ensuring cooperation. Sharing "reflected glory" from successful projects also earns you "favors" that may be useful in future projects. For example, development of a cervical spine clearance protocol for your ED should involve the radiology, trauma, and neurosurgical departments. A review of the literature, audit of present practice, and post-implementation review could result in publications and presentations, which will bring kudos to your department and the other units involved. Improved outcomes, with reduction in radiology, fewer missed diagnoses, and faster patient processes can be "owned" by the whole organization. Most importantly, by coordinating the effort and undertaking the "leg work," you will have most control over the outcome.

## Democratization

The most effective means of managing your own group is to make the group feel that they are controlling the outcome. Ensure that there are team meetings, where staff can have their say and be listened to. It is good if major decisions can be voted on. Make time to listen to staff in the corridor or at tea breaks. If there is a complicated issue, ask them to put it in writing and follow it up. Delegate key tasks to different members of the team, so that decision making is "horizontal," not "vertical." For example, implementation of a new information technology system may be delegated to a senior staff member to chair the project team.

The concept of a rotating chair of department (to make everyone equal) has been suggested. However, there are some personalities that manage this role well, and generally a competitive process to select the best person (including outside candidates) will result in the most effective chair. Time-limited positions (e.g., 5 years with a 10-year maximum) are a useful way of reducing the risk of prolonged incumbency and ensuring the highest possible caliber of person for the job.

## Mistakes

It is inevitable that you will make mistakes and that the people under you will make mistakes. There is always the temptation to attribute the problems to those around you. As a general rule, the safest approach is to accept all blame (as the leader), then work out why the problem occurred and how it could be done better next time. As a clinical example, in a busy shift one of the juniors might have discharged a patient unsafely, resulting in a complaint from an inpatient unit. The best approach is to acknowledge the problem and state that you will explore what happened. Then speak with the junior concerned, look at supervision, staffing, etc. If there is a real problem, the recommendation might be better training, better supervision, better access to investigations or referral (all of these issues are departmental and relate to you). Unless there is criminal negligence, targeting a junior for public criticism as the cause of the problem should not happen.

At a departmental/administrative level, there will be issues such as cost overruns, poor staff performance, and so on. The best thing is to accept responsibility but then come up with the answers. Starting the conversation with "That's not my problem" will always get managers off side.

## Strategy

It is not enough to work in a "good ED." Each ED must develop a strategy to enable continuing improvement towards specific goals. These will depend on the specific role of each ED. For example, an inner-city ED serving indigent poor might have a very different mission than a state trauma center. Some EDs will have difficulty attracting good staff, inadequate finance, inadequate physical facilities, or a poor public image. A three- to five-year strategy mapping out a mission statement, departmental priorities, and key tasks will enable staff to see what they need to do and what they should be focused on. This is usually best undertaken in a workshop environment or during a retreat over a couple of days. Even a few hours away from the ED each year by senior staff can be useful in framing strategy.

In framing strategy, it is essential to be sensitive to the culture/values of the department, and not to bring in foreign dogma and force this onto the staff. Do some homework before the strategy meeting and work out what the issues are and what is important to the staff. A few anecdotes, especially relating to patients, are useful, as well as some basic statistics to show that you have done the background work. Having wonderful vision/mission statements that are not owned by the staff is useless.

## Succession planning

A successful team requires forward planning. Key positions such as the departmental director/chair, the director of training, and the director of research should have a succession plan and time-limited appointments. Senior physicians may still play a role even after moving out of the director positions, and the experience of senior clinicians should not be lost. There is a temptation in large departments to favor internal candidates, but most departments benefit from a regular infusion of new, outside talent. In small centers, this is not always possible.

One approach to getting new ideas and ways of doing things, while also giving internal candidates a chance to work in their alma mater, is to encourage young graduates to travel to other institutions and internationally. Once they have learned alternative approaches and new methods, they can return to a more senior position.

# Key designations on the leadership team

The required designations and tasks in the leadership team will vary according to the size and function of the ED. An ED with only one doctor will have many functions vested in one individual, whereas an emergency group with 50 specialists will have a large number of delegated tasks. The key designations are listed below. A weekly/monthly meeting of the group greatly enhances coordination and helps the department to function smoothly.

## Director/chair of department

Depending on the role of the ED and whether there is a major academic component, the chief of service holds the title of director or chair. There may also be site directors if there are multiple hospitals in a network or group. Increasingly, business responsibilities are held by non-medical personnel, and the director may be under the financial authority of a business director or "divisional head." This person may have been trained as a nurse or business analyst. Alternatively, the business manager may be a part of the ED team under the ED director.

In general the director of a large department should aim to delegate key roles to other senior staff so that most operational details are managed by others.

The question of clinical participation by the director is often debated. As a clinical director it is important to maintain a clinical presence and clinical credibility. It is important that the clinical director is seen as part of the team. Undertaking less clinical work than others will inevitably mean some decay in clinical skills, and if this is not managed well it may result in lack of clinical competency. However, 25% of the normal working week (e.g., 10–15 hours) spent on active clinical duty should be enough to maintain basic skills. This can be supplemented by regular updates for specific skills if necessary. The clinical work should involve some after-hours participation, so that the director is aware of how the ED operates at all times of the day.

## Training director

Training of doctors in emergency medicine is now highly structured, with international recognition of the curriculum needed for specialist training. Every ED should have one doctor designated and accountable for the overall teaching program. This will usually require a minimum of 0.5 FTE for a residency program. This person is responsible for ensuring that the teaching is delivered, that training materials are available, and that assessments are undertaken and fed back to trainees. This person should not be the director. In addition, training of non-specialist trainees rotating through the ED, medical students, and senior staff should be considered. If there are sufficient senior staff, then one person can be allocated to each of these roles.

The increasing specialization of nursing training in emergency medicine has meant that many of the teaching modules and training packages can be shared between nursing and medical trainees. This can markedly increase resources for training in terms of staff and content. This is especially important for online material and packaged courses such as advanced cardiac life support/advanced pediatric life support (ACLS/APLS).

## Quality

Developing a coherent quality-improvement program for the ED is essential for a high-functioning department. Although resources restrict the size and depth of activities undertaken, some basic structural components are essential (see Chapter 7). One senior medical staff member should be designated to take responsibility for the overall program and coordinate departmental meetings such as morbidity and mortality meetings. For complaints and incident reports, a single point of contact and accountability will help to ensure appropriate follow-up and feedback to staff and complainants. There are multiple priorities for audit and review of activities within the ED, and it is important that one senior staff member ensures that all the important matters are adequately dealt with.

## Research

In larger academic departments, research output is a key measure of success. Success is usually measured by the number and impact of published papers and the number, source, and size of research grants. An important "byproduct" of a research-intensive department is the promotion of evidence-based practice within the department.

Key functions of the research director are to make sure that the research effort is focused on relevant clinical topics, that research projects are coordinated and feasible, and that staff members are engaged. In addition, sourcing and coordinating grant applications to fund key projects is a major task. Research training should be seen as a central role of academic departments. A good research program should ensure that staff members actively question current practice and have an evidence-based approach to delivery of clinical programs. An active journal club will assist with this. The director of research will require a minimum of 0.5 FTE to be effective. This can be financed through grants, or it may be seen by more enlightened hospitals to be cost-effective in promoting evidence-based practice and attracting high-quality staff.

## Emergency medical services

The responsibility for emergency medical services (EMS) varies in different countries. In many countries, the EMS is coordinated from the hospital, although this is becoming less common with the professionalization of the paramedic workforce and greater central coordination of dispatch. When the EMS is independent of the hospital it is still useful to appoint one person to act as the contact for EMS issues. This person follows up on clinical problems, assists with protocol development, deals with coordination across sites, and oversees the management of system overload in times of ED overcrowding.

## Other physician roles

Many of the senior physicians will have special interests in important clinical areas such as pediatrics, geriatric medicine, toxicology, and disaster medicine. In many departments it will be necessary to have a separate head of pediatrics, to ensure that protocols, training, equipment, and so forth are adequate. Similar arguments can be made for other subspecialty areas, if there is sufficient volume of patients and/or subspecialty interest. These should not be seen as separate EDs, but as domains of activity within the overall ED.

## Nursing

Generally it is useful for the major medical designations to be mirrored by equivalent appointments for nurses. The terms will vary in different countries: for example, in Australia, the nurse director is called a "nurse manager." For major domains such as quality and training, it is particularly important to have a senior nurse identified and responsible to assist in engagement by the nursing group.

## Allied health

This group is often not seen as a crucial part of the ED function, but when they are fully integrated as a part of the ED team they can greatly facilitate patient throughput and patient experience. Physiotherapists, occupational therapists, social workers, and others have skills that are very useful in the ED. Having a spokesperson for this group will greatly assist the team.

## Clerical/administrative

Clerks are also often overlooked, but appointing a head clerk to bring issues to the management meetings is very useful.

## Key leadership tasks
## Getting the right people

Most of the time you will be appointed to a leadership position with staff already in place. Thus, getting a team together is as much about making the most of incumbents as it is about appointing new people. The first step is to make sure that everyone is aware of your expectations in terms of behavior, work ethic, and outcomes. Every team member should feel ownership of the shared goals for the department. It is important to speak to each team member, to work out what they want, what their skill sets are, and what their aspirations are. Just by going through this process, a number of staff will leave and move on to a different ED or position outside emergency medicine.

There are usually obvious deficiencies in the "mix" of people that you need to make a good department. You might need someone with research or teaching experience, an IT guru, pediatrics or other skill sets. Think carefully about each appointment and what benefit it will bring to the team. Never appoint someone just because that person is available, or because no one else applied. It is better to have a vacant position than a non-performer who is hard to move on.

Identify potential candidates for specific jobs in advance and let them know that you are interested in their career development. The most important skill set for any potential employee is the ability to work in the team (i.e., personality). This is usually evident from previous work experience. Having personally worked with someone previously is very useful in assessing personality, and personal recommendations from friends may also be helpful. Interviews are generally unhelpful in assessing personalities.

When you are unsure of the suitability of a candidate, it is sometimes helpful to mutually agree to a short-term contract with agreed outcomes at the conclusion of the probation period. This is only useful for junior staff. A short period of observership, with leave of absence from the current employer, may also be helpful for more senior appointments, avoiding potential mutual embarrassment if the candidate does not fit with the group. A further approach is to undertake a joint project together, which will give insights into teamwork, flexibility, compromise, and other traits. It is also worth remembering that candidates may work well in one team and not in another, because of the different mix of personalities. It is not always possible to predict how people will behave, so it is inevitable that you will make mistakes.

---

**Case study 4.1.  Managing underperformers**

Staff specialist Peter is notorious amongst nursing staff for his shifts. Patients wait a long time to be seen and his shifts are always the "busiest." How do you manage this?

It is important to have factual information – how many patients are seen each shift, waiting times, and casemix. Feeding this back in a non-judgmental way (relative to peers), is often sufficient to improve performance. Regular review (at least annual) and encouragement is important. Getting 360-degree assessments from all staff can be helpful in allowing senior staff to reflect on how others see them. If all else fails, then allocation to other tasks, such as teaching or review clinic, can allow an "honorable" exit. In general, confrontational performance reviews are counterproductive to the individual and to the ED team as a whole.

---

## Mentoring junior staff members

During training, the director of training will often assume the role of mentor for junior residents. This may work well but can become confused with assessments and clinical oversight. Mentoring can also occur by default, when juniors look up to particular individuals and model their behavior accordingly. Many departments have an active mentorship program, where juniors are allocated to a specific mentor who gives career advice and encouragement and acts as an advocate for the trainee. Clearly the selection of mentors should be agreed on by both parties – because, for it to be useful, both mentor and mentee have to be compatible and enthusiastic participants.

Mentoring of doctors following training is equally important, as frequently this group is forgotten and their potential is not maximized. Giving junior doctors roles in assisting with training, research, and administrative tasks allows them the chance to experience different aspects of extended emergency physician roles.

## Managing underperformers

Even in the best department, with careful selection of staff members, there will be some staff performing at a suboptimal level. Failure to manage this effectively decreases productivity of the individual – and, more

importantly, brings down the team. In much the same way that a stellar performer will spur staff on to produce better outcomes, a staff member performing badly will create a negative attitude and "permit" negative behaviors for the group as a whole.

The starting point for managing performance is to ensure that all staff have at least annual performance reviews with adequate documentation. Ideally performance issues should be discussed regularly and frequently (e.g., weekly) so that there are no surprises regarding good and bad aspects of individual performance. This can be done both formally and informally. Performance reviews also reassure staff who are performing well, as frequently it is the best performers who are most anxious about being seen as underperformers! For example, regular issues such as timeliness, documentation, and speed of patient assessments should be fed back to the staff member. Ideally performance should be benchmarked with others, so that there is a degree of objectivity, rather than subjective labels such as "laziness."

It is more difficult when the issues are related to personality or interpersonal skills. Again, it is much more straightforward to manage if this is presented in an objective manner. Having a structured assessment form with key traits that are reviewed and scored at each appraisal helps. Other examples of structured feedback include patient satisfaction surveys and "360-degree assessments" (where staff members receive anonymous feedback from all staff they interact with).

Most staff members will respond positively to assessment and feedback, but there will always be a small percentage who continue to perform poorly despite counseling. The rules of employment vary between countries, but as a general rule, for serious underperformance, three briefings with a third party (usually a human resources officer) present are adequate to ensure procedural fairness before termination. For all positions, especially senior staff, the best outcome is for the staff member to realize that he or she does not fit the expectations of the organization and move on. It can help if you provide such staff with alternatives and where their strengths and weakness lie, so that they apply for the most suitable positions. If staff can leave with a mutually agreed outcome of alternative employment, this is good for you, the staff member, and the organization. A disgruntled employee can have disastrous effects on your ability to employ good people into the future. Therefore "sacking" staff should be avoided if at all possible. Importantly, however, if the staff member shows blatant disregard for the organization and its values (e.g., "sloppy work," absenteeism, etc.), then terminating employment may actually show other employees that you are serious about maintaining a high-quality organization.

Clearly where there are documented criminal or professional issues such as theft, sexual harassment, illicit drug taking, or bullying, then involvement of the appropriate authorities should occur early. Trying to manage these issues internally is problematic. They are always best managed in conjunction with external expertise.

## Measuring and benchmarking

This will be considered in more detail in Chapter 7. For high-achieving health professionals, there is an innate degree of competitiveness. This becomes a powerful driver for change. Something that was "impossible" to change or improve because of lack of resources or because it was too difficult will suddenly become possible. This is more plausible if a like institution has already achieved the goal. Used well, with credible data, benchmarking changes behavior. Benchmarking can be done at an organizational level or at an individual level. The principal message in using these tools is to work out what your aim is first – then work out how you are going to monitor progress toward this aim. Do not develop a random suite of indicators that look good and then present fancy graphs to the board or the ED group. Decide on a program (e.g., improved analgesic administration), then work out what indicators will best track the impact of your improvement program.

For individual staff member feedback, some basic numbers such as the number of patients seen, complexity/casemix, and consumer satisfaction can be helpful to the individual, and as a means of adding objectivity to performance reviews (see above). It is best to do this with other staff de-identified.

## Work–life balance

It is almost inevitable, as a leader of a department that works 24 hours a day, 7 days per week, that a director will be tempted to be available *all* the time. This is often accentuated by issues that arise after

hours such as staff shortages, disasters, complaints, and media inquiries. Arriving on Monday morning to find that a series of disasters has occurred over the weekend further exacerbates the problem and encourages directors to make themselves universally available. Most clinical directors should have some clinical load and be involved in the after-hours roster – but this makes it even more difficult to get time off.

To function effectively, think strategically, and make balanced decisions, a leader should not be tired, irritable, and unapproachable. Taking adequate time off and having other interests is in the department's interest and your own. Rostering at least one day per week when you are not at work and uncontactable (apart from disasters) is one approach. Going week-about (for on-call issues) or sharing the position with a deputy is another. There is no magic number of hours or days that one should work, but consideration of "balance" is crucial.

The key to this is having a good team. This means that if you work the weekend and want Monday off, you know that there is someone available to deputize for meetings and other issues that might arise. As director, you should not feel that your presence is essential. It is gratifying – and it helps your ego – when staff welcome you with open arms and say "Thank God you are here." However, this demonstrates failure in some ways – as it demonstrates that the ED does not function well without you. The ultimate aim is to make yourself redundant!

Being director of an ED has a time limit, and most people should limit their tenure to 5–10 years maximum. This does not preclude a further position after a gap of some years.

---

**Case study 4.2. Rostering**

You have been asked to provide better after-hours cover for your ED with senior staff. Staff specialists are happy with their current 0800–1800 shift, but with increasing expectations from the hospital you now need to cover 24 hours per day. What options do you have?

Although commonplace in the USA, the practice of 24-hour senior specialist on-site cover is less common elsewhere. Rostering senior clinicians to see patients overnight is associated with burnout and decreased satisfaction. It is important that there are sufficient numbers of staff to support a 24-hour roster – more than a few nights per month for each senior staff member will generally fail. Overnight shifts should be shorter – no more than 10 hours.

It is possible to cover the majority of the 24 hours by extending the evening shift until 0200 and starting the morning shift at 0600. This may be sufficient in many EDs to cover the vast majority of attendances. If full 24-hour coverage is mandated then a "casino shift" is another option – evening shift until 0300–0400 hours and morning shift starting at 0400 hours. Using a senior fellow/trainee to cover a significant percentage of night shifts can work (short-term rotational appointment). Also, some staff specialists prefer night shifts and will take a larger percentage of the shifts.

As an interim solution, many EDs have trialed using an overnight specialist who sleeps on the premises and is woken for any major cases. This may be useful for a low-volume ED.

## Conclusion

Developing a high-functioning emergency department team is challenging but rewarding. The basic principles can be gleaned from any leadership text. The content knowledge specific to emergency medicine has been learned many times over by hundreds of like-minded individuals in many countries. By talking to and collaborating with others who have experienced similar trials and tribulations, one can hopefully avoid the common pitfalls and advance the clinical practice of emergency medicine internationally.

Chapter

# 5

# Establishing the emergency department's role within the hospital

Thomas Fleischmann

## Key learning points

- Describe the vision and the mission of an emergency department.
- Define the role of an emergency department within a hospital.
- Identify the medical tasks of the emergency department.
- Understand the relationship between the emergency department and other departments and facilities of the hospital.

## Introduction

Emergency care around the world is organized in many ways, mainly because of differences in the respective countries' healthcare systems, economic status, and history. While there are differences among countries, there have been three major trends globally that have had a strong impact on emergency care in many countries. These are:

- the growing number of patients who seek emergency care in a hospital
- the tremendous increase in the standard of knowledge in emergency medicine
- the rising expertise in how emergency care in a hospital can best be organized to match the needs of the acutely ill and injured

Following these solid trends over the years, emergency departments (EDs) in many countries are becoming better organized, and at the same time increasingly similar. Lessons learned in other countries are very helpful in shaping a clear idea of an effective and efficient ED.

Regardless of how the care is organized in various countries, the first and most important step is to look at the needs of the emergency patients – as they are uniformly the same all over the world. The economic status, the medical history of the country, and the interests of medical organizations are to be acknowledged, but they fall in line after the needs of the patients.

## A brief history of emergency medicine

Seen from a historical perspective, hospital-based emergency medicine is a very recent institution.[1] For a long period of time in the history of medicine, emergency care was delivered mainly in an outpatient setting and by laypersons or aides often willing to help but poorly trained. For centuries medical treatment of an acutely ill or injured person inside a hospital was the exception rather than the rule. This may have been due to limited access to hospitals and an apparently high acceptance of fate in case of an emergency. Even doctors seemed to be at peace with the idea of treating critically ill or injured patients at home or not at all.

The next step in history was that it became more and more common for a doctor to take care of medical emergencies, although at first only in the outpatient setting. This change was supported by a more generous coverage of medical costs in those countries which started to provide social security systems, but there was still a way to go until it became common behavior to seek emergency medical care in a hospital. Some countries tried to restrict immediate access to a hospital to very severe or life-threatening emergencies only. In Germany or the Netherlands, for example, acutely ill or injured patients were until recently advised to call their primary care physician services first, except in the case of a severe emergency. But even in these countries patients have increasingly

*Emergency Department Leadership and Management*, ed. Stephanie Kayden, *et al.* Published by Cambridge University Press.
© Cambridge University Press 2015.

decided to go to a hospital even for a minor emergency. The tremendous spread of EDs over the past few decades, and of professional medical care delivered there, has inspired both patients and providers to install well-organized emergency care systems within the hospitals in even more countries.

There are four main ways to take care of acutely ill or injured patients in a hospital:[2]

- direct ward admission
- decentralized admission areas
- central emergency departments but subdivided by specialties
- interdisciplinary emergency departments

## Direct ward admission

Direct admission to a ward was often the first approach to deal with an emergency in a hospital. This was due to the fact that some hospitals had no outpatient area at all. Even if they had one, it was often closed after normal business hours. With the growing number of emergency patients coming to the hospital, however, it was soon realized that emergency care can easily compromise the regular work of a ward. Another disadvantage of this system is that it is not an easy task to discharge a patient with a minor condition once that patient has been admitted to a ward. This system is therefore rarely seen today, or is limited to hospitals with a very low number of medical emergencies and countries with less well established healthcare systems.

## Decentralized admission areas

After realizing the disruptive potential of direct ward admission, some medical specialties began to set up designated areas for emergency patients. These admission areas were often installed in the premises of the respective specialty, often close to their wards. These areas therefore belong to the particular specialty and often operate independently from other specialties. As a result, large hospitals with a high number of medical specialties can have up to 20 or more independently organized and operating admission areas.[3]

This creates a number of serious problems, of which one of the most important is that the triage and the decision about which admission area might be the most appropriate is the responsibility of the least medically trained person, such as the doorman or receptionist of the hospital. Based on the description

of the complaint, a decision has to be made as to which specialty might be appropriate to send the patient to, often without medical training. A second major disadvantage is that the attendants of an admission area might send the patient to another specialty, arguing that they are not responsible for the medical problem in question. It is not unusual for this to result in an appalling tour of several admission areas until someone accepts responsibility. Patients' complaints of being sent around the hospital and taken care of reluctantly are common in this system. Thirdly, it is very expensive and inefficient to sustain several admission areas within a hospital at the same time.

---

**Case study 5.1**

Mr. Pheffer is brought to the hospital by ambulance. He has been found with a slightly altered level of consciousness and a scalp wound. Because of the injury the ambulance workers decide to bring him to the surgical admission area. He is awake but uncooperative. He talks and acts strangely. The surgeon on call notices alcohol on his breath. The scalp wound is superficial and needs no further treatment. The surgeon decides to send the patient to the admission area of the psychiatric department, which is in another part of the hospital. After an hour of transportation and waiting, the psychiatrist notices an alcohol level and liver enzymes too high to keep him in the psychiatric ward. Mr. Pheffer is sent to the admission area of the medical department, in another part of the hospital, for medical clearance and further evaluation. After another hour of transportation and waiting he is seen by the gastroenterologist on call. During this the patient has an epileptic seizure. He is then rushed to the neurological department, which is in another part of the building. The neurologist on call finds that Mr. Pheffer is now unresponsive. He is then brought to the radiology department, which is in another part of the building. The CT scan of the brain reveals a large subdural hematoma. Mr. Pheffer is then transported to the neurosurgical department, which is in another part of the building. The subdural hematoma is operated on immediately, but it is more than 5 hours since the patient entered the hospital.

---

## Central but subdivided emergency department

Some hospitals started to design special areas to receive all or at least most of the acutely ill or injured patients, but because of the political leverage and power of some specialties these central EDs were subdivided into specific treatment areas by specialty. Another reason for this subdivision by specialties is the shortage of trained emergency physicians in some places. A not atypical form of organization is that some rooms of the ED are reserved for a certain specialty only; another common setup is that a room can be used by several specialties, but the patient is seen by the resident of a certain specialty only, whichever seems to be the most appropriate at admission.

One advantage of this system is that travel over several admission areas is discouraged. Another is that the decision which resident to call is taken by a nurse and not by a layperson. But there are disadvantages, too. An important one is that at the initial presentation of an emergency it is often far from clear which specialty the patient might fall to in the end. Additionally, a large number of patients have more than one medical condition, and it is unclear again which specialty should eventually take care of the patient. These issues account for a large proportion of the patients in a medical emergency, if not the majority. The identification of the specialty which the patient should be referred to takes place at the end of the process of emergency care much more often than at the start of it.

This again leads to the fact that patients in a central but subdivided ED are often seen by many doctors. It is not infrequent that the patient is seen by doctors of several specialties and different ranks. The length of stay in subdivided EDs is often severely prolonged by this, and the process of decision making can be tedious. Patients often complain about a loss of clarity concerning which doctor is responsible for them. This loss of clarity is often shared by the doctors and nurses involved, too.

---

**Case study 5.2**

Mrs. Omidyar comes to the ED because of midline abdominal pain for several hours. There are no emergency physicians in this hospital, and the nurses have to call the doctor of the specialty thought to be appropriate for the complaint. The nurses decide to call the cardiologist on call. The ECG is non-specific, and the first troponin is unremarkable. Another ECG and a lab test 3 hours later are unremarkable, too. But the epigastric pain is still present, and now there is some midline tenderness. The cardiologist calls for a gastroscopy to rule out a gastric ulcer. This is done almost 2 hours later and shows no signs of illness. The gastroenterologist who performed the gastroscopy recommends a urological consultation to exclude ureteral obstruction. This is done 1 hour later. The urologist performs an ultrasound examination of the kidneys and finds nothing specific. He then asks for a gynecologist to rule out a gynecological cause of the ongoing pain. The gynecologist responds to the call 90 minutes later and performs an endovaginal ultrasound, which reveals nothing. He then asks for a surgeon to rule out a bowel obstruction. The surgeon orders a CT scan of the abdomen by phone. This is done 90 minutes later and shows gallstones and an acute cholecystitis. The diagnosis is made almost 7 hours after the patient entered the hospital and after examinations by six doctors (cardiologist, gastroenterologist, urologist, gynecologist, radiologist, surgeon).

## Interdisciplinary emergency department

Hospitals with modern EDs typically hold the big advantage of having a single entry point for all medical emergency patients. They avoid the disadvantage of attributing patients to a specialty too early in the course of emergency care, i.e. at a stage when the true nature of the medical emergency is often far from clear.[4] The vision of this type of ED is best described by the well-known and widely accepted principle of EDs worldwide: "anyone, anything, anytime."[5]

These EDs prove to be effective and efficient at the same time, too. It is very expensive to have several doctors of different specialties present in the ED or in the hospital at all times.[2] In many countries medical specialization has reached a high degree, and more than 40 different specialties and subspecialties are not unusual. It is neither reasonable, affordable, nor necessary to have them present in the early stages of medical care, provided there is a professional emergency physician in the ED who takes care of the patient at short notice. Doctors of a specialty can be called in the event that they are needed. The advancement of emergency medicine and designated training in emergency medicine is supported by the fact that the principles of dealing with a medical emergency are very similar, regardless whether it is an illness, injury, or intoxication.

Within the past few decades, EDs of this type have spread around the world, and they have proved to be

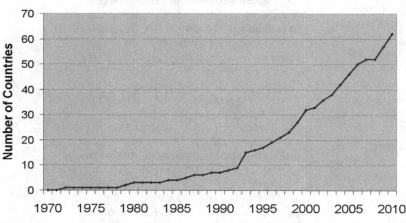

**Figure 5.1** The growth in emergency medicine. Reproduced with permission from Anderson PD, Hegedus A, Holliman CJ, *et al.* Worldwide growth of emergency medicine as a recognized medical specialty (manuscript in submission).

useful in the care of emergency patients every day and night, reducing the time spent by patients in the hospital, the performance of needless and duplicative tests, and the chance that mis-triage to a wrong service leads to a patient not being treated in a timely manner for a life-threatening illness.

## The future of emergency medicine

The mission of an ED is to deliver appropriate care to patients in any kind of medical emergency, based on proven knowledge and sound experience, providing the same good quality at all times.

The vision shared by many practitioners in emergency medicine is to prepare an area solely devoted to the care of patients in any type of medical emergency, be it an illness or an injury, where well-trained nurses, doctors, and other staff deliver emergency care at a highly scientific and empathetic level.

Some but not too many conditions are required to reach this ambitious target. First, there has to be a space within the hospital, specially designed to receive patients in a medical emergency. Some decades ago this was often only a single room, hence the term "emergency room." With the growing number of emergency patients seeking help in a hospital it became necessary to provide more than one room and to design the area specially to match the needs of emergency care. Therefore the emergency room became an emergency department. It is worthwhile to note that the design of this facility is very different than that of a ward or an ambulatory area, for example.

Second, there must be nursing staff devoted to taking care of emergency patients.[6] Emergency nursing is obviously different than the care in a ward or in an outpatient department. Emergency nursing is best practiced in an ED. Classroom training is needed to perform this duty, but the best place to learn this is the ED.

Third, doctors with training and experience in emergency medicine are needed to provide good care to patients in an emergency. Amongst others, two important reasons account for this: (1) the principles of medical action in an emergency are very different from other kinds of practice, and (2) the proven and partly even evidence-based knowledge in emergency medicine has grown rapidly and vastly over the past few decades. High-quality emergency care cannot be delivered without knowledge, training, and experience in this very special form of medical care. The knowledge needed to take care of patients in an ED is well described and approved.[7,8] The growth of what can be described as emergency medicine has been remarkable, as shown in Figure 5.1.

It is important to acknowledge that the presence and action of doctors in an ED must not be compromised by other medical duties, for example in the operating theater or on a ward. The true nature of an emergency demands the undivided attention of the doctors taking care of it, often "right now on the spot." Mixing the duties of the doctors in the ED with other medical tasks – ward duty, responding to emergencies throughout the hospital, etc. – invariably leads to dissatisfaction on the part of patients, doctors, nurses, and administrators at many levels.[9]

Fourth, clear leadership of the ED is essential to assure a high level of care for emergency patients.[10] The leader of the ED has to conduct a set of tasks specific for an ED, for example patient flow management, quality assurance, and risk management. In larger EDs this task often requires an individual to be assigned to the position as his or her main duty. EDs are often the largest departments in a hospital in respect of the number of patients. In many hospitals a large fraction or even the majority of the patients enter the hospital by the ED. It, too, has a vast number of links to other facilities of the hospital. It also relies heavily on good interactions with them to secure seamless patient care from admission to discharge. To cultivate these interactions takes time and attention. A certain state of independence is necessary to comply with these tasks properly.

Fifth, the procedures in the ED, both medical and operational, have to be clearly described, followed, and observed.[11] Many operations in an ED are highly time-dependent, either because of the critical condition of the patient or because of a large number of patients. Skilled time and flow management is highly important, and this again is a permanent and time-consuming challenge for the leader and the staff of an ED.[12]

---

**Case study 5.3**

After getting a substantial number of complaints from patients and relatives about long waiting times and prolonged stays in the ED, the director of the Southwest Hospital decides to have a closer look at the ED. He realizes that there are sometimes junior doctors at work with no training in emergency medicine and little or no supervision. At times the doctors have to serve the ED and a ward, or even the operating room, at the same time. There is little interdisciplinary thinking and acting on the medical side. Because of this, many patients in the ED are seen by five or more doctors of different specialties and ranks. He concludes that long waiting times, unclear responsibilities when a large number of doctors are involved, and a high consumption of resources are closely linked with these procedures.

Impressed by this and inspired by descriptions of well-organized EDs by other hospital directors, he decides to act. He determines the ED to be a department of its own at the same level as the other medical departments of the hospital. He looks for an experienced leader of an ED, and assigns her as the medical director of the ED. He makes clear that he expects a well-functioning ED with a clear mission and well-described procedures within a pre-assigned period of time. In order to achieve this he provides his support and the resources necessary. This includes hiring some doctors experienced in emergency medicine to work in the ED on a permanent basis, but also the mentoring of junior doctors and those not trained in emergency medicine.

Within less than a year the ED is said to be one of the best in the city. More patients than ever before seek help in the ED. They are seen in a timely fashion and well treated according to established guidelines. The revenues of the ED increase, and consumption of resources is controlled at the same time.

---

# The medical role of the emergency department

The operational role of an ED can be easily defined as a place to receive all patients in a medical emergency, where treatment begins immediately, and as a point where the decision is made concerning whether to discharge or admit the patient.

On the other hand, the medical role can be subdivided into five assignments:[13]

- assessment and stabilization
- diagnosis
- therapy
- risk stratification
- disposition

Assessment and stabilization of the patient's vital functions are core competencies of emergency physicians. In order to perform at the high level of pressure regularly experienced in the ED they have to be well trained and used to this special kind of work. The process of finding a diagnosis can be a challenge in an emergency, as most patients present with a symptom, not a diagnosis. Many key presentations in an emergency are ambiguous, and atypical presentations even of life-threatening conditions are often more common than typical presentations. To find the right diagnosis in a stressful situation can be demanding even for senior emergency physicians. By having physicians trained in a comprehensive emergency medicine program that includes training in all specialties, the chance of having to send a patient from specialty to specialty is lessened.

Once the patient has been stabilized and a diagnosis has been reached, therapy is often easy in emergency medicine. But not infrequently emergency physicians face the predicament of taking care of a patient who is declining rapidly when a diagnosis has not been established yet. Then the doctors are forced to perform diagnostic and therapeutic procedures concomitantly to stabilize the patient. Sometimes they have to start treatment even before having a clear diagnosis. This again makes EDs very special places where the practice of medicine differs from that in other fields of care. This is not to say that from time to time other specialties will not be called to the ED. Even the most progressive EDs have established relationships with other specialties in the hospital for occasional consultations on difficult cases.

Risk stratification is another key competency of emergency medicine. In many cases it is not possible to establish a diagnosis for the presentation at hand. The first task then is to rule out a life-threatening or otherwise dangerous condition. The risk of an adverse event in the near future has to be assessed to determine whether the patient has to be admitted or can be sent home for further treatment in the outpatient setting. The knowledge regarding risk stratification in emergency medicine has grown considerably in recent years and supports these sometimes difficult decisions in the ED.

The last step in the process of delivering care in the ED is to either admit the patient to a ward suited best for his or her condition or discharge the patient. In either case, the doctor who takes over the care of the patient needs to be informed about the findings and actions in the ED, to assure seamless medical care.

There are some issues concerning what ED cannot or should not do. It is no substitute for a primary care physician. Nor is it the place to ask for a second opinion. Nor can it provide continuous medical care to patients with chronic conditions. This can be done via faxing of the chart to the primary care doctor post discharge, via phone call, or via email – and it is essential to building good relations with the primary care community.

There is another medical task which the ED cannot and should not peform: it is not the place for patients with scheduled consultations. The needs and expectations of a patient with an appointment are completely different from the needs and expectations of the patient in a medical emergency. Those two groups of patients should be completely separated and never mixed. Scheduled patients and emergency patients compete with each other for resources if they are processed through the same pathways or even through the same rooms. Dissatisfaction of many patients, if not all, then becomes inevitable.

In conclusion, there are specific roles that EDs are best suited for, but there are others that an ED should not fulfill. The local ED should be viewed as a place where patients in a given community feel comfortable attending as a competent, efficient, and well-organized facility in case of a medical emergency.

# Organization within the hospital

As discussed above, there is a clear role for the ED as the sole entry point for all emergency patients within the hospital, and as such it fills a unique position within the hospital. For many reasons the ED is different from other facilities in the hospital. First, it receives patients with all kinds of illnesses and injuries and is therefore a truly interdisciplinary facility. Most of the departments of a hospital are defined according to a specialty or an organ, whereas the ED is geared to a condition: the emergency.

Second, the ED is often the first, but only rarely the final department to care for the patient. Doctors in the ED do not work alone but are a vital link in the care of patients. They prepare the patient either for the primary care physician, if the patient is discharged, or for the specialty doctors in the hospital, if the patient is admitted.

These issues influence not only the medical work but also the organization of the ED. Looking at the structure of the hospital, the medical specialty departments can be seen in parallel alignment, whereas the ED is a broad but thin layer in front of all of them.

Given the interdisciplinary nature of the ED, it has to be an independent facility in the hospital. Independence assures a neutral position both toward the patient and toward the different specialties the doctors in ED are constantly working with. If the ED is part of one specialty, this neutral position can easily be compromised.

Different countries have tested several organizational forms of EDs in the hospital. The lessons learned are much the same even in different healthcare systems and in different countries. There is no other widespread and widely accepted form of providing good care in a medical emergency other than a true interdisciplinary ED. For that reason EDs are becoming more and more similar in many countries of the world.[14–16]

The interdisciplinary nature of the ED, the importance of its neutrality toward all specialties and facilities, and the fact that the ED often has by far the largest number of patients in a hospital, mean that the status of an ED as a single and independent facility is a matter of importance.

## Relationship with other departments

Emergency care is the first step in the care of a patient with an acute condition, but it is seldom the only one. Because of this, the ED relies heavily on close and good relationships with all other departments and facilities of the hospital. Once again, the alignment of the medical specialties may be looked at as parallel columns, with the ED as a thin but broad layer in front of them.

Administratively, the ED should be responsible for every patient in the ED, and also involved in the laboratory and radiology for a significant number of them. Consultants from cardiology, neurology, pediatrics, and orthopedic and general surgeons, are often called into the ED, but every other specialty may be called from time to time as well. Only about 5–10% of the patients of the ED are admitted to an intensive care unit eventually, but these transfers can be very urgent.[17] In order to provide a safe and easy course for the patient after leaving the ED it is very important to establish close and trusting links to every other specialty and department in the hospital.

The ED is closely linked with all other departments through the patients they share. The medical care is often just started in the ED, to stabilize the patient, and that care needs to be continued in another department of the hospital. Every ED needs every other medical facility eventually, and this works both ways: every medical department needs the ED as a source of patients. These close links should be respected and nourished. This can be done by concerted work on hospital committees regarding quality assurance, the development of specific clinical pathways, patient safety, or service capacity, for example. Mutual medical education and training should be regular events. Cross-training opportunities, especially at the resident level, can serve both sides, both regarding the transfer of knowledge and contributing toward mutual appreciation.

The idea of an interdisciplinary ED is spreading rapidly in many countries of the world. But it has to be realized that emergency care existed in hospitals before any EDs were set up. In addition, in every hospital there was someone who took care of emergencies in earlier times, mostly in addition to other positions and duties. In many countries several specialties tried to secure an influential role in emergency care.

An ED as an independent institution in a hospital can provide not only good emergency care but also good service to all specialties and to the hospital as a whole. The advantages of this way of organizing emergency care are evident, but sometimes an orientation to the past, or perhaps individual interests, might hamper this insight. It is therefore not surprising that in most countries emergency medicine as a specialty was not at first greeted enthusiastically by other specialties. But in no country did the skepticism of other specialties stop the advancement of EDs and emergency medicine in the long term.

In some countries emergency medicine was set up as a specialty not by insight but by government decree. This did not always help its acceptance by other medical authorities. But in all of the many countries around the world which have now recognized emergency medicine as a specialty there were farsighted doctors who had a clear vision of how EDs could provide good emergency care. Pioneer work is never easy. But the clear evidence of what this institution can do for patients, doctors, and hospitals – combined with the lessons learned from those countries who have walked this path before – can greatly help to secure and advance the vision of an ED.

## Communication and the community

People generally view EDs favorably. They may not like to enter them as patients, but as citizens of a community they are happy to know that there is always a place to go to in case of an emergency. Politicians, too, are often proud of their contribution to the existence of this service to the public.

The notoriety of an ED, and sometimes its fate, relies strongly on the trust of the citizens who seek help there. Rumors and stories about an ED spread fast, whether good or not so good. It is therefore one of the tasks of the leaders of an ED to establish and foster close and trustful bonds with the community it serves. This is a constant challenge which needs enthusiasm, tact, and ingenuity. A good way to achieve this is to hold regular meetings with citizens and the media. The media can act as a link between the department and the public. Fostering good connections with the media may even help in a crisis, for example when a patient in the ED turns out to be a celebrity or when a major disaster brings a lot of attention to the department. Having earned trust and respect with the public beforehand goes a long way with the media and politicians then.

## Conclusions

Emergency care around the world is organized in many different ways, mainly arising from differences in the respective countries' healthcare systems, economic status, and history. But what is common to the entire world is the medical need of the acutely ill and injured.

Starting from unequal points of origin, and following different paths, EDs are becoming more highly organized and more similar in many countries. To provide high-quality emergency medicine it is essential to establish a clear idea of how emergency care in a hospital can best meet the needs of the patients.

Establishing an ED in a hospital is a worthwhile journey, but a long one – but lessons learned from other countries which have traveled the same path previously can be a tremendous help.

## References

1. Fleischmann T. A history of emergency medicine. In T Fleischmann, ed., *Clinical Emergency Medicine*. Munich: Elsevier, 2012; 3–12 [German].

2. Fleischmann T, Walter B. Interdisciplinary emergency departments. *German Medical Journal* 2007; **104**: A-3164–6 [German].

3. Moecke H, Lackner C, Altemeyer K. No way back: central emergency departments are increasingly popular in German hospitals. *Preclinical and Clinical Emergency Medicine* 2007; **5**: 321 [German].

4. Kahrer C. *Patient Flow in the Emergency Department.* Saarbrucken: VDM, 2009 [German].

5. Zink B. *Anyone, Anything, Anytime: a History of Emergency Medicine*. Philadelphia, PA: Mosby Elsevier, 2005.

6. O'Hara S. The nursing perspective and role in planning a simulation modeling: historical, experimental, and future applications of complex adaptive system thinking. In J Shiver, D Eitel, eds., *Optimising Emergency Department Throughput*. New York, NY: Taylor & Francis, 2010; 67–107.

7. Thomas H, Beeson M, Binder L, *et al*. The 2005 model of the clinical practice of emergency medicine: the 2007 update. *Annals of Emergency Medicine* 2008; **52**: e1–17.

8. UEMS Multidisciplinary Joint Committee on Emergency Medicine, European Society for Emergency Medicine. *European Curriculum for Emergency Medicine*. http://www.eusem.org/assets/PDFs/Curriculums/European_Curriculum_for_EM-Aug09-DJW.pdf. (accessed May 26, 2011).

9. Fleischmann T. Prerequisites for doctors in an emergency department. In W von Eiff, M Brachmann, T Fleischmann, *et al.*, eds., *Management of an Emergency Department*. Stuttgart: Kohlhammer, 2011; 376–83 [German].

10. Baker S. Building the case for service: evidence based leadership. In S Baker, *Excellence in the Emergency Department*. Gulf Breeze, FL: Studer, 2009; 17–30.

11. Fleischmann T. Managing an emergency department. In T Fleischmann, ed., *Clinical Emergency Medicine*. Munich, Elsevier, 2012; 707–35 [German].

12. Mayer T, Jensen K. Emergency department flow: the hospital's front door. In T Mayer, K Jensen, *Hardwiring Flow: Systems and Processes for Seamless Patient Care*. Gulf Breeze, FL: Studer, 2009; 149–85.

13. Fleischmann T. Missions of emergency medicine. In T Fleischmann, ed., *Clinical Emergency Medicine*. Munich: Elsevier, 2012; 9–11 [German].

14. Arnold J. International emergency medicine and the recent development of emergency medicine worldwide. *Annals of Emergency Medicine* 1999; **33**: 97–103.

15. Fleischmann T, Fulde G. Emergency medicine in modern Europe. *Emergency Medicine Australasia* 2007, **19**: 300–2.

16. World Health Organization. *Emergency Medical Services Systems in the European Union*. http://www.euro.who.int/__data/assets/pdf_file/0016/114406/E92038.pdf (accessed December 12, 2011).

17. Fleischmann T. Pathways out of the emergency department: to discharge, refer, admit to a ward or send to an intensive care setting? *Hospitalist* 2009; **38**: 26–30.

Chapter

**6**

# Strategies for clinical team building: the importance of teams in medicine

Matthew M. Rice

## Key learning points

- Understand the philosophy and basic concepts of teams and teamwork.
- Review strategies to deploy successful teams.
- Consider difficulties in developing and managing teams.

## Introduction

Medicine is facing significant challenges. Even the most sophisticated health systems are being forced to look again at how medicine is practiced and what new approaches may be useful to enhance the provision of care.[1,2] There are increasing pressures focused on cost, quality, efficiency, and access to care.[3–5] With the advent of economic concerns there has also been a focus on topics, some long taken for granted, that are often overlooked in medical cultures. Among these topics are patient safety, workforce provider tasks, technology, transparency, research, and even non-scientific medical practices that often challenge the traditional logic of allopathic medicine.[6,7] With these challenges come tremendous opportunities that must be considered when mixing science with sociology, and the inevitable cultural hurdles that are faced in the application of the theory to the practice of medicine. Coupled with diverse social and individual expectations, it is important to consider strategies that will be useful to enhance medical care.[8–10]

One of the seemingly simple concepts that have been successful in other industries, and most recently in medicine, relates to teams and teamwork.[11–13] Rather than just looking to solve challenges through more dollars, equipment, buildings, or personnel, effective teamwork is capable of providing synergies

for health care in both sophisticated and basic health delivery systems.[14] This chapter explores the philosophy and basic concepts of teams and teamwork, examines why teams make sense, and discusses some strategies to deploy successful teams as well as obstacles that get in the way of teams being successful. Many of these team concepts are universal, and they are often applied in non-medical industries, but the challenges and complexities of medicine, and the inherent mix of cultural diversity in medical systems and medical economics, make implementation of team strategy more difficult in the medical environment.[15–17] Yet it is essential to explore the exciting opportunities presented by successful team concepts, as a partial solution to some of medicine's current and future challenges. There is no better place to implement team principles and strategies than the emergency department (ED), where the success of teams and teamwork can contribute to the success of patient outcomes, staff efficiency, and staff and patient satisfaction.

### Case study 6.1

A city hospital ED is a busy and chaotic institution with daily patient needs overwhelming the staff. This leads to a chaotic and often difficult work environment, with high patient and staff dissatisfaction. Although the clinical skills of all the health professionals are excellent, each shift is difficult and tiring, leading to high worker turnover in an unhappy workplace. As the new ED director, you realize that more resources are not forthcoming, and that to be successful a new approach is necessary. You just read some medical references relating to the concept of teams in the workplace. But what is "teamwork" really about in the context of the ED?

*Emergency Department Leadership and Management*, ed. Stephanie Kayden, *et al.* Published by Cambridge University Press.
© Cambridge University Press 2015.

# What is a team, and teamwork?

Being inherently social, people generally do not choose to live or work alone. Most of our time is spent interacting with others. People are born into family groups, worship in groups, work in groups, and play in groups. Much of our identity is based on the ways that other individuals and groups perceive and treat us. Because of this, at least some competencies in communication and interpersonal dynamics are vital to everyone, especially to the organizations where we work.[18] From the recognition of the benefits of group behavior there is intuitively recognition of the value of teams. Various military, sports, aviation, and business analogies spring to mind when we consider how teams can improve effectiveness and efficiency. The "Toyota" model revolutionized the business world. Likewise, teamwork is recognized as being critical to the success of many businesses. Police special weapons and tactics (SWAT) teams and military special operations teams are common to our understanding of teams and teamwork. In medicine, operating room teams, intensive care unit (ICU) teams, rapid response teams (RRTs) and ED teams are commonly referred to and organized, with varying degrees of success. Interestingly, in medicine, we are not traditionally trained in teamwork and thus have little understanding of how teams form and work together.

Over the past decade, various resources and tools have been developed to assist in better understanding teams and teamwork, and how they can be applied to medicine.[19,20] Aviation analogies, especially cockpit resource management (CRM), sometimes referred to as "crew resource management," are infamous now in healthcare management training.[21,22] Over the years airplane crashes have resulted in large losses of life, reputation, and treasure. These tragedies triggered research and practical programs to limit such high losses. Much success in preventing accidents and improving efficiency was related to programs developed to enhance teamwork within well-structured teams.

During the past 20 years, experience shows that working with well-formed and functioning teams can provide efficiencies and a great sense of satisfaction in work environments. This includes medicine, and particular success with teams has been shown in emergency medicine. Medical professionals want to be part of the winning "A team" so that they can be acknowledged, and they appreciate being part of a quality team during routine work. Some teams seem to come together naturally, but their formation usually involves great leadership and hard work to develop and sustain team successes. Being part of the less successful "B team" has probably been a negative experience for many in their workplace, and medical professionals typically want to avoid being part of an ineffective team. Despite best efforts, some teams may never be successful at teamwork, but we all look forward to being part of the "A team."

Medical professionals naturally develop a concept of working together because assisting each other in often challenging situations makes work easier and better. Interestingly, it is unusual for medical training programs to build specific team training into the curriculum of the future practitioners and medical leaders. It is even more unusual for senior medical mentors to grasp and adapt practical team concepts in effective ways. There are likely many reasons for this. The concept of working in a "group" is standard in medicine, but it is often different than working together in a "team." The two need to be distinguished. A group can be any number of people who work together but who may lack mix, focus, and commitment to a common set of values. By their very nature a group is less efficient, interacting through individual contributions rather than through a collective effort. A team is usually a small number of people with complementary skills who are committed to a common purpose, share common performance goals, and have an understood approach to problem solving. Team members hold themselves mutually accountable. A team recognizes the value of collective effort beyond what is right for any individual member, and in a team all members recognize the importance of a greater good. They function dynamically, interdependently, and adaptively toward a common and valued goal (Table 6.1).[21,23] Most effective teams range in size from 2 to 24 individuals, with approximately 12 members considered ideal. Having more than 12 members creates less sense of shared commitment and more difficulty in maintaining team unity and focus. Larger groups have difficulty in agreeing on actionable specifics, and thus

**Table 6.1** Essential elements of a team

1. A common purpose and shared goals
2. Interdependent action among members
3. Accountability as a functioning unit
4. Value for collective effort (synergy)

**Table 6.2** Elements leading to team effectiveness

1. Clear team goals and objectives
2. Clear accountability and authority
3. Diversity of skills and personalities
4. Clear individual roles for members
5. Shared tasks
6. Regular internal formal and informal communication
7. Full participation by members
8. The ability to change and develop
9. The confronting of conflict
10. Feedback to individuals
11. Team rewards
12. Monitoring of team objectives
13. Outside recognition of a team
14. Two-way external communication
15. Feedback on team performance.

groups of particularly large size are most effective only when broken down into smaller teams.

There are five attributes of an effective team: a meaningful common purpose; specific, valued-added performance goals; a common approach through a collective effort; complementary skills with interdependent action; and mutual accountability.[24,25] Working together as a team in a predictable and effective manner is referred to as teamwork. It occurs when interactions and coordination between team members occur, with products derived from the team's collective efforts. A successful team requires empowerment. This refers to the degree to which its members perceive the group as capable of being effective (potency), performing important and valuable tasks (meaningfulness), and having independence and discretion (autonomy) in performing the work. Experiencing a sense of importance and significance (impact) in the work performed and goals achieved leads to more effective success with teamwork.[26,27] An effective team, then, is merely the means to create enhanced performance through teamwork (Table 6.2). If there is a lack of vision, a failure to make decisions, a failure to accept a common goal, or an inability to hold each other mutually accountable, teams are ineffective, since the very nature of a team requires these skills. An inability to interact and collaborate leads to an inability to process work. Failure to achieve recognized attributes of teams means that teams will typically be ineffectual groups, and thus will fail to perform more efficiently in attaining team goals. But effective teams lead to teamwork and enhanced performance, as repeatedly demonstrated in team-oriented practices.[28,29]

# Developing teams: stages of team development

The formation of teams is not automatic, and does not always happen the same way, by any means. But research has found that there are at least four stages of team development, sometimes referred to as the forming, storming, norming, and performing stages.[30,31]

## Forming stage

Team members focus on defining or understanding goals and developing procedures for performing their tasks. Team development in this stage involves getting acquainted and understanding formal leadership and other member roles. Socially it means getting to understand members' feelings. In this stage there is a tendency for some members to depend on one or two other team members rather than contributing themselves. Appropriate early interactions and sharing is important to prevent individuals from keeping feelings to themselves. Some members may act more secure than they actually feel, experience confusion and uncertainty about what is expected of them, and attempt to be polite while sizing up the personal benefits relative to the personal costs of being involved with the team.[32]

## Storming stage

During this stage conflicts may emerge between group members over work behaviors, relative priorities of goals, and responsibility for tasks, and even challenges to the leader's task-related guidance and direction may arise. Social behaviors can be experienced through a mixture of expressive hostility and strong feelings. Competition over leadership and conflict over goals may dominate feelings, and some members may withdraw or isolate themselves from the emotional tensions. Informal leaders may emerge. The key is to manage conflict during this stage, not to suppress it or withdraw from it. Suppressing conflict will likely create bitterness and resentment, which will last long after team members attempt to express their differences and emotions. Withdrawal from addressing any conflict may cause the team to fail. This stage may be shortened if all agree to a team-building process from the beginning even if conflict and controversy arise. Facilitators may assist in this stage to mentor those with concerns and to mediate differences of opinion and style.[33]

## Norming stage

Work behaviors at the norming stage evolve into a sharing of information, acceptance of different options, and positive attempts to make decisions that may require compromise. During this stage, team members set the rules by which the team will operate. Social behaviors and expressions of feelings will lead to a sense of cohesion. Cooperation and a sense of shared responsibility develop among team members. Norms are rules and patterns of behavior that are accepted and expected by members of the team. They help define behavior that members believe to be necessary to help them reach their goals. Over time this establishes and adapts norms while the team enforces them on its members. These norms should be consistent with appropriate organizational rules. Teams form norms with respect to behaviors that they believe to be particularly important. These norms aid in survival, simplify and make predictable expected member behaviors, avoid embarrassing interpersonal situations, and express central values and goals of the team to clarify the team's distinctive identity. Compliance and conformity are helpful in reflecting a team's desired behaviors due to real or imagined pressure, and lead to personal acceptance of group norms by individuals.[34–37]

## Performing stage

In this stage, team members show how effectively and efficiently they can achieve results together. The roles of individual members are accepted and understood. The members have learned when they should work independently and when they should work with each other. Excessive self-oriented behaviors, development of ineffective behaviors, inefficient task completion, and poor leadership are recognized as hurting productivity. Following the progress in achieving initial goals, teams should work to identify new goals that are critical to allowing teams to succeed and progress.[38–41] Success breeds success, and effective teams tend to remain together. A sense of cohesiveness, defined as the strength of a team member's desire to remain in a given team, develops in most effective teams. A team member's commitment is greatly influenced by compatibility between team goals and individual members' goals, and is often influenced by real

and perceived team successes. Progress in maintaining cohesive performance may be maintained and improved through the use of technology, value orientation and reorientation of members, improvement in working conditions, demonstration of best management practices, and fair and equitable organizational rules enforcement. The best teams remain as high performers and cohesive when leadership recognizes successes and provides organizational rewards and punishments in a fair and focused manner.

### Case study 6.2

With full buy-in by the physician and nursing staff, and with the attention of hospital leadership, the challenge to the ED leader is to better understand and plan how to form, and incorporate the ED staff into, functioning teams. Some thoughtful insight into staff, their skills and personalities, and how patient care can be best provided under this new teamwork concept has opened up some ideas on how "teams" just might come together.

## Getting started with teams

Medical work is very complex.[42] The price of failure is very high in lost wealth, chances for improvement, and lost individual and social well-being. Failure can often lead to the steep costs of lost chances in efficiency and lost opportunity to alleviate suffering and prevent unnecessary disability and death. Understanding the basic principles of teams and implementing teamwork is important in improving organizations large or small. But implementing teams in health care is often more complex than it may seem. Hoping that teams will form and teamwork will naturally occur is fraught with a high risk of failure. Hope is not a strategy. Without specific strategies and plans to implement teams, considerable time and resources may be wasted with little improvement in the practice environment, and with potential damage to the existing healthcare organization

Fundamental in team building is determining team size, membership, leadership, composition, identification, and distribution. Also important is determining what type of team is expected in the work environment. Part of early team formation is to understand that various types of teams can be defined in various ways. Functional teams can include: problem-solving teams – these teams focus on specific issues in areas of responsibility, develop potential solutions, and take action within defined limits; cross-functional teams – these teams draw members from various specialties to deal with problems that cut across department and functional lines; self-managed teams – these teams must work together effectively daily to ensure an entire product or service, perform managerial tasks, rotate tasks and assign members, order needed materials, decide on team leadership, set key team goals, recruit new team members, and sometimes evaluate performance. In medicine many types of teams may be formed, but most practical long-lasting care teams will be considered self-managed teams that raise productivity and change how work is organized and practiced.[16,42] It is important to understand what a team needs to accomplish, how it might develop, and how best for the team to implement teamwork. It is also important to successfully start and then carefully develop teams so there is a reasonable chance of early success.

Structured teams do not just occur; they must be formed. Fundamental in team building is determining organizational philosophy, deciding on leadership, and determining team size, composition, membership, and distribution in the work environment. One of the earliest steps in moving towards successful teams is to have an understanding of organization culture and to determine team leadership structure. The complexity of medical work requires that careful planning occurs, with thoughtful leadership, strong commitment to purpose, and application of time and resources. The belief that any change is easy or obvious will often lead to failure.[43] Critical in the initial step of developing teams is leadership at various levels. Teams cannot form, develop, and be successful in a vacuum. Senior leadership, the "C-suite" (senior hospital administration), boards of directors, department chairs, and nurse managers are just some of the health-organization leaders who must really understand and support – both in theory and with resources – the concept of teams. These healthcare senior leaders can help create support and enthusiasm that should drive team formation and allow teamwork.

Team development begins with, and its success is ultimately dependent upon, a supportive culture. A very basic understanding of organizational cultures is a good starting point to approach the development and ongoing management of medical teams. Organizational culture represents a complex pattern of beliefs, expectations, ideas, values, attitudes, and behaviors shared by members of an organization. Routine behaviors occur when people interactively relate to norms and common values. In emergency medicine, routine behaviors that foster joy in work, concern for others including both patients and other team members, respect for skills, and a focus on a job well done go a long way in supporting quality in care and performance. Successful teamwork is often reflected through a philosophy of getting things done in culturally approved interactions between team members and customers.

Organizational culture develops as a response to the challenges of external adaptation and survival of internal integration. The formation of organizational culture is also influenced by the culture of the larger society within which the organization must function. Organizations maintain and change organizational culture by: (1) noting what managers and teams pay attention to, measure, and control; (2) observing the ways managers and employees react to crisis; (3) ensuring remodeling, teaching, and coaching; (4) setting criteria for allocation of rewards; (5) determining criteria for recruitment to, selection and promotion within, and removal from the organization; (6) establishing the organization's rites, ceremonies, and stories.[44]

The feeling or climate conveyed in an organization as reflected through enactment of its dominant values, philosophy, and policies guides an organization in its relationship with patients and employees. Established guidelines help form team values, as well as an understanding of the rules of the game that serve to enhance each team member's ability to get along with the organization.[16] If the culture of an organization strongly supports teams, they are likely to succeed and thrive. Thus an understanding of institutional culture, and a consideration of how organizations will influence teams, is important background information prior to team planning.[45] But the key to transferring cultural values is picking appropriate team leaders.

Team building is a key component of leadership. Likewise, leadership is a key to building and managing successful teams. This is true in any small or large healthcare organization. A conscious decision is often necessary to agree that teamwork will occur. This is often the responsibility of a designated leader, often the department chair. But the real day-to-day work of a team or multiple teams requires the presence and active participation of a leader for each

**Table 6.3** Effective team leaders

1. Organize the team and resources to maximize performance
2. Articulate clear goals with delegation of tasks
3. Make decisions through collective input of members
4. Empower team members to speak up and challenge the leader when appropriate, using group norms to guide behavior
5. Actively promote and facilitate good team processes.
6. Are skillful at conflict resolution

**Table 6.4** Qualities of effective team members as followers

1. Understand team role
2. Provide information for decision making
3. Adapt work skills and team tools for success
4. Accept ownership of team decisions
5. View feedback as an opportunity to learn

**Table 6.5** Teamwork competencies

1. Leadership
2. Team orientation
3. Shared vision
4. Team cohesion
5. Mutual trust
6. Collective orientation
7. Understand the Importance of teamwork
8. Collective efficacy of team as a unit
9. Communication skills
10. Information exchange
11. Open feedback and assessment
12. Conflict resolution
13. Flexibility and adaptability
14. Mutual performance monitoring
15. Task-specific responsibilities
16. Knowledge of team mission, norms and resources
17. Shared task models and situational assessment
18. Understanding strategies to reach goals

team. Team leaders may emerge naturally or be trained and coached by existing role models. Leveraging leadership skills to create a realistic vision and encourage others to adopt a shared vision is a mark of a true leader. A successful leader's vision is one that is inspirational and requires the contributions and "buy-in" of each individual in the team. In addition, leaders enhance communications, foster the education and development of team skills, and create ownership and accountability. Finding or developing the "right" leader to manage a team is a critical early step in team formation and development. Good leaders recognize accomplishments, provide rewards, and celebrate efforts with a focus on team successes. The most effective team leaders are recognized for their professional excellence and specific technical skills, but also are known to be thoughtful, fair, insightful, caring, and trustworthy (Table 6.3).[21]

## Selecting team members

Selecting and developing team members is critical in establishing teams. While there must be leaders, teams are successful when formed with members who are also successful followers (Table 6.4).[21] Selecting team members with the right set of skills, competencies, temperament, enthusiasm, and commitment is essential to enhance efficient adhesion by members to the team (Table 6.5).[46,47]

Some individuals naturally fit into teams because of inherent skills. Most dedicated health professionals can be trained to team proficiencies if they are motivated and believe in the process. Successful teams possess special skills. Some of these attributes and skills include respectful interaction. This is a social skill through which one individual's interpretation is respectfully communicated to another individual, and through this communication a shared interpretation

is generated. Respectful interacting requires the presence of trust, honesty and self-respect. Heedful interrelating is also an important competency. This social skill is a competency in which individual action contributes to a larger pattern of shared action and in which individuals understand how their actions fit into a larger action. Team members must be selected according to their skills and understanding of how a particular system is configured to achieve agreed-upon goals. This requires the team members to be able to subordinate their own goals for the purpose of success in shared goals. Perhaps the most important criteria for selecting team members are their dedication to patient care, their dedication to patient comfort, and their dedication to patient concerns. Many successful teams make the patient the focus of core care teams.[48] Often overlooked, the patient should not just be a focus of the team, but should also be considered part of the team.[49]

Where social/cultural structures and values will not allow teams to organize or function because of broad deficiencies in key team principles, teamwork will likely not succeed. Key individuals either ignored or placed on a "pedestal" by the team, or arrogance among team members, defeats team purpose and can destroy the key principles that allow teams to achieve exceptional performance. Thus choosing team participants should include a reference to their professionalism and personal values. The best teams are serviced by good managers who help shape values and encourage appropriate behaviors. Such behaviors include selflessness, work sharing, and maturity, allowing team members to avoid misperceptions about roles and responsibilities. Enhancing knowledge and technical skills in a permissive way is critical to a sharing of values that are consistent with vision. Thus a willingness to teach and to learn is important for all team members. In medical teams, understanding the short- and long-term goals – i.e. saving lives and alleviating suffering, while ensuring dignity of patients and team members – is critical for team members, who often face competing social and cultural norms. Allowing various team members to have appropriate authority allows the development of situational leaders, which enhances team skills and team missions. Sharing appropriate team skills can strengthen and energize teams, while an egotistical and self-centered focus can destroy teams.

**Case study 6.3**

Once teams are formed, you as the ED director realize that some team tools would be useful. As you search references on teamwork you come up with some ideas on how to enhance team skills and you learn more about the risks to the performance of medical teams.

## Team tools to enhance teamwork

Once teams have appropriate leadership, and are functionally structured, their performance is enhanced through the use of various "tools." These tools, developed from different industries, including those of high reliability organizations (HROs), are quite helpful. Many of the tools focus on team monitoring, communication, and mutual support. Monitoring of teamwork through *situational awareness*, *cross-monitoring*, and the *STEP technique* is helpful. For effective communication, using concepts such as *SBAR, call-outs, check-backs*, and *hand-offs* is incredibly valuable. And concepts such as *advocacy, assertion, DESC script, the two-challenge rule*, and *task*

**Table 6.6** Suggested teamwork tools for individual reading research

1. **Situation monitoring**
   a. Situational awareness
   b. Cross-monitoring
   c. STEP

2. **Communications**
   a. SBAR
   b. Call-outs
   c. Check-backs
   d. Hand-offs

3. **Mutual support**
   a. Advocacy
   b. Assertion
   c. DESC script
   d. Task assistance
   e. Two-challenge rule

*assistance* contributes to mutual support among team members. Including these tools in the work of the team, combined with appropriate management, mentoring, and coaching, will be one of the most useful and practical practices, allowing exceptional team performance. The most effective team training and orientation programs have bundled sets of tasks and organized training information to enhance team members' performance and teamwork success. Some of these tools are listed in Table 6.6. Access to the details of how to implement and use these tools should come through reading and/or in-depth participation with the programs referenced, including MEDTEAMS, Team STEPPS, and other human performance research.[23,50]

## Challenges and risk to medical teams: considerations of socialization

There are many challenges to what seems logical in concepts surrounding teams and teamwork.[51–53] This is especially true in complex and multidimensional medical environments. Some of these challenges include: medical specialty focus, with varying perspective on what is most important; competition for limited resources; and personalities, including egocentric behaviors that clash with team values. When cultural or other social variables enter the formation and management of teams, difficulties arise in team function and performance.

As medical professionals become "socialized" or even co-opted into the practice patterns of medicine, some interesting challenges develop to the concept of teams and teamwork. Medical education, training, and practice is not just about acquiring and then providing medical care. Rather, such care takes place in a culture that is related to the socialization of the providers, institutions, and overall society where the care is provided. Therefore the manner in which socialization takes place, particularly during formative times of professional development, has a tremendous influence on the ideas, habits, and styles of medical professionals. The Western model of medical education has traditionally focused on individual excellence, personal performance, and achievements. Often there is little recognition of or effective communication with other members of parallel schools of thought or contributions made by others to the overall success of patient outcomes. Thus physicians as a group, and in particular subspecialists, along with nurses, technicians, and administrators, often communicate poorly. This leads to compartmentalizing of information, a loss of sharing, and often confusion. Such "siloing" can lead to dysfunction through the lack of insight and the power of collaboration. In many medical cultures specialty training often creates apprentice-style career paths in which mentoring relationships encourage trainees to emulate and assimilate the attitudes, demeanor, and behaviors of their mentors. Unfortunately dissident attitudes and dysfunctional behaviors help create and may even define how the professions act, and the result is not always conducive to effective teamwork. Such behaviors can lead to adversarial relationships that are inevitably destructive to team building and patient care.[54] Also, when there is a wide diversity of training and technical knowledge there is a natural tendency for teams to be less effective, especially if those with the greatest knowledge do not share and allow other team members to participate in an important, sharing way.

Great challenges also exist in medical teamwork when cultural approaches to ethnicity, gender, religion, and/or professional status are disruptive to the concepts of forming teams and performing work. Such cultural patterns can lead to authority gradients. The term *authority gradient* applies to authority figures (through title, culture, law/regulation, and other means of influence, including fear or even earned respect) who hold power or influence over others. In medicine, physicians are often considered a "higher level" of authority because of their respected skills, or through structure, resident–attending, generalist–specialist, or through sheer intimidation in relation to others in the medical environment. For example, in some cultures, the senior physician is considered the "master" of all decisions and practices. In some cultures, religion and gender norms determine who will make final decisions. Such hierarchies in many cultures can develop between physicians, nurses, pharmacists, clerical personnel, or other members of the care group.

Authority and structure are not inherently bad, and in fact both are critical to effective teams. But the authority must be respected through experience or expertise and focused on the agreed-upon values of any medical team. Disorder and harm may occur in teams when authority figures use their position with impunity and without regard to the respect and trust necessary for teams. To be effective in forming teams, and in managing effective teamwork, there needs to be mutual commitment and congruence of role expectations in order to increase productivity. Recognizing these realities and appropriately including medical team members in decision making is critical to the success of the team. These facts do not denigrate the role of physicians. Physicians are typically leaders of teams because of their knowledge and skills, and are naturally considered to be in a leadership role. There is a human desire to comply with leaders through authority gradients that if managed correctly can lead to stronger teams, but that if mismanaged can lead to corruption of principles, especially when inexperienced team members are fearful of contradiction or afraid to challenge their superiors.

## Summary

Teams and teamwork can make a difference in health care. Understanding how a team is superior to a group and how it can be successful through teamwork will make a difference for medical providers and patients. Having successful teams means having the right leadership and support at all levels of an organization. It also requires hard work and commitment to achieve common goals. Specific training and team tools are available for those who want to start and develop effective teams. Maintaining teams requires continuous education, monitoring, and adaptability. Danger of failure exists in improperly establishing and monitoring teams, and a haphazard approach often leads to unsuccessful teams. Failures can lead to cynicism, and to a waste of time and resources. But successful teams will make a difference in productivity, as well as in staff and patient satisfaction, and can be an integral part of successful change in medical organizations. Teams and teamwork are worth exploring and adopting, as we face the evolving challenges to medicine.

# References

1.  Patient Protection and Affordable Care Act, Pub. L. 111–148, 124U. Stat. 119, March 30, 2010.

2.  Institute of Medicine. *The Healthcare Imperative: Lowering Costs and Improving Outcomes.* Washington, DC: National Academies Press, 2011.

3.  Fuchs VR. Government payment for health care: causes and consequences. *New England Journal of Medicine* 2010; **363**: 2181–3.

4.  Newhouse J. Medical costs and medical markets: another view. *New England Journal of Medicine* 1979; **300**: 855–6.

5.  Goldman D, Sood H. Rising health care costs: are we in a crisis? *Health Affairs* 2006; **25**: 389–90.

6.  Shortwell S. Health care reform requires accountable care systems. *JAMA* 2008; **300**: 95–7.

7.  Royal College of Physicians and Academy of Medical Royal Colleges. *The Future of Academic Medicine: Five Scenarios to 2025.* London: The Colleges, 2004.

8.  Mountford J, Davies C. Towards an outcomes based health care system: a view from the United Kingdom. *JAMA* 2010; **304**: 2407–8.

9.  Kaplan JP, Fleming D. Current and future public health challenges. *JAMA* 2000; **284**: 1696–8.

10. Connors E, Goston L. Health care reform: an historic moment in U.S. social policy. *JAMA* 2010; **30**: 2521–2.

11. Dynamics Research Corporation. *Emergency Team Coordination Course.* Andover, MA: Dynamics Research Corporation, 1997.

12. Risser DT, Rice MM, Salisbury ML, *et al.* The potential for improved teamwork to reduce medical errors in the emergency department. The MEDTEAMS research consortium. *Annals of Emergency Medicine* 1999; **34**: 373–83.

13. Brannick M, Prince C. An overview of team performance measurement. In MT Brannick, E Salas, CW Prince, eds., *Team Performance Assessment and Measurement.* Mahway, NJ: Erlbaum, 1997; 3–16.

14. Institute of Medicine. *Leadership Commitments to Improve Value in Healthcare: Finding Common Ground.* Washington, DC: National Academies Press, 2010.

15. Jay GD, Berns SD, Morey JC, *et al.* Formal teamwork training improves teamwork and reduces emergency department errors. *Academic Emergency Medicine* 1999; **6**: 408.

16. Hellriegel D, Slocum J, Woodman R. Organizational culture. In *Organizational Behavior*, 9th edn. Cincinnati, OH: South-Western Publishing, 2001.

17. Spear, S, Learning to lead at Toyota. *Harvard Business Review* 2004; **82** (5): 78–9.

18. Katzenbach JR, Smith DK. *The Wisdom of Teams: Creating the High-Performance Organization.* New York, NY: Harper Collins, 1994.

19. Helmreich RL, Wilhelm JA, Gregorich SE, Chidester TR. Preliminary results from the evaluation of Cockpit Resources Management Training: performance ratings of flight crews. *Aviation, Space, and Environmental Medicine* 1990; **61**: 576–9.

20. Helmreich RL, Schaefer HG. Team performance in the operating room. In MS Bogner, ed., *Human Error In Medicine*. Hillsdale, NJ: Erlbaum, 1994: 225–53.

21. Rice M. Teams and teamwork in emergency medicine. In P Croskerry, KS Cosby, SM Schenkel, RL Wears, eds., *Patient Safety in Emergency Medicine.* Philadelphia, PA: Lippincott Williams & Wilkins, 2009; 177–80.

22. Henry H. *Lessons from Team Leaders: a Team Fitness Companion.* Milwaukee, WI: ASQ Quality Press, 1998.

23. Ratliff RL, Beckstand SM, Hanks SH. The use and management of teams: a how-to guide. *Quality Progress* June 1999: 31–8.

24. Kirkman B, Rosen B. Beyond self-management: antecedents and consequences of team empowerment. *Academy of Management Journal* 1999; **43**: 58–74.

25. Wetlaufer S. Organizing for empowerment: an interview with AFS's Roger San and Dennis Bakke. *Harvard Business Review* January–February, 1999: 110–23.

26. Firth-Cozens J. Celebrating teamwork. *Quality in Healthcare* 1998; **7**: S3–7.

27. Morey JC, Simon R, Jay GD, *et al.* Error Error reduction and performance improvement in the emergency department through formal teamwork training: evaluation results of the MedTeams project. *Health Services Research* 2002; **37**: 1553–81.

28. Gersick CJ. Time and transition in work teams: toward a new model of group development. *Academy of Management Journal* 1988; **31**: 9–41.

29. Tuckman B, Jensen M. Stages of small group development revisited. *Group and Organization Studies* 1977; **2**: 419–27.

30. Montebello AR. *Work Teams That Work*, Minneapolis, MS: Best Sellers, 1994.

31. Herbelin S, Guiney P, eds. *The Do's and Don'ts of Work Team Coaching*. Riverbank, CA: Herbelin, 1998.

32. Ezzamel M, Willmott H. Accounting for team-work: a critical study of group-based systems of organizational control. *Administrative Science Quarterly* 1998; **43**: 358–96.

33. Feldman DC. The development and enforcement of group norms. *Academy Management Review* 1984; **9**: 47–53.

34. Spich R, Leleman R. Explicit norm structuring process: a strategy for increasing task-group effectiveness. *Group and Organization Studies* 1985; **10**: 37–9.

35. Besser TL. *Team Toyota*, Ithaca, NY: State University of New York Press, 1996.

36. Cannon-Bowers J, Salas E, eds. *Making Decisions Under Stress: Implications for Individual and Team Training*. Hyattsville, MD: American Psychological Association, 1999.

37. Denton DK. How a team can grow. *Quality Progress* June 1999: 53–8.

38. Gibson CB. Do they do what they believe they can? Group efficacy and group effectiveness across tasks and cultures.

*Academy of Management Journal* 1999; **42**: 138–52.

39. Xaio Y, Hunter WA, Mackenzie CF, Jefferies NJ, Horst RL. Task complexity in emergency care and its implications for team coordination. *Human Factors* 1996; **38**: 636–45.

40. Rose E, Buckley S. *50 Ways to Teach Your Learner: Activities and Interventions For Building High-Performance Teams*. San Francisco, CA: Jossey-Bass, 1999.

41. Purser R, Cabana S. *The Self Managing Organizations: How Leasing Companies are Transforming The Work of Teams for Real Impact*. New York, NY: Free Press, 1999.

42. Senders JW. On the complexity of medical devices and systems. *Qualty and Safety in Health Care* 2006; **15** (suppl.1): 41–3.

43. Martin J. *Cultures in Organizations*. New York, NY: Oxford University Press, 1992.

44. Hellriegel D, Jackson SE, Slocum JW. *Management*, 8th edn. Cincinnati, OH: South-Western Publishing, 1999; 624–8.

45. Kraft R. *Utilizing Self-Managing Teams: Effective Behavior of Team Leaders*. Hamden, CN: Garland, 1999.

46. Vogus TJ, Sutcliffe KM. The safety organization: development and validation of a behavioral measure of safety culture in hospital nursing units. *Medical Care* 2007; **45**: 46–54.

47. Vogus TJ, Welbourne TM. Structuring for high reliability:

HR practice and mindful process in reliability-seeking organizations. *Journal of Organizational Behavior* 2003; **24**: 877–903.

48. Schulman P. The negotiated order of organizational reliability. *Administration and Society* 1993; **25**: 353–72.

49. TeamSTEPPS. *Strategies and Tools to Enhance Performance and Patient Safety*. Agency for Healthcare Research and Quality. http://teamstepps.ahrq.gov.

50. Murphy K. *Individual Differences and Behavior in Organizations*. San Francisco, CA: Jossey-Bass, 1996.

51. Hackman JR. Group influences on individuals. In MD Dunnette, LM Hough, eds., *Handbook of Industrial and Organizational Psychology*, 2nd edn., vol. 2. Palo Alto, CA: Consulting Psychologists Press, 1992: 199–267.

52. Edmondson A. Psychological safety and learning behaviors in work teams. *Administrative Science Quarterly* 1999; **44**: 358–83.

53. Hambrick DC. Fragmentation and the other problems CEOs have with their top management teams. *California Management Review* Spring 1995; P110–127.

54. Harrison D, Price KH, Bell MP. Beyond relational demography: time and the effect of surface and deep level diversity on work group cohesions. *Academy of Management Journal* 1998; **41**: 96–108.

Chapter

# 7

# Quality assurance in the emergency department

Philip D. Anderson and J. Lawrence Mottley

## Key learning points

- Review key concepts related to peer review, including adverse events, errors, and standard of care.
- Discuss metrics used to measure quality of care.
- Describe how to set up a new quality assurance program: selecting committee members, cases to review, and a review process.

## Introduction

Emergency department (ED) leaders around the world face a growing public awareness and demand for improved quality in emergency care delivery. The US Institute of Medicine (IOM) report from 2000, *To Err is Human: Building a Safer Health System*, dramatically focused worldwide attention on the magnitude of the problem of medical errors and the adverse events that result from them.[1] Citing two large studies of hospitalized patients, the IOM reported that adverse events occurred in roughly 3% of all hospitalizations, that between 7% and 14% of adverse events led to death, and that over half of these adverse events resulted from medical errors that could have been prevented.[2–4] When these data were extrapolated to all hospital admissions in the USA, it was suggested that between 44 000 and 98 000 patients die each year as a result of preventable medical errors. One of the studies cited in the IOM report found that only 3% of adverse events detected in hospitalized patients occurred in the ED; however, 70% of these adverse events were judged to be negligent.[2,3] Other studies looking at the occurrence of error in the ED have reported higher error rates of 13–33% in cases

involving return visits to the ED within 72 hours;[5,6] 18–26% in cases involving deaths in the ED;[7,8] and up to 60% in cases of unanticipated death following discharge from the ED.[9]

Although the science of detecting errors in the ED is still evolving, and overall baseline error rates in the ED are not known, it is quite clear that successful ED leaders must be focused on understanding and improving the quality of care that is delivered. Regulatory agencies and payers in many countries have become increasingly focused on measuring ED performance, and on quality metrics that can have implications for hospital accreditation and reimbursement. In order to successfully advocate for our departments within the hospital administrative environment, we need mechanisms in place to reliably address any questions about the quality of care in ED cases, using accurate data and review processes.

This chapter will explore the issues of defining and measuring quality of care in the ED and describe strategies for establishing a successful quality assurance peer review program.

## Defining quality in emergency care

Quality, like beauty, is conceptually ethereal in nature and can therefore be difficult to define specifically. As a result, it may mean different things to different stakeholders. For example, payers, patients, and providers may each assign different value to different aspects of healthcare delivery or health outcomes. Over the past several decades, the way in which quality in healthcare is defined has evolved to become increasingly more specific and actionable.

In 1990, the IOM first defined quality of care as being "the degree to which health services for

*Emergency Department Leadership and Management*, ed. Stephanie Kayden, *et al.* Published by Cambridge University Press. © Cambridge University Press 2015.

**Table 7.1** Dimensions of healthcare quality

| Institute of Medicine dimensions of quality | |
|---|---|
| Safety | Avoiding injuries to patients from the care that is intended to help them |
| Effectiveness | Providing services based on scientific knowledge to all who could benefit and refraining from providing services to those not likely to benefit |
| Patient-centeredness | Providing care that is respectful of and responsive to individual patient preferences, needs, and values, and ensuring that patient values guide all clinical decisions |
| Timeliness | Reducing waits and sometimes harmful delays for both those who receive and those who give care |
| Efficiency | Avoiding waste, including waste of equipment, supplies, ideas, and energy |
| Equity | Providing care that does not vary in quality because of personal characteristics such as gender, ethnicity, geographic location, and socioeconomic status |
| **Simplified dimensions of quality** | |
| Clinical quality | Degree to which clinical care matches evidence-based guidelines (corresponds to safety, effectiveness, timeliness, equity) |
| Service quality | Degree to which care meets patient expectations (corresponds to patient-centeredness, timeliness) |
| Cost efficiency | Amount of medical benefit divided by cost (corresponds to efficiency) |

*Sources*: Institute of Medicine. *Crossing the Quality Chasm*, 2001;[11] James, 1989.[12]

individuals and populations increase the likelihood of desired health outcomes and are consistent with current professional knowledge."[10] In 2001, this definition was expanded to highlight six more specific dimensions of quality that provide a clearer focus for measuring and improving quality.[11] In a 2002 article by Graff *et al.*, these dimensions of quality were further sharpened in relation to emergency care delivery to include clinical quality, service quality, and cost efficiency (Table 7.1).[13]

## What is quality assurance?
### The measurement imperative

In order to achieve consistently high quality ED care delivery, we need mechanisms for managing the quality of that care. Florence Nightingale is quoted as having once said, "The ultimate goal is to manage quality. But you cannot manage it until you have a way to measure it, and you cannot measure it until you can monitor it."[14] The concept that successful management depends on the measurement and tracking of quantitative performance data lies at the center of all modern industrial management theories and is essential for the successful management of an ED.

## Quality assurance versus quality improvement

Overall quality management in the ED depends on two inter-related sets of activities, quality assurance (QA) and quality improvement (QI). QA activities are related to monitoring and evaluating the delivery of care in the ED to ensure that the care delivered meets the applicable standards for that department and to identify opportunities for improvement. This involves both peer review activities and metric-based reporting. Peer review is a way to audit selected cases to determine whether the standard of care was met and whether there are opportunities for improvement (preventable adverse events, near misses, and so on). Metric-based reporting gathers data to meet reporting requirements on quality and performance metrics that may be required by external regulatory agencies as well as hospital and departmental administration.

QI activities are related to improving the quality of care delivered in the ED through systems improvements geared towards standardizing practice, optimizing processes, improving flow, enhancing patient safety and satisfaction, and education of staff. These topics are discussed in more detail elsewhere in this book.

QA and QI activities are often handled by a single individual or committee in smaller EDs, while in larger departments the responsibilities for these activities may be delegated to different groups. In the latter case, it is important that the two efforts be closely integrated, as each activity informs the other.

## A fair and just culture

In his 1997 book, *Managing the Risks of Organizational Accidents*, James Reason characterized the environment necessary for conducting effective quality assurance activities as being a "just culture," that is, one in which there is "an atmosphere of trust in which people are encouraged, even rewarded, for providing essential safety-related information, but in which they are also clear about where the line must be drawn between acceptable and unacceptable behavior."[15] Because many employees fear they could be penalized for reporting adverse events, errors, or unsafe working conditions, it is the responsibility of ED leadership to actively promote a fair and just culture, by setting clear expectations and rewarding good behavior.

## Measuring quality in emergency care
### External and internal drivers for measuring quality

National and regional healthcare systems may use a variety of interconnected mechanisms for monitoring and ensuring the quality of care throughout the healthcare system, including licensure and accreditation of hospitals, licensure and credentialing of providers, pay-for-performance mechanisms, and requiring malpractice insurance as a condition for licensure. The specific organizations that are responsible for these functions may vary by country or region, but the concepts are similar. The oversight and regulatory bodies within the healthcare system have the authority to require reporting of specific data from healthcare institutions as a requirement for maintaining licensure, accreditation, insurance, and, in some cases, receiving full funding or bonuses. Often, the external reporting of quality and performance data is coordinated at the hospital level, but it is of the utmost importance for the ED leader to understand and approve the data that are being reported about the ED to external agencies. At the hospital level, there may be additional reporting requirements related to healthcare quality or performance monitoring that are placed upon the ED by hospital administration.

### Licensure

A license to operate a hospital facility is generally required in all countries. This regulatory function often rests at the state or regional level. In the US state of Massachusetts, for example, this function is carried out by the state's Department of Public Health (DPH), which requires hospitals to maintain a risk management program that monitors and reports certain types of incidents that seriously affect the health and safety of patients. Examples of these types of adverse events are listed in Table 7.2. The DPH may refuse to renew, or even revoke, a hospital's license for non-compliance with reporting. Licensure of physicians and other healthcare providers is commonly used in most countries to regulate the practice of medicine. The agency that issues physician licenses may also have the authority to require hospitals to check and confirm the credentials of physician applicants ("credentialing"), to monitor physician performance, and to report on incidents where patient safety may be compromised.

### Accreditation

Increasingly, hospitals in many countries are seeking, or are required to undergo, a further level of regulatory oversight called accreditation, which is usually carried out by a separate agency that is focused on assessing the level of performance in relation to established standards. Accreditation organizations typically require hospitals to report data on a range of indicators as a requirement for accreditation, and make periodic inspection visits to hospitals to ensure that standards are maintained. The accredited institutions are expected to identify and respond appropriately to certain types of adverse events, and even to report these to the accreditation agency.

### Pay for performance

Regardless of whether health care is financed through public or private funds, or a combination, payers may require hospitals to report on specified quality measures as a condition for receiving reimbursement for services. An example of this can be seen with the US Centers for Medicare and Medicaid Services (CMS), which coordinates all of the federally funded health insurance programs in the USA and is responsible for over 60% of all US healthcare expenditures. CMS established a Physician Quality Reporting System (PQRS) in 2006, which includes an incentive payment

**Table 7.2** Serious reportable events as defined by the National Quality Forum

| | |
|---|---|
| Surgical or invasive procedure events | • Surgery or other invasive procedure performed on the wrong site<br>• Surgery or other invasive procedure performed on the wrong patient<br>• Wrong surgical or other invasive procedure performed on a patient<br>• Unintended retention of a foreign object in a patient after surgery or other invasive procedure<br>• Intraoperative or immediately postoperative/postprocedure death in an ASA class 1 patient |
| Product or device events | • Patient death or serious injury associated with the use of contaminated drugs, devices, or biologics provided by the healthcare setting<br>• Patient death or serious injury associated with the use or function of a device in patient care, in which the device is used or functions other than as intended<br>• Patient death or serious injury associated with intravascular air embolism that occurs while being cared for in a healthcare setting |
| Patient protection events | • Discharge or release of a patient/resident of any age, who is unable to make decisions, to other than an authorized person<br>• Patient death or serious injury associated with patient elopement (disappearance)<br>• Patient suicide, attempted suicide, or self-harm that results in serious injury, while being cared for in a healthcare setting |
| Care management events | • Patient death or serious injury associated with a medication error (e.g., errors involving the wrong drug, wrong dose, wrong patient, wrong time, wrong rate, wrong preparation, or wrong route of administration)<br>• Patient death or serious injury associated with unsafe administration of blood products<br>• Maternal death or serious injury associated with labor or delivery in a low-risk pregnancy while being cared for in a healthcare setting<br>• Death or serious injury of a neonate associated with labor and delivery in a low-risk pregnancy<br>• Patient death or serious injury associated with a fall while being cared for in a healthcare setting<br>• Any stage 3, stage 4, and unstageable pressure ulcers acquired after admission/presentation to a healthcare setting<br>• Artificial insemination with the wrong donor sperm or wrong egg<br>• Patient death or serious injury resulting from the irretrievable loss of an irreplaceable biological specimen<br>• Patient death or serious injury resulting from failure to follow up or communicate laboratory, pathology, or radiology test results |
| Environmental events | • Patient or staff death or serious injury associated with an electric shock in the course of a patient care process in a healthcare setting<br>• Any incident in which systems designated for oxygen or other gas to be delivered to a patient contains no gas, the wrong gas, or is contaminated by toxic substances<br>• Patient or staff death or serious injury associated with a burn incurred from any source in the course of a patient care process in a healthcare setting<br>• Patient death or serious disability associated with the use of physical restraints or bedrails while being cared for in a healthcare setting |
| Radiologic events | • Death or serious injury of a patient or staff associated with the introduction of a metallic object into the MRI area |

**Table 7.2** *(cont.)*

| Potential criminal events | • Any instance of care ordered by or provided by someone impersonating a physician, nurse, pharmacist, or other licensed healthcare provider<br>• Abduction of a patient/resident of any age<br>• Sexual abuse/assault on a patient or staff member within or on the grounds of a healthcare setting<br>• Death or serious injury of a patient or staff member resulting from a physical assault (i.e., battery) that occurs within or on the grounds of a healthcare setting |
|---|---|

*Source*: National Quality Forum. Serious reportable events.[16]

for eligible physicians who satisfactorily report data on quality measures for covered professional services. In 2012, the PQRS incentive payment for individual emergency physicians or group practices amounted to 0.5% of the total estimated Medicare allowed charges for covered services during 2012.[17] CMS has also created a consumer-oriented website in collaboration with the Hospital Quality Alliance that provides information on how well hospitals provide recommended care to patients.[18] CMS incentivizes hospitals to report designated quality measures for this website by paying hospitals that successfully report all measures at a higher rate (2% as of 2005).[19]

### Malpractice insurance

Both hospitals and individual physicians are required, in many countries, to have malpractice insurance as a condition for maintaining licensure. The malpractice insurance provider may require hospitals to report certain types of incidents, especially if there is a potential for future malpractice claims or compensations. The malpractice provider may be required to report malpractice claims against physicians and hospitals to the respective licensing authorities.

## Framework for measuring quality within healthcare systems

Donabedian offered a framework for assessing quality in 1988 in which he proposed that in order to fully understand and improve quality within complex systems such as health care, information is needed from three categories: structures, processes, and outcomes. Structures include the resources used and the conditions under which care is delivered (material resources, human resources, organizational structures). Processes include everything that happens to patients during care delivery, as well as

patients' activities in seeking care and implementing care plans. Outcomes describe the result of our delivering care to patients and includes both health status measures (morbidity, mortality, disability) and patient satisfaction. Donabedian argued that because outcomes can be influenced by many factors, it can be difficult to know, even after extensive adjustment for differences in case mix, to what extent observed outcomes are attributable to the antecedent processes of care. In order for process and structural measures to be valid, however, there must be clear pre-existing evidence supporting the link between structure and process, and between process and outcome.[20]

Michael Porter has recently proposed a fundamentally new and different approach for understanding performance and driving improvement in health care, in which the pursuit of value is the pre-eminent goal.[21] Porter defines value as "patient health outcomes achieved per dollar spent." In contrast to Donabedian, he argues that successful risk adjustment of outcomes is feasible and that properly risk-adjusted outcome measures are the only relevant measures of performance that ultimately matter for patients, providers, payers, and suppliers, and for the purpose of driving innovation in health care. Process or structure measures are potentially useful as strategies for improvement and may correlate with certain outcomes, but are not direct measures of the actual health results achieved.

Under this value-based framework both outcomes and costs need to be defined and measured for specific medical conditions or defined patient populations with similar needs, over the full cycle of care for that specific medical condition, and not just for any one intervention or care episode. Porter argues that the quality of care for a patient is the full set of relevant outcomes, which have been appropriately adjusted for individual patient circumstances. The full spectrum of outcomes that are proposed includes three tiers, encompassing (1) health status achieved or retained, (2) process of recovery, and (3) sustainability of health. Outcomes need to be carefully risk-adjusted taking into account patient demographics, pre-existing conditions, patient compliance with treatment, as well as concurrent or associated medical conditions. Interestingly, patient satisfaction with the health status achieved is included as an important outcome measure; however, patient satisfaction with the process of care is considered a process measure and not an outcome.

As with outcomes, costs need to be aggregated around the individual patient, rather than for discrete services related to the care delivery. The challenge of cost accounting in health care is to allocate the shared or indirect costs to an individual patient based on that patient's actual use of the resources involved, instead of the average use across all patients. The method for carrying out this type of cost accounting is called time-dependent activity-based costing, and it is widely used in other industries, but rarely applied in health care.[22,23]

By measuring value this way, Porter argues that we gain an effective tool for comparing innovations in care delivery with current practice, something we currently lack most everywhere in the world. Porter notes that "to reduce cost, the best approach is often to spend more on some high-value services, frequently including . . . earlier-stage care, in order to reduce the cumulative cost of care over the full care cycle."[24]

## Market basket approach to measuring quality

While the Porter–Kaplan approach to measuring value may represent a new paradigm that will change how we measure performance in health care in the future, most healthcare systems are still taking a market basket approach to measuring quality today. Because emergency care delivery, like all of health care, consists of a complex set of processes, and because we care for a complex population of patients with a wide variety of conditions and acuities, we need to use a sufficiently broad array of quality measures to provide a meaningful picture of the overall quality of care delivered; this constitutes our market basket of indicators. Ideally, we would want to include an array of measures that would give us insight into the performance of each aspect and

phase of the emergency care delivery process and also into our performance in taking care of each level of patient acuity and type of condition seen in the ED. However, we also have to balance the cost of gathering quality assurance data with the value of those data to the organization. In practice, this means selecting a limited number of measures that are representative of key processes and patient groups or conditions.

The key process elements of hospital-based emergency care delivery have been well described in national and international emergency medicine curricular documents.[25–27] Lindsay et al. proposed criteria for selecting clinical conditions upon which to base emergency care quality indicators (Table 7.3). Based on a modified Delphi approach, they arrived at a set of disease entities representative of the spectrum of ED patients (Table 7.4). This represents one approach to selecting a representative array of target areas for evaluating care in the ED. However, in many, if not most, healthcare systems, the selection of ED quality metrics will be made at the governmental, regulatory body, or payer level. Often the selection of quality metrics will be agenda-driven, based on specific healthcare quality challenges that have been identified. As old challenges are met and new challenges are identified, it should be expected that metrics focusing on areas where improvement has been achieved will be retired, and metrics focusing on new challenges will be implemented.

Whether or not we have a direct role in selecting the quality metrics that are used to evaluate the care

**Table 7.3** Criteria for selecting clinical conditions upon which to base emergency care quality indicators

| |
|---|
| They must be treated in most EDs |
| They must relate to a wide spectrum of age groups |
| They must represent different degrees of patient acuity |
| They must be common reasons for which emergency care is sought |
| Evidence must exist to suggest that best-practice clinical care in the ED may have a significant impact on patient outcome or lead to enhanced clinical efficiency (for example, more appropriate diagnostic test utilization) |
| Conditions that are rare, or where improving ED care is unlikely to change patient outcomes, should be excluded |

Source: Lindsay et al., 2002.[28]

provided in our departments, it is also important for ED leaders to think critically about the suitability of individual quality metrics by which they are evaluated. Graff *et al.* described a range of factors to consider in selecting quality measures (Table 7.5).[13]

## Benefits and pitfalls of QA measures

QA metrics clearly influence the behavior of healthcare providers and organizations. Recent studies show both desirable and undesirable effects on healthcare delivery resulting from the implementation of quality metrics.

In 2006, CMS introduced a quality metric tracking the percentage of patients with ST-elevation myocardial infarction (STEMI) who have door-to-balloon (D2B) times below 90 minutes, with the goal of at least 75% of hospitals meeting this target. Krumholz *et al.* examined improvements in D2B times in the USA since the implementation of CMS AMI-8.[31] They reviewed all patients reported by US hospitals to CMS for inclusion in the AMI-8 inpatient measure from January 2005 to September 2010 (approximately 50 000 patients per year). They found that the median D2B time decreased from 96 minutes to 64 minutes over this period, and the percentage of patients with D2B below 90 minutes increased from 44.2% to 91.4%. The greatest improvements in D2B times were in groups with the worst initial performance: patients over 75 years old, women, and African-Americans.

Poorly designed quality metrics can cause unintended consequences that may harm patients. In 2003, CMS introduced a quality metric tracking the percentage of hospital patients admitted with pneumonia who receive antibiotics within four hours of hospital arrival (PN-5). Kanwar *et al.* studied a total of 518 patients with an admission diagnosis of community-acquired pneumonia (CAP) before (2003) and after (2005) the institution of the CMS PN-5 measure.[32] They found no difference in pneumonia severity scores or mortality between the two periods, but in 2005 more patients were admitted with the diagnosis of CAP without radiographic evidence of pneumonia (28.5% vs. 20.6%, $p = 0.04$) and fewer patients had a final discharge diagnosis of CAP (58.9% vs. 75.9%, $p < 0.001$) than in 2003. They also found that more patients with the admission diagnosis of CAP in 2005 received antibiotics within the four-hour window than in 2003 (65.8% vs. 53.8%, $p = 0.007$). Their conclusion was that during the period after the start of CMS PN-5, there was a greater tendency to overdiagnose pneumonia in patients and inappropriately administer antibiotics.

Another potential risk of using poorly designed performance targets is that the focus of innovation

**Table 7.4** Example of a set of disease entities representative of the spectrum of ED patients

| Asthma |
| Pneumonia |
| Acute myocardial infarction |
| Deep vein thrombosis/pulmonary embolism |
| Chest pain |
| Minor head trauma |
| Ankle/foot trauma |

*Source*: Lindsay *et al.*, 2002.[28]

**Table 7.5** Factors in selecting process-of-care measures

| Factor | Definition |
| --- | --- |
| Level of evidence for process–outcome link | There should be good evidence in the medical literature of the link between the process of care measured and outcome (mortality, morbidity, patient satisfaction) |
| Abstractability | There should be an ability to abstract data relevant to the measure |
| Opportunity for improvement | There should be a clinically significant gap between present practice and best practice |
| Barriers to change | There should be limited barriers to change |
| Applicability | There should be applicability of the measure to the population at large or significant subgroups |

*Sources*: Graff *et al.*, 2002;[13] Jencks *et al.*, 2000;[29] Krumholz *et al.*, 2000.[30]

**Table 7.6** Emergency department clinical quality indicators (United Kingdom)

| | |
|---|---|
| Ambulatory care | Ambulatory care for emergency conditions: the percentage of ED attendances for cellulitis and DVT that end in admission |
| Unplanned re-attendance rate | Unplanned re-attendance at ED within 7 days of original attendance (including if referred back by another health professional) |
| Total time spent in the ED | The median, 95th percentile, and single longest total time spent by patients in the ED, for admitted and non-admitted patients |
| Left without being seen | The percentage of people who leave the ED without being seen |
| Service experience | Qualitative description of what has been done to assess the experience of patients using ED services, their carers and staff, what the results were, and what has been done to improve services in light of the results |
| Time to initial assessment | Time from arrival to start of full initial assessment, which includes a brief history, pain, and early warning scores (including vital signs), for all patients arriving by emergency ambulance |
| Time to treatment | Time from arrival to start of definitive treatment from a decision-making clinician (someone who can define the management plan and discharge the patient) |
| Consultant sign-off | The percentage of patients presenting at type 1 and 2 (major) EDs in certain high-risk patient groups (adults with non-traumatic chest pain, febrile children less than 1 year old, and patients making an unscheduled return visit with the same condition within 72 hours of discharge) who are reviewed by an emergency medicine consultant before being discharged. |

*Source*: Department of Health A&E clinical quality indicators data definitions, 2010.[35]

can become solely on hitting the mark rather than addressing underlying inefficiencies. In a 2006 article in the *BMJ* examining the benefit of the four-hour length-of-stay rule for EDs in the UK National Health Service (NHS), it was noted that while the percentage of patients spending more than four hours in the ED decreased from 23% in 2002 to only 5.3% in 2004 – with associated improvement in overall patient satisfaction – subsequent evidence of gaming to achieve these results raised questions about the overall benefit to patients resulting from the target. Examples of gaming included the practice of pulling staff from other parts of the hospital to the ED, cancelling elective surgeries during the period where performance was being measured, having patients wait in ambulances outside the ED until staff were confident they could meet the four-hour target, and ambiguity in reporting of data.[33]

Quality metrics are powerful tools for influencing the way health care is delivered, but – as these examples illustrate – thoughtfulness in the design and selection of quality metrics is needed, in order to decrease the potential for unintended consequences and gaming, and to increase the likelihood of desired systems improvements.

## Examples of quality metrics used in different countries

Many countries around the world have begun to develop and track QA measures specific to emergency medicine.

Healthcare quality monitoring in the United Kingdom is carried out by the NHS through its Information Centre for Health and Social Care.[34] In April 2011, the NHS released a new set of clinical quality indicators to replace the previous four-hour rule, with the goal of presenting a more comprehensive and balanced view of the care delivered in British emergency departments (Table 7.6).[35]

In Australia, healthcare quality monitoring is carried out both by the Australian Institute of Health and Welfare (AIWH),[36] a governmental agency, and also by an independent, not-for-profit organization, the Australian Council on Healthcare Standards (ACHS).[37] In 2008 the Australian Health Ministers' Conference commissioned the AIHW to develop an updated set of performance indicators to be used for public performance reporting across the entire health and aged care system.[38] Many of the 40 performance indicators are relevant to care delivery in the ED

**Table 7.7** Australasian Council on Healthcare Standards indicators specific to emergency medicine

| |
|---|
| ATS Category 1 patients attended to immediately |
| ATS Category 2 patients attended to within 10 minutes |
| ATS Category 3 patients attended to within 30 minutes |
| ATS Category 4 patients attended to within 60 minutes |
| ATS Category 5 patients attended to within 120 minutes |
| Thrombolysis initiated within 1 hour of presentation for AMI |
| AMI patients who have percutaneous transluminal coronary angioplasty (PTCA) as their primary treatment, having balloon inflation within 1 hour of ED presentation |
| Access block, ED time exceeding 8 hours |
| Access block, ED time exceeding 4 hours |

Source: Australasian Council on Healthcare Standards, 2011.[39]

(adverse drug events, falls resulting in patient harm in care settings, intentional self-harm in hospitals), and three indicators are specific to ED care:

- access to emergency department services by triage category
- potentially avoidable hospital emergency department attendances
- waiting times for emergency departments

The ACHS includes an indicator set specific to emergency medicine in its *Australasian Clinical Indicators Report 2003–2010*.[39] These indicators focus on waiting time, acute myocardial infarction, and access block (Table 7.7).

In the USA, multiple governmental and non-governmental organizations are involved in healthcare quality monitoring. The CMS is the US government agency responsible for managing the Medicare and Medicaid programs for elderly and disabled persons, respectively, and is the largest healthcare payer in the USA. CMS has sets of quality measures for the inpatient (National Hospital Inpatient Quality Measures) and outpatient (Hospital Outpatient Quality Reporting Program) settings, both of which contain measures that apply to care delivered in the ED. The inpatient ED measures focus on management of acute myocardial infarction (AMI), pneumonia, and ED throughput. The outpatient ED measures focus on AMI, antibiotic use in pneumonia and

before surgery, imaging in the ED, cardiac enzyme turnaround time in chest-pain patients, ED throughput, and pain control in ED. The CMS quality indicators that apply to ED care delivery are shown in Table 7.8.[40]

## Performance and benchmarking metrics

Emergency care professional organizations have begun to develop standardized measures of processes and activity in EDs that can be used for comparing departments.[41,42] While these do not necessarily represent quality standards as such, they do provide an opportunity for identifying outliers in performance that may represent either errors or examples of care that should be emulated.

## Key concepts in peer review
### Goals

The goals of peer review are to determine:

- if the care delivered in a specific case failed to meet the agreed-upon standard of care for that hospital setting (error in management)
- if there was an adverse event that was caused by an error (preventable adverse event)
- if there was no adverse event, whether there were any errors that could potentially have led to an adverse event (near miss)

## What is the standard of care?

Generally, the "standard of care" in medicine refers to the set of expectations within the medical community about how a reasonable physician within that medical community would think and act in caring for a particular patient under the circumstances of a particular case. However, in many countries and legal systems, the standard of care also has a specific legal definition in determining whether a defendant was negligent in medical malpractice cases. Establishing negligence is one of several conditions that must be met in the US legal system for a plaintiff to recover damages in a malpractice lawsuit.[43]

Generally, the standard of care is not precisely defined and must be judged on a case-by-case basis. As a result, the standard of care in particular cases may be different in different countries and even in different settings within countries. Within the US

**Table 7.8** CMS quality metrics

| Inpatient CMS metrics relevant to emergency medicine | |
|---|---|
| AMI 1 | Aspirin at arrival |
| AMI 7 | Median time to fibrinolysis (within 30 minutes of arrival) |
| AMI 8 | Median time to primary PCI (within 90 minutes of arrival) |
| PN 3b | Blood culture performed in the ED before initial antibiotic received in hospital |
| PN 6 | Empiric antibiotic consistent with guidelines |
| **Outpatient CMS metrics relevant to emergency medicine** | |
| OP-1 | Median time to fibrinolysis |
| OP-2 | Fibrinolytic therapy within 30 minutes |
| OP-3 | Median time to transfer to another facility for acute coronary intervention |
| OP-4 | Aspirin at arrival |
| OP-5 | Median time to ECG |
| OP-6 | Timing of antibiotic prophylaxis (surgical care) |
| OP-7 | Prophylactic antibiotic selection for surgical patients |
| OP-8 | MRI lumbar spine for low back pain |
| OP-14 | Simultaneous use of brain CT and sinus CT |
| OP-15 | Use of brain CT in the ED for atraumatic headache |
| **CMS metrics for ED throughput** | |
| OP-16 | Troponin results for ED patients with AMI or chest pain (with probable cardiac chest pain) within 60 minutes of arrival |
| OP-18 | Median time from ED arrival to ED departure for discharged ED patients |
| OP-19 | Transition record with specified elements received by discharged patients |
| OP-20 | Door to diagnostic evaluation by a qualified medical professional |
| OP-21 | ED – median time to pain management for long bone fracture |
| OP-22 | ED – patient left without being seen |
| OP-23 | ED – head CT scan results for acute ischemic stroke or hemorrhagic stroke who received head CT scan interpretation within 45 minutes of arrival |
| ED-1 | Median time from ED arrival to ED departure for admitted ED patients |
| ED-2 | Admit decision time to ED departure time for admitted patients |

*Source*: CMS Hospital Quality Initiative, 2012.[40]

legal framework, the standard of care is also viewed as being specific to the defendant doctor's particular field of medicine, or specialty.[43,44] Individuals called upon to provide expert medical testimony on whether the standard of care was met in particular cases must be recognized experts in the specialty area that the case concerns. The American College of Emergency Physicians policy statement on expert witnesses recommends that expert witnesses in emergency medicine cases should be board certified emergency medicine specialists.[45] Likewise, in the domain of QA within the hospital setting, it is important that peer review of ED cases be conducted by individuals with relevant expertise in emergency medicine, which in most cases will be the physician leadership and staff in the ED.

**Table 7.9** Agency for Healthcare Research and Quality harm scale

| | |
|---|---|
| Death | Dead at time of assessment |
| Severe harm | Bodily or psychological injury (including pain or disfigurement) that interferes substantially with functional ability or quality of life |
| Moderate harm | Bodily or psychological injury adversely affecting functional ability or quality of life, but not at the level of severe harm |
| Mild harm | Minimal symptoms or loss of function, or injury limited to additional treatment, monitoring, and/or increased length of stay |
| No harm | Event reached patient, but no harm was evident |

*Source*: AHRQ Common Formats Event Description Hospital Version 1.2, 2012.[48]

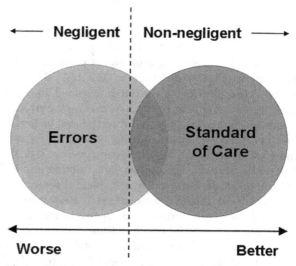

**Figure 7.1** Relationship between errors and standard of care.

From a QA perspective, it is important to emphasize that the standard of care should not be thought of as being the same as care that is "average." If we define the standard of care in terms of what is average, then by definition half of all care must be substandard or negligent, making it impossible to ever achieve acceptable care in the majority of cases. The standard of care should be thought of as being the "minimum safe standard" that is acceptable within an organization.

Lastly, it is also important to note that the standard of care should not be thought of as the absence of all error. Although errors are, by definition, present when the standard of care is not met, cases may contain minor errors (such as documentation errors) and still meet the standard of care. In order for errors to violate the standard of care, they must exceed a certain threshold of severity (Fig. 7.1).

The individual or committee tasked with performing QA within the ED acts on behalf of the department to determine whether the standard of care has been met in the cases that are reviewed in the peer review process.

## What is an adverse event?

While there is a seemingly infinite variety of undesirable occurrences that can happen, only a subset of these are considered to be "adverse events" from the perspective of healthcare quality improvement in general and peer review in particular. The definitions used in the major studies that have determined the incidence of adverse events in health care include the following key elements:[2-4,46,47]

- An *unintended* or unexpected injury or complication
- which results in death, disability, or additional treatment (including prolonged hospitalization) – that is, some type of *harm* happens to the patient (in some countries "harm" is broadly interpreted to include psychological distress) – and
- is *caused by healthcare management* rather than simply being a result of the natural course of the patient's disease (for example, a patient who suffers cardiac arrest after a massive myocardial infarction).

Severity scales and classification schemes for healthcare-related adverse events have been developed by various entities including the Agency for Healthcare Research and Quality (AHRQ) in the USA. The AHRQ harm scale for classifying the severity of adverse events is included in the AHRQ Common Formats Events Description Hospital Version 1.2, which also categorizes the types of healthcare events that are considered to be adverse events (Table 7.9).[48] Regulatory agencies in some countries require hospitals to report certain types of adverse events such as:

- sentinel events[49]
- serious reportable events[16]
- hospital-acquired conditions[50]

## What is an error?

Most current definitions of error in health care refer to the work of James Reason, professor of psychology at the University of Manchester in the UK. Reason described two theories by which to understand human error: the *person approach*, which focuses on the errors of individuals, blaming them for forgetfulness, inattention, or moral weakness; and the *systems approach*, under which errors are viewed as consequences rather than causes, and which focuses on the conditions under which individuals work and tries to build defenses to avert errors or mitigate their effects.[51] Reason also described two basic error forms: *errors in planning* (mistakes) and *errors in execution* (slips and lapses).[52] He also described the concept of *chains of errors* leading to an adverse event whereby a series of steps (or missteps) leads to a proximal event. The chain of errors may occur in the context of a number of contributing factors.

The most commonly cited definition of error in the US medical literature is based on the work of Reason and first appeared in the 2000 IOM report *To Err is Human*. The IOM report defines error as "the failure of a planned action to be completed as intended (error of execution) or the use of a wrong plan to achieve an aim (error of planning)."[1,52] The Harvard Medical Practice Study (1991) and the Australian Healthcare Quality Study (1995) both used this definition but further defined error in terms of the "preventability" of an adverse event. In other words, if an adverse event occurred and was preventable, then there was, by definition, an error in management. If there was no adverse event, but there was an error in management that had the potential to cause an adverse event, then this would be considered a "near miss" (Table 7.10). Errors in management in these studies were considered a failure to follow accepted practice at an individual or system level, which is the current level of expected performance for the average practitioner or system that manages the condition in question. It includes acts of omission (delay or failure to diagnose or treat) and acts of commission (incorrect treatment or management).[2,3,46]

**Table 7.10** Combinations of adverse events and errors

|  | – Error | + Error |
| --- | --- | --- |
| – Adverse event | Adequate care | Near miss |
| + Adverse event | Non-preventable adverse event | Preventable adverse event |

Because errors ultimately involve breakdowns in the process of emergency care delivery, they can be categorized according to the types of processes in which the breakdown occurs. Leape *et al.* described five major categories of medical error, based on process type, in the Harvard Medical Practice Study:[3]

- procedural performance
- prevention and monitoring
- diagnosis
- medication
- system and other

Why do errors happen in the first place? As James Reason observed, answers to this question can be complex, and a complete explanation usually requires a formal root-cause analysis. Kachalia *et al.* described several categories for factors contributing to medical errors:[53]

- cognitive factors
- communication factors
- systems factors
- patient-related factors
- normative factors

Our assumption in QA is that in the vast majority of cases, healthcare providers are well intentioned and try their best to deliver the highest-quality care in the conditions in which they work. However, given that human beings are, by our nature and despite our best intentions, prone to error, our focus in seeking to reduce errors and the adverse events that result from them must be to identify and fix the underlying conditions in our emergency care delivery systems that predispose towards human error.

## Data sources that support QA programs

Effective peer review and QA processes require sufficient internal data-gathering mechanisms to easily access relevant documentation as well as other clinical and operational data to understand the delivery of care in specific cases and for the ED as a whole.

The questions that QA evaluation tries to answer include:

- Were specific steps or actions (diagnostic or therapeutic) carried out in patients with particular conditions?
- Was there timely recognition and treatment of time-sensitive conditions?

## Individual case documentation

Retrospective peer review activities evaluate the care delivered in specific cases and depend on documentation to reconstruct and understand what happened in a given case. When available documentation is not sufficient, reviewers need to go back and interview care providers. However, providers' ability to recall details of specific cases may fade with time or be influenced by the outcome, so it is always desirable to have real-time documentation. In addition to understanding what actions occurred in a specific case, peer reviewers need to understand the thought processes and medical decision making of the care providers in the case. Ideally, all paper documentation for an individual case should be gathered and scanned electronically before these documents are sent to medical records, so that a copy of the documentation is readily accessible for all ED cases.

## Electronic timestamp data

As hospitals shift from paper-based systems to electronic medical records, computerized provider order entry systems, laboratory and imaging data management systems, inventory control systems, and other computerized systems for managing workflow, QA opportunities for gathering and utilizing timestamp data that are automatically generated in the routine course of carrying out work in the ED are becoming more common. Collectively, this information provides a concrete representation of the actions that occurred during the case. The more data are electronically gathered and available for subsequent review, the more care providers can focus on documenting their thought processes and medical decision making instead of documenting what happened in a case. Whenever possible, QA data should be gathered electronically to facilitate analysis and reduce administrative burden.

## Setting up an ED peer review program
## Types of models

When setting up a QA peer review program, EDs must balance efficiency and bias. Efficiency means the volume of cases reviewed with a given amount of administrative and personnel effort. Having a single individual from the ED (such as the ED director) carry out all peer review activities can be highly efficient, because that person is a content expert in the area, understands the clinical processes and how they are supposed to work, is able to interpret the documentation and data sources, and does not need to discuss the case with others. On the other hand, there is a limit to how many cases one person can review, especially if that individual has many other duties, as is often the case with the ED director. There is also the risk of individual biases resulting in a tendency to either over- or under-identify problems or issues with the quality of care provided by peers.[54,55] Having a committee of clinicians from the ED, both physicians and nurses, is perhaps the most common solution to carrying out QA peer review. This approach spreads the work among many individuals and can help limit individual bias.

While individuals from the same specialty may be best equipped to understand what the standard of care is in a given clinical area, such as emergency medicine, there is also a risk that staff from the same specialty or department may have a tendency to overlook errors or suboptimal care by their peers. While it may not be practicable to involve clinicians from other specialties in the routine QA peer review work of the ED, many institutions use a multispecialty hospital QA peer review committee for cases that involve multiple departments or involve errors or adverse events of such severity that they require external reporting to regulatory agencies.

## Selecting cases for peer review

Cases are typically selected for peer review based on either reactive or proactive criteria. Reactive criteria include referrals of a case by other healthcare providers, patients, or family members, who question the quality of care in a case. It is essential for the ED to respond to every complaint raised, even those that appear trivial or unfounded. Taking all complaints seriously sends a clear message that the ED leadership is concerned about quality.

Proactive criteria include screening criteria that identify cases that may have a higher than average potential for errors or adverse events, or that are being closely monitored for other quality measurement purposes. Examples of proactive criteria include deaths in the ED or within 24 hours of admission, and returns to the ED within 72 hours that are admitted on the second ED visit. Other examples include cases that involve high-risk procedures (intubation, procedural sedation) or specific institutional protocols that dictate specific ED management steps (STEMI, stroke, sepsis, trauma). Departments may also review randomly selected cases to estimate the baseline rate of errors and adverse events in the ED. And lastly, cases involving particular diagnoses that are the focus of externally reported quality metrics (pneumonia, AMI, stroke) may need peer review, especially cases that are judged not to be in compliance with those metrics.

## The review process

After being selected for peer review by one of the criteria above, cases will typically undergo an initial review by an individual member of the QA committee to determine whether there is any possibility of errors, adverse events, or other management issues in the case that warrant discussion by the full QA committee. Cases ideally should be assigned randomly to peer reviewers who were not involved with the care of the patient. Reviewers should have access to sufficient documentation and data to be able to reconstruct the relevant aspects of the case and to understand the medical decision making of the providers. The focus of this initial review should primarily be on identifying systems issues that may contribute to the occurrence of adverse events or errors, and not primarily on assigning blame for errors to individuals.

Numerous studies have found that inter-rater reliability scores in peer review tend to be low, especially when unstructured review processes are used.[56] The more structured the review, the greater the inter-rater reliability. However, more structured review processes also are difficult to develop and tend to be specific to particular types of cases, thereby limiting the scope of their applicability.[57] Simple examples of how to provide structure to the review include using a series of specific, standardized questions that reviewers answer about each case, such as:

- Were there any adverse events?
- Were there any errors in management?
- Was the standard of care met?

Given that the available documentation for a case may not be sufficient for reviewers to determine with certainty whether, for example, an error occurred, many studies based on peer review have used likelihood scales rather than yes-or-no answers when asking reviewers to make these determinations.[2,3,58]

In addition, questions about the level of performance (using Likert scales) in specific domains can provide additional feedback for providers and ED leadership. Examples of these domains can include documentation, medical decision making, resource utilization, performance of procedures, and coordination of care.

Cases in which a question of adverse event or error arises in the initial review should be discussed by the larger QA committee to come to a consensus on whether adverse events or errors occurred and to determine what follow-up actions, if any, are needed to address identified problems. These actions may include individual remediation and education of providers, fixes to address systems issues identified in the review process, presentation at departmental morbidity and mortality conference, or referral of the case outside the department.

The morbidity and mortality (M&M) conference is an important tool for continuing medical education of ED physicians and nursing staff, as well as for maintaining a common standard of care across all providers in the ED.[59] The M&M conference should be educational in nature and attended by all ED staff and trainees. M&M cases are chosen either because of the nature or severity of the management errors, or because of the complexity of the management and the educational value that the case may have for ED staff.

Specific cases may need to be reported to entities outside the ED if they meet certain criteria. For example, if the case involves providers from other departments, it may need to be referred to that department's QA committee. If the case involves certain types or categories of events (sentinel events, serious reportable events, major incidents), these may need to be reported to regulatory agencies. The specific types of events that need to be reported will vary by region and country.

### Case study 7.1. Does an adverse event always indicate an error?

At an emergency department M&M conference, a case was discussed involving a 60-year-old man who presented to the ED with a history of fever, malaise, and productive cough for the past week. Vital signs showed heart rate 110, systolic blood pressure 80, respiratory rate 28–30; $O_2$ saturation 85% on room air. Lung exam revealed diffuse rhonchi. Chest x-ray showed multilobar pneumonia, and serum lactate was 4.2 mmol/L. The patient was started on intravenous fluids and antibiotics. After 2 liters of normal saline, the patient remained hypotensive. Based on the working diagnosis of septic shock, the ED physician decided to place a central venous line according to the departmental protocol for early goal-directed therapy. The ED physician used a right subclavian approach and standard Seldinger technique to place a triple-lumen catheter; the wire advanced easily and there was good return of blood from all ports. The post-procedure chest x-ray showed a 10% right pneumothorax. The QA committee agreed that the pneumothorax represented an adverse event, but some questioned whether this also represented an error. Pneumothorax is a known complication of central venous line placement that occurs in 1–3% of cases, even when it is performed properly. Based on the available information in this case, it appeared that

the ED physician followed standard operating procedure for placing the central line. Therefore, the pneumothorax cannot be considered to be an error, only a non-preventable adverse event.

## Conclusions

Quality assurance in the emergency department depends on both data gathering and measurement of indicators that provide an overview of the quality of care delivered by the ED. In addition, peer review of selected cases can address potential problems in care delivery and identify opportunities for improvement. A robust quality assurance program is an essential administrative tool for developing and maintaining a high-performing ED.

## References

1. Institute of Medicine. *To Err is Human: Building a Safer Health System*. Washington, DC, National Academies Press, 2000.

2. Brennan TA, Leape LL, Laird NM, *et al*. Incidence of adverse events and negligence in hospitalized patients. Results of the Harvard Medical Practice Study I. *New England Journal of Medicine* 1991; **324**: 370–6.

3. Leape LL, Brennan TA, Laird N, *et al*. The nature of adverse events in hospitalized patients. Results of the Harvard Medical Practice Study II. *New England Journal of Medicine* 1991; **324**: 377–84.

4. Thomas EJ, Studdert DM, Burstin HR, *et al*. Incidence and types of adverse events and negligent care in Utah and Colorado. *Medical Care* 2000; **38**: 261–71.

5. Lerman B, Kobernick MS. Return visits to the emergency department. *Journal of Emergency Medicine* 1987; **5**: 359–62.

6. Keith KD, Bocka JJ, Kobernick MS, *et al*. Emergency department revisits. *Annals of Emergency Medicine* 1989; **18**: 964–8.

7. Lu TC, Tsai CL, Lee CC, *et al*. Preventable deaths in patients admitted from emergency department. *Emergency Medicine Journal* 2006; **23**: 452–5.

8. Nafsi T, Russell R, Reid CM, Rizvi SM. Audit of deaths less than a week after admission through an emergency department: how accurate was the ED diagnosis and were any deaths preventable? *Emergency Medicine Journal* 2007; **24**: 691–5.

9. Sklar DP, Crandall CS, Loeliger E, *et al*. Unanticipated death after discharge home from the emergency department. *Annals of Emergency Medicine* 2007; **49**: 735–45.

10. Committee to Design a Strategy for Quality Review Assurance in Medicare (Institute of Medicine). *Medicare: a Strategy for Quality Assurance, Volume I*, Dallas, TX: National Academies Press, 1990.

11. Committee on Quality of Health Care in America (Institute of Medicine). *Crossing the Quality Chasm: a New Health System for the 21st Century*, Dallas, TX: National Academies Press, 2001.

12. James BC. Improving quality can reduce costs. *QA Review* 1989; **1** (1): 4.

13. Graff L, Stevens C, Spaite D, *et al*. Measuring and improving quality in emergency medicine. *Academic Emergency Medicine* 2002; **9**: 1091–107.

14. Eagle CJ, Davies JM. Current models of "quality": an introduction for anaesthetists. *Canadian Journal of Anaesthesia* 1993; **40**: 851–62.

15. Reason J. *Managing the Risks of Organizational Accidents*. Burlington, VT: Ashgate, 1997.

16. National Quality Forum. Serious reportable events. http://www. qualityforum.org/Publications/ 2008/10/Serious_Reportable_ Events.aspx (accessed March 18, 2012).

17. Centers for Medicare and Medicaid Services (CMS). Overview: Physician Quality Reporting System. http://www.cms.gov/PQRS// (accessed March 26, 2012).

18. Medicare. Hospital Compare. US Department of Health and Human Services. http://www. hospitalcompare.hhs.gov (accessed May 15, 2012).

19. Centers for Medicare and Medicaid Services (CMS). Hospital Inpatient Quality

Reporting Program. http://www.cms.gov/Hospital QualityInits/08_Hospital RHQDAPU.asp#TopOfPage (accessed March 26, 2012).

20. Donabedian A. The quality of care: how can it be assessed? *JAMA* 1988; **260**: 1743–8.

21. Porter ME. What is value in health care? *New England Journal of Medicine*. 2010; **363**: 2477–81.

22. Kaplan RS, Porter ME. How to solve the cost crisis in health care. *Harvard Business Review* 2011; **89**: 46–52, 54, 56–61.

23. Kaplan RS, Anderson SR. Time-driven activity-based costing. *Harvard Business Review* 2004; **82**: 131–8, 150.

24. Porter ME. Value in health care. Supplementary Appendix 1 to Porter ME. What is value in health care? *New England Journal of Medicine* 2010; **363**: 2477–81.

25. Perina DG, Beeson MS, Char DM, *et al*. The 2007 model of the clinical practice of emergency medicine: the 2009 update. *Academic Emergency Medicine* 2011; **18**: e8–26.

26. Hobgood C, Anantharaman V, Bandiera G, *et al*. International Federation for Emergency Medicine Model Curriculum for Emergency Medicine Specialists. *Emergency Medicine Australasia* 2011; **23**: 541–53.

27. Petrino R. A curriculum for the specialty of emergency medicine in Europe. *European Journal of Emergency Medicine* 2009; **16**: 113–14.

28. Lindsay P, Schull M, Bronskill S, Anderson G. The development of indicators to measure the quality of clinical care in emergency departments following a modified-Delphi approach. *Academic Emergency Medicine* 2002; **9**: 1131–9.

29. Jencks SF, Cuerdon T, Burwen DR, *et al*. Quality of medical care delivered to Medicare beneficiaries:

profile at state and national level. *JAMA* 2000; **284**: 1670–6.

30. Krumholz H, Baker DW, Ashton CM, *et al*. Evaluating quality of care for patients with heart failure. *Circulation* 2000; **101**: e101–40.

31. Krumholz HM, Herrin J, Miller LE, *et al*. Improvements in door-to-balloon time in the United States, 2005 to 2010. *Circulation* 2011; **124**: 1038–45.

32. Kanwar M, Brar N, Khatib R, *et al*. Misdiagnosis of community-acquired pneumonia and inappropriate utilization of antibiotics: side effects of the 4-h antibiotic administration rule. *Chest* 2007; **131**: 1865–9.

33. Bevan G, Hood C. Have targets improved performance in the English NHS? *BMJ* 2006; **332**: 419–22.

34. NHS Information Centre for Health and Social Care. http://www.ic.nhs.uk (accessed May 28, 2012).

35. Department of Health. Urgent & Emergency Care. A&E Clinical Quality Indicators Data Definitions. London: Department of Health, 2010.

36. Australian Institute of Health and Welfare. http://www.aihw.gov.au (accessed May 28, 2012).

37. Australian Council on Healthcare Standards. http://www.achs.org.au (accessed May 28, 2012).

38. Australian Institute of Health and Welfare. *A Set of Performance Indicators Across the Health and Aged Care System*. Canberra: AIHW, 2008.

39. Emergency Medicine, version 4. Clinical Indicators. In *Australasian Clinical Indicator Report 2003–2010*. 12th edn. Australasian Council on Healthcare Standards, 2011.

40. Centers for Medicare and Medicaid Services (CMS). Hospital Quality Initiative. https://www.cms.gov/Medicare/ Quality-Initiatives-Patient-

Assessment-Instruments/Hospital QualityInits/index.html (accessed July 23, 2012).

41. Welch S, Augustine J, Camargo CA, Reese C. Emergency department performance measures and benchmarking summit. *Academic Emergency Mediine*. 2006; **13**: 1074–80.

42. Welch SJ, Asplin BR, Stone-Griffith S, *et al*. Emergency department operational metrics, measures and definitions: results of the Second Performance Measures and Benchmarking Summit. *Annals of Emergency Medicine* 2011; **58**: 33–40.

43. Moffett P, Moore G. The standard of care: legal history and definitions: the bad and good news. *Western Journal of Emergency Medicine* 2011; **12**: 109–12.

44. McCourt v Abernathy. in., S.C.; 1995: 603.

45. American College of Emergency Physicians (ACEP). Expert witness guidelines for the specialty of emergency medicine. *Annals of Emergency Medicine* 2010; **56**: 449–50.

46. Wilson RM, Runciman WB, Gibberd RW, *et al*. The Quality in Australian Health Care Study. *Medical Journal of Australia* 1995; **163**: 458–71.

47. Vincent C, Neale G, Woloshynowych M. Adverse events in British hospitals: preliminary retrospective record review. *BMJ* 2001; **322**: 517–19.

48. Agency for Healthcare Research and Quality. AHRQ Common Formats Event Description Hospital Version 1.2. https://www.psoppc.org/c/ document_library/get_file? p_l_id=375679&folderId=409252 &name=DLFE-14073.pdf (accessed July 24, 2012)

49. Sentinel events. In *Comprehensive Accreditation Manual for Hospitals: the Official Handbook*. The Joint Commission, 2011.

50. Centers for Medicare and Medicaid Services (CMS). Hospital-acquired conditions. http://www.cms.gov/Hospital AcqCond/06_Hospital-Acquired_ Conditions.asp#TopOfPage (accessed March 18, 2012).

51. Reason J. Human error: models and management. *BMJ* 2000; **320**: 768–70.

52. Reason J. *Human Error*. Cambridge: Cambridge University Press, 1990.

53. Kachalia A, Gandhi TK, Puopolo AL, *et al.* Missed and delayed diagnoses in the emergency department: a study of closed malpractice claims from 4 liability insurers. *Annals of Emergency Medicine* 2007; **49**: 196–205.

54. Goldman RL. The reliability of peer assessments of quality of care. *JAMA* 1992; **267**: 958–60.

55. Thomas EJ, Lipsitz SR, Studdert DM, *et al.* The reliability of medical record review for estimating adverse event rates. *Annals of Internal Medicine* 2002; **136**: 812–16.

56. Smith MA, Atherly AJ, Kane RL, *et al.* Peer review of the quality of care. Reliability and sources of variability for outcome and process assessments. *JAMA* 1997; **278**: 1573–8.

57. Lilford RJ, Mohammed MA, Braunholtz D, *et al.* The measurement of active errors: methodological issues. *Quality and Safety in Health Care* 2003; **12** (Suppl 2): ii8–12.

58. Studdert DM, Mello MM, Gawande AA, *et al.* Claims, errors, and compensation payments in medical malpractice litigation. *New England Journal of Medicine* 2006; **354**: 2024–33.

59. Seigel TA, McGillicuddy DC, Barkin AZ, *et al.* Morbidity and Mortality conference in Emergency Medicine. *Journal of Emergency Medicine* 2010; **38**: 507–11.

## Further reading

Welch SJ. *Quality Matters: Solutions for a Safe and Efficient Emergency Department*. Oakbrook Terrace, IL: Joint Commission Resources, 2009.

Jensen K, Kirkpatrick DG. *The Hospital Executive's Guide to Emergency Department Management*. Marblehead, MA: HCPro, Inc., 2012.

## Chapter

# 8

# Emergency department policies and procedures

Kirsten Boyd

### Key learning points

- Emergency department policies and procedures are used to standardize practice and ensure quality care.
- There are essential steps in writing, implementing, and evaluating policies.
- Successful policy and procedure implementation is supported and driven by leadership.

## Introduction

Policies and procedures are an instrumental foundation of any successful business or organization. These structured, approved organizational tools form the basis for setting expectations within the organization about standardized protocols, practice, operations, and accountability. A well-written and implemented policy can improve communication and standardize practice in the fast-paced world of emergency medicine.[1]

A *policy* is a rule adopted by the organization after it has gone through an appropriate approval process, which serves to assist frontline providers in decision making. A *procedure* is the methodology used to carry out specific tasks on a daily basis. A procedure is one way to implement a policy in practice.[2]

Some policies and procedures may be specific to one department, while others involve many departments within an organization. Those that reach across departmental boundaries will require more input and greater collaboration to ensure communication among specialties as well as consistent practice throughout the organization.

In this chapter, we will discuss how policies are written, approved, implemented, and evaluated. A critical component of the chapter will be to focus on your role as the leader of the department to ensure your team is knowledgeable and consistently practicing within the scope outlined.

## Role of policies and procedures in an emergency department

### Standardizing clinical practice

Clinical pathways have become an increasingly common strategy for ensuring evidence-based practice for conditions where there is significant benefit to be gained by following standardized diagnostic and treatment protocols.[3] Physician and nursing training programs expose their trainees to this approach as a standard of care for certain populations. Policies and procedures function in much the same way to introduce a standard to support clinical and operational functions in an organization.[4]

The role of policies and procedures is to frame the practice of the department or the organization. This standard is intended to support and guide clinicians in their patient management and decision making. When new physicians or nurses join the organization, a review of the policy and procedure manual is critical to their orientation and training.[5] This review will set the foundation for practice in your institution.

## Building a structure for operations

Getting started is often the most challenging aspect of policy or procedure development. If your organization has a policy coordinating office, you should work with them to get information on templates, language, and approval process.[5] However, if, like many organizations, you are just starting to build a structure for operations or a department-specific clinical practice,

*Emergency Department Leadership and Management*, ed. Stephanie Kayden, *et al.* Published by Cambridge University Press.
© Cambridge University Press 2015.

then creating your own policy and procedure development team will be an important first step.

The responsibilities of the team will include providing input to policy creation, implementation, and evaluation. There will need to be "section owners" who will have responsibility for specific policy and procedure areas. These individuals, who are identified by your organizational leaders, are typically selected based on individual expertise. Putting this structure in place will facilitate the development of new policies by having content experts in place and ready to lead the process.[6]

## The process of writing a policy

The overall goal of writing a policy or procedure guideline is to keep it simple, consistent, and easy to locate. The best-written policies have two major characteristics. First, the frontline staff clearly understands the policy, which is written in simple language. Second, the policy reflects the care provided. One of the most common errors that healthcare regulatory agencies cite with regard to polices or procedures is that policies have been implemented that are too complicated, are not consistently implemented from provider to provider, or do not match actual practice.[3]

A departmental committee to review policies, procedures, and other practices is standard in most organizations.[2] Members of this committee often include the emergency department (ED) director, the chief nurse, and other ED leaders, such as nurse managers, physicians, and nurses in charge of departmental operations, quality assurance, medical informatics, and clinical training programs. Approval of a policy is the responsibility of a governing committee, not an individual. As many policies and procedures will impact other specialties or areas of the organization, it is critical to be mindful and inclusive to ensure standard practice and minimize confusion among providers.

## Tips for writing a policy

- A good policy will be written in clear, concise, simple language.
- The policy statement should address the rule, not how to implement the rule (implementation is part of a procedure).
- The policy should be accessible to all providers easily. Many organizations have adopted online manuals to ease access and the ability to update or edit existing policies, so that frontline providers have the most up-to-date information.[7]

- Authors should use a template that is standardized by your institution and is user-friendly so readers can find the policies they are looking for with ease.

## Tips for writing a procedure

- All written procedures are linked to organizational policies. This link provides clear guidance to physicians and nurses for clinical and operational decision making and bridges communication.
- The language used is simple and clear – much like the writing of a policy. The authors can test this by having frontline providers read and verbalize their understanding as a method to test readability as well as understanding.[7]
- Procedures should be linked to owners. This establishes a link for frontline physicians and nurses to question the content of the procedure as well as gain more information on a subject.
- Double-check accuracy – to establish credibility, ensure that you are factual and correct in what you are putting forward. This is applicable to the writing of any document that will be rolled out to staff or clinicians.

## Design and layout of policy and procedure documents

Building a template for your policy index that is clear, structured, and readable for your physicians and nursing staff is another critical component to ensure ease of use as well as speed of access to the information. Organizations typically adopt formats or templates to ensure consistency. Labels are often utilized to introduce key points and structure the document into segments required for each policy.[5] An example of an institutional framework for administrative policy and procedure development can be found in Table 8.1.

The title of the policy clearly indicates what the policy will be about. This is most commonly the header of the relevant format, followed by a number. This number will help to classify the document in an organized way. For example, an administrative policy may be numbered as ADM-01, to be followed by ADM-02. A clinical policy may be numbered as CL-01.[6] This is solely up to the organization and should be based on the system that is in place to organize a large number of documents. A sample template for starting a policy or procedure is shown in Table 8.2.

**Table 8.1** An example of an institutional framework for administrative policy and procedure development (Source: Beth Israel Deaconess Medical Center)

**Name of medical center or institution**
**Manual**

**Title**: Policy, procedure, guideline, and directive (PPGD) sponsorship, formulation, approval and implementation in the medical center

**Number**: According to medical center standards

**Policy statement/purpose:** this policy establishes the process for the development, revision, approval and dissemination of medical center policies, procedures, guidelines and directives (PPGD). Implementation of this policy is designed to:

- Result in an appropriate and consistent set of Medical Center PPGDs,
- To ensure timeliness, accuracy, ownership, historical tracking, appropriate approval, and
- Ease of access/use by Medical Center staff

**A. PPGD development and plan for implementation**

Organization policy, procedure, guideline and directive manuals are inter- and intradepartmental PPGDs. The PPGD manuals are on-line in the PPGD section of the Institution's portal or the department should maintain a written copy of their respective manual. Email directives that are issued by Institution Communications or a Vice President must include the effective dates. The process for managing and posting a PPGD will be implemented by the Health Care Quality Professional Staff Affairs Office (PSA).

**The Institution Policy Manual** is the core set of hospital-wide PPGDs that sets the standard for all other inter- and intradepartmental PPGD manuals throughout the medical center.

**Senior Leadership Sponsorship** – All PPGDs must be sponsored by an Institution's vice president or department chief. "Sponsorship" indicates that the proposed new PPGD has received the endorsement of a vice president or department chief who has assured that the PPGD is appropriate, that appropriate content expert persons are involved in new PPGD formulation, and a plan is in place to educate staff and implement the PPGD and monitor compliance. The PPGD is reviewed and revised at appropriate times by the author/owner. The sponsor must approve both the PPGD and implementation plan.

**Regulatory Compliance and Monitoring Plan** – The requestor and sponsor of a PPGD must ensure that the new PPGD is consistent with the Institution's mission and values as well as all relevant regulatory and accreditation requirements. The PPGD must reflect the actual work practices of the Medical Center. In addition, the sponsor is responsible for developing and implementing a plan to monitor compliance with the PPGD.

**PPGD Oversight Committee** – The PPGD Oversight Committee will be managed by the PSA Office. The Committee will advise the Operations Council on the management of all PPGDs and maintain the content of the Institutions Policy Manual. The committee will regularly review any requests for new PPGDs that cross departments or services and will provide guidance on the content, format and use of the "Content Management System" in the tracking and formal review process for all such approved PPGDs. The primary purpose of the oversight committee will be to manage the content of the Institution's Policy Manual as the guiding source for other PPGDs in the Medical Center. The committee will ensure that PPGDs are not duplicative or conflicting in content and will ensure that appropriate review for new PPGDs has occurred by the content experts and that all renewals or revisions are undertaken in a systematic manner.

No PPGD may be written, posted, disseminated or implemented in the Medical Center unless it has been processed according to these requirements. Any reference to a particular PPGD on the web portal site, or elsewhere, outside of the original placement within the respective PPGD manual, must be hyperlinked to the original source document.

**B. PPGD review process**

Depending upon the content of the PPGD, the following process will be implemented for the review and approval of the respective PPGD. If any such PPGDs are identified to become part of the Institutions Policy Manual, the draft will be reviewed by the PSA Office and appropriate content experts (see Appendix F) prior to final approval.

1. **Clinical Care PPGD/Clinical Practice Guidelines** – All must be reviewed by the appropriate Clinical Chief(s) or clinical committee chair who will make or be delegated the authority to approve and make a

**Table 8.1** *(cont.)*

| Name of medical center or institution |
| :--- |
| **Manual** |

recommendation for final approval to the Medical Executive Committee, Operations Council and/or the Institution's Board of Directors. (Regulations require Board approval of some policies; the Legal Office will advise as to whether the policy requires Board approval.)

2. **Administrative PPGD** – All must be reviewed by the appropriate department head and respective vice president to make a recommendation for final approval to the operations council (and, if required by the Institution's Board of Directors and MEC).

3. **Research PPGD** – All must be reviewed by the vice president, research operations to make a recommendation for final approval by the research advisory committee (ReAC) and/or further by the Institution's Board of Directors, if required.

4. **Graduate Medical Education PPGD** – All PPGDs that govern the academic programs of the medical center must be reviewed and approved by the GME committee, and reviewed by the chief academic officer to make a recommendation for final approval to the medical executive committee (and, if required, by the Institution's Board of Directors).

**C. Implementation of the approved policy**

Upon full approval by the authorities outlined above, the author/owner will ensure that any medical center wide or interdepartmental PPGD is placed into the on-line content management system (CMS). Placement of intradepartmental PPGDs on the CMS will be at the discretion of the sponsor. The sponsor for the PPGD will assist the author/owner to then implement the plan for dissemination, staff training and monitoring of compliance with the new or revised PPGD within a reasonable time frame. It is recommended that whenever possible, direct observation and Lean organizational principles are applied to PPGD development and/or revision to insure that the PPGD reflects actual work practices and identifies opportunities to improve implementation and education.

**D. Frequency of review**

All PPGD's will be reviewed a minimum of at least every three (3) years. However, revisions should occur at such time as the content is no longer relevant, as when governing regulations or accreditation standards have changed or the evidence-based clinical practice guidelines have been revised. The sponsoring vice president, in collaboration with, the content owner/author will be responsible for identifying the frequency on the tracking form for each PPGD.

**E. PPGD revisions**

All revisions to the Institution's Policy Manual shall be reviewed by the all appropriate stakeholders and content experts (see Attachment F). While revisions may be initially proposed by anyone, the revision must be reviewed by the VP sponsor of the relevant policy prior to sending it to the PSA Office. The PSA Office will determine if the proposed revision is minor or major.

- *Minor revision:* If determined to be minor, the sponsoring VP can approve such revisions and disseminate appropriately to update web site and existing documents though the PSA Office. *The "Next Review Date" will remain unchanged.*

- *Major revision:* If determined to be major, approval to such revisions will go through the same process as outlined above for proposed new policies. All interdepartmental PPGD revisions will be reviewed by the responsible department/committee *who will make their recommendations to their supervising leader/committee. The "Next Review Date" will be changed as for all PPGDs.*

**F. PPGD elimination**

All Institution Policy Manual changes that recommend elimination shall be reviewed by the sponsoring VP and must be approved through the same process as outlined above for proposed new PPGDs. All interdepartmental PPGDs will be reviewed by the responsible department/committee.

**G. Retention**

Any old (i.e., revised) or eliminated policy manual PPGDs shall be archived through the CMS system or kept by the respective department in writing. In addition, the department of Health Care Quality, PSA office, will have a backup copy of the current Institutions Manual for reference. All other collections will be automatically archived once placed on CMS or have the respective department keep a copy that is not on the CMS system. The individual department is

**Table 8.1** *(cont.)*

| |
|---|
| **Name of medical center or institution**<br>**Manual** |

responsible for their collection/manual and will keep a written copy, if not on-line. All previous versions must be saved for a period of seven (7) years after its revision or elimination date. The Legal Office shall notify hospital administration of any request to retain a policy for more than seven (7) years.

**H. Definitions/glossary of terms**

   **1. Policies**

      **a. Medical center-wide policies**

         1. high-level, embracing the mission, core values and general goals to be followed by all staff of the medical center
         2. typically effect several departments
         3. establish a standard practice (e.g. clinical practice or research standard based on accepted standards of care or administrative practice: industry standards, efficient use of system resources; federal, industry and other grant sponsoring agency standards)
         4. establish the scope for decision making and action
         5. refer to associated procedures and guidelines that serve to facilitate policy compliance
         6. typically required by regulatory or accrediting authorities

      **b. Interdepartmental policies** – apply to more than one department for implementation but are **not** medical center-wide

      **c. Intradepartmental policies** – refer to those within one department. Those PPGDs that apply only to a single department may follow the minimum requirements regarding sponsorship and approval outlined in Attachment A: Minimum requirements for single department.

   **2. Procedures** – procedures are sets of instructions or specific steps that MUST BE FOLLOWED in order to achieve compliance with a policy requirement or intended result.

   **3. Guidelines** – guidelines provide parameters or ranges of action to be used, based upon the discretion of the department head(s) or identified content expert; and/or address specific methods by which to operationalize a requirement. **Clinical practice guidelines (CPG)** represents "evidence-based best practice" for patient care or treatment that has been approved for use in the medical center by MEC. Such guidelines govern all supporting PPGDs across all other clinical disciplines.

Clinical practice guidelines (CPGs) are considered, based on established criteria, for use in designing or improving patient care processes within the medical center. The clinical practice guideline author, sponsor and medical executive committee use criteria consistent with the institution's mission/vision, in line with current professional practice and technology – based recommendations as well as relevant to the annual operating and strategic plans in the selection/development and approval of clinical practice guidelines.

   Based on prioritized aspects of care and service provided, the medical executive committee reviews and approves CPGs that will be utilized in populations of:

   - High volume, and/or
   - New service/equipment/resources, and/or
   - High risk for serious consequences or of deprivation of substantial benefit when care is not provide when indicated/correctly, and/or
   - High cost

Sources for clinical practice guidelines may include, but are not limited to:

   - National Guideline Clearing House
   - Agency for Healthcare Research and Quality
   - Professional organizations (American Heart Association, Society for Critical Care, American Gastroenterological Association etc.)
   - Internal expert practitioners
   - Interdepartmental subcommittees of institution's medical executive committee

The medical executive committee considers the steps and changes or variations needed to encourage use, dissemination and implementation of chosen CPGs throughout the medical center. This includes staff communication, training, implementation, feedback and evaluation as outlined in this policy.

**Table 8.1** (*cont.*)

| Name of medical center or institution<br>Manual |
| --- |

\* Clinical practice guidelines can be viewed as standards to be considered in an attempt to individualize treatment for each patient. The ultimate judgment regarding the care of a particular patient must be made by the physician in light of all of the circumstances that are relevant to that patient.

4. **Directives** – an interim instruction that is issued based upon an urgent or emergent operational matter that must be known immediately for implementation. Directives can only remain posted for up to 90 days and must either be incorporated into a PPG or eliminated.

5. **Sponsor** – every PPGD must be sponsored by a Vice President or Department Chair. Any revisions to PPGD shall be approved by the appropriate committee and/or Vice President. Any proposed revision to the Institutions Policy Manual must be submitted to the PSA office by its sponsor.

6. **Author/owner** – every PPGD must have an identified author and owner of the content of the policy. This may be an individual, a committee or workgroup, specifically, identified as the author/owner by the sponsoring Vice President or Chief. The **author/owner** will be identified and develop the new draft or revision to an existing PPGD in the required PPGD format (if possible), The author/owner initially ensures that the content is in compliance with all regulatory and accreditation standards (e.g. The Joint Commission, DPH, OSHA, etc.) consulting the panel of identified content experts as necessary.

7. **Content experts** – all departments are available to consult on PPGD content as appropriate. (Refer to Attachment F).

8. **Content management system** (CMS) – CMS provides the format, linking, key word searching and historical tracking for all PPGD placed on the web. Each department will assign a staff person to be trained to use CMS. This person will be responsible to maintain the "manual" on the web under the direction of their departmental designated person/committee chair/VP/chief.

9. **PPGD format** (if possible), includes:
   a. **Title** – concisely describes the scope of the PPGD
   b. **Purpose** – succinctly describes the goal(s) that the policy addresses
   c. **Numbering system** assigned for the document (usually alpha-numeric; max of 3 alpha description and 4 numeric)
   d. **Policy statement** – provides a summary description of the intentions of the PPGD
   e. **Content formatting** – numbering sequence should follow a capital alpha/number/small alpha/italicized number format (e.g., A-1-a-i.) A sample of the policy format that can be copied is included as Attachment B
   f. **Attachments of forms** that are related to the PPGD will be identified by its form number. All medical record electronic or paper forms related to the PPGD should be approved by the forms committee prior to PPGD approval (see ADM-06).

Attachment A: minimum requirements for department ppgd manual (single department only)
Attachment B: policy and approval sections hospital-wide/interdepartmental template (title and approval sections)
Attachment C: intradepartmental template (approval section)
Attachment D: clinical practice guideline template
Attachment E: PPGD tracking summary form
Attachment F: resources for content expertise
Attachment G: development and approval flow for policies, procedures, guidelines and directives
Vice president sponsor: name, title of vice president sponsor
Requestor: name and title of person and department requesting this policy
Approved by:
☐ Committee or council: date
Original date approved:
Revisions: dates of all revisions
Next review date:

The body of the policy has a critical function to clearly establish standard practice. This may be based on clinical practice, research standards, federal requirements, or other standards. If the policy is department-based, it needs to be approved by that department's leadership. When a policy crosses to other departments, it needs a larger group to approve it, as it involves other parties. Medical center-wide policies

**Table 8.2** Sample template for policies and procedures (Source: Beth Israel Deaconess Medical Center)

| |
|---|
| **Institution name**<br>**Clinical practice guideline – (service area)** |
| **Title:**<br>Number (grouping-section # categorized by department/service area. e.g., CC, ED, GenMed):<br>Purpose: |
| **Guideline introduction statement/rationale:**<br>The ultimate judgment regarding the care of a particular patient must be made by the physician in light of all of the circumstances that are relevant to that patient. These practice guidelines can be viewed as standards to be considered for each patient in an attempt to individualize treatment for each patient.<br>Key parameters<br>Outcome metrics/effectiveness measures<br>References:<br>Related forms/attachments: (process flowchart/algorithms/decision tree, etc. . .)<br>Author/owner/chair name:      Title:<br>**Approved by**:<br>Chief: _____ Date: _____<br>Clinical department head: _____ Date: _____<br>Clinical division head: _____ Date: _____ |
| **Approved by:**<br>☐ Operations council/date: _____<br>Chief operating officer<br>☐ Medical executive committee/date: _____<br>Chairman, MEC<br>And if applicable:<br>☐ Board of directors/date: _____<br>Chair |
| **Origination/review**<br>Original date approved:<br>Revisions (dates):<br>Next review date:<br>Eliminated (date):<br>Reference (including all forms approved by forms committee – see ADM-06): |

are typically required by regulatory or accrediting authorities and impact many departments. Defining the scope of the impacted audience initially will ensure that the correct people are involved in building, implementing, and evaluating the success of the policy to support the work from the initial stage.[8]

## Approval process for policies and procedures

Organizations use different methods to track policy review and updates. It is also important to track the audiences who have been informed of a new policy, changes to a policy, or retiring a policy. There are many different styles and formats, but the essential components remain the same.

The "owners" of the policy have the obligation for reviewing, updating, and disseminating the information to the appropriate people in the department.

The owner may be determined by the department or, if cross-departmental, by a higher governing board.[9]

For new policies and procedures, it is imperative that the leader of the development of the policy or procedure considers the input of all parties who will be impacted, at the beginning of development, to ensure all aspects are considered. Once the policy or procedure is drafted, it will require those impacted to approve it, and, if necessary, perhaps a higher governing committee if teams cannot reach a desirable outcome.

The highest governance board in an organization typically defines the level of policy or procedure approval, both at the department level and across departments.[3] This board, often referred to as the medical executive committee (MEC), is made up of all senior hospital administrators as well as physician chiefs of service.[9]

**Table 8.3** Policy, procedure, guideline, and directive (PPGD) tracking summary form (Source: Beth Israel Deaconess Medical Center)

| 1. PPGD | | | |
|---|---|---|---|
| | Author/owner: | | Date: |
| 2. Purpose of request | ☐ Triennial/annual review – no significant changes<br>☐ New policy | | ☐ Triennial/annual review – significant changes (list below)<br>☐ Other (needed because of change to policy that could not wait until triennial/annual review) |
| 3. If new policy, rationale (why it is needed – by regulation, etc.) | | | |
| 4. If revision, highlight changes from old to new | | | |
| 5. List of reviewers and provide names | List reviewers (in order of approval)<br>Senior VP<br>Chiefs/VPs<br>Key context expert input (as per ADM-01 attachment F)<br>Committee(s) approval<br>Forms committee approval (for all forms – see ADM-06) | Complete<br><br>☐<br>☐<br>☐<br><br>☐<br>☐ | Date approved |
| 6. Process of disseminating information (ID posting, mailings, online) | Check off all that are applicable:<br>☐ HR newsletter/leadership/monthly PPGD Update<br>☐ Email to be sent out to applicable staff<br>☐ Other: | | |
| 7. Training and implementation | Responsible dept/ person for training and implementation: | | How will training be implemented?<br>☐ Training module (web portal or other site – list:<br>☐ Live session (at departmental or other meeting)<br>☐ Other (please list below): |
| 8. Request for committee approval | | | |

For review of policies and procedures that have been approved and are up for re-approval, the owner should review the entire content to ensure it is current and meets standards of care. The timing of review is determined by the organization, but typically department polices are reviewed annually, and organizational policies every three years.[10] Again, this is determined by the organization and should be consistent across all departments. A tracking tool for policies can be found in Table 8.3.

## Implementation of policies and procedures

Just as important as how the policies and procedures are written is how they are implemented within your department or organization. The best-written policy or procedure is of no use if physicians and nurses are not educated and are not able to demonstrate understanding of the content. As mentioned, this is how many regulatory agencies are now verifying organizational structure – by speaking with staff and asking them about specific policies.[3]

Faculty and staff meetings are commonly used to disseminate policy and procedure information. This is often an interactive meeting in which there can be discussion, time for questions, and feedback. Many organizations keep a staff attendance list to verify real-time education; other organizations may use email or online modules to verify participation in the roll-out of a policy or procedure.[10]

Department experts on the content of a policy or procedure are a benefit to frontline physicians and nurses. This provides physicians and nurses with a contact person with whom to discuss a specific case or event and learn how best to apply the departmental policy or procedure. In some instances, this may lead the department expert to make changes to a policy or procedure or provide clarification.[6]

As a leader in the department, it is important to understand the process in place for education of all physicians and staff on policies and procedures. Records of staff meetings, email communications, or compliance logs may serve as a method of "proof" of roll-out and may serve well in assessing the success of a policy or procedure.[10] If you find that the roll-out was not inclusive of those making errors, leaders will need to re-educate clinicians. This is also an opportunity to look at the process in your department for the purposes of education and information sharing.

## The role of the emergency department leader

The leadership of the ED is responsible for building, implementing, sustaining, and evaluating clinical pathways, operational structures, and systems to support patient care. Often ED leaders are called upon to make administrative and organizational decisions related to policy and procedure that can directly impact the care of patients as well as the affiliated organization.[11] The direct role that leaders have in policy approval and in requesting new policies is important in building the foundation for operations and clinical practice.

This aspect of leadership regarding policies and procedures requires knowledge of the delivery of care and adherence to regulatory standards. With physicians and nurses, there is a clinical expertise that develops through education, training, and practice.[4] Equally important in leadership is the role of ensuring that all clinicians are meeting regulatory standards, as well as ensuring that the department is aligned with the mission of the organization.

## Meeting regulatory standards

Survey visits by government and regulatory agencies often produce a list of items to improve, correct, or audit. Many of the standards against which healthcare organizations are measured are now assessed by talking with staff to see if they have the knowledge they need to do their jobs.[3] Years ago, what was written was often sufficient. Today, leaders need to ensure that policies and procedures are introduced to staff, that education related to policies occurs, and that frontline physicians and nurses clearly understand not only what they are supposed to do in specific situations, but also where to find relevant policies and procedures.

The Joint Commission is one example of an accrediting body that seeks to standardize, measure, and evaluate patient safety standards for hospitals, long-term care, ambulatory clinics, and other healthcare operations. This organization dates back to 1910, and it has evolved from a vehicle for data collection to one for setting patient safety goals and standards for organizations to achieve.[6]

When an organization is audited by a regulatory body, it is a time for the leadership as well as frontline staff and physicians to showcase the work they do to provide excellent patient care. There are standards to meet as well as interviews to pass. A regulatory visit may involve interviewing employees or physicians, reviewing medical records for documentation standards, inspecting work sites, and interviewing patients.[8]

Tracing patients through different care sites has become a very helpful method to evaluate processes in place to ensure smooth transitions. In the United States, this focus has evolved into the development of the National Patient Safety Goals.[6] During a patient tracing visit, a patient or family member may be interviewed to check the work of the organization. Observation of work is also an essential component of the survey visit that surveyors use to establish whether the written policies or procedures are in place and match clinical practice.

---

**Case study 8.1. Alignment of policy and practice**

One academic medical center instituted a policy for the waiting room of the ED, which stated that every 30 minutes a member of the support or technician staff should re-evaluate patients in the waiting room. The goal of this re-evaluation was to ensure that the vital signs and initial chief complaint had not changed, and to check on any new needs the patient may have. Shortly after initiating this process, the Joint Commission visit for this medical center started. During the two-week visit by the regulatory body, the waiting room was observed by the surveyor. Aware of the policy the department had drafted and approved, there was interest in the actual process of waiting room surveillance. Upon review, the surveyors witnessed patients in the waiting room who were not checked after 40 minutes, falling outside of the policy standards the department had set in place. All of the patients checked had no clinical changes in their presentation or needs. However, the policy as written was not being adhered to, based on the standard set by the department.

This is an example of setting a standard that cannot be met at all hours of the day and on all days of the week. Practice does not reflect the policy – a red flag for surveyors. On the day of the survey, the ED was saturated with volume and acuity. The ED personnel were working diligently to see all patients and look after all needs. There was no governing body that stated this policy needed to exist; it had been set by the leadership of the department as a standard they wanted to achieve.

# Evaluation and review of policies and procedures

Annually, leaders of departments will review their active policies to ensure that they are applicable, that they reflect practice, and that they are clearly understood by staff.[9] Developing a process to review policies and procedures as a leadership team on an annual basis can serve your department and hospital organization very well.

Policies or procedures that cross departmental lines should be brought to the appropriate committees to ensure all providers are updated on changes or refreshed with the information. At the end of the written document, list all committees that approved the policy, to show collaboration, ownership, and cross-implementation.[12]

Administrative assistants are very helpful in the organization of a schedule covering which polices are ready for review. Depending on the policy, there may be no changes or large changes. In addition, it is always best to first ask your review team, "Do we need this policy?" Over time, a range of policies may be created for good reasons. However, the annual review is an opportunity to merge policies, update policies, or simply cancel a policy that is no longer helpful or applicable to a departmental practice or operation.[12]

# Measuring success
## Quality assurance

Once a policy or procedure is implemented in an organization, it is imperative to have a sound process to ensure the clinicians are meeting the standards of care and following the protocols in place. There are many strategies by which to ensure this process is carried out both locally in the department and on a larger scale within the organization.

At a departmental level, there should be a formalized process whereby a committee meets regularly to review cases that may potentially deviate from the accepted standard of care, or in which systems, judgment, or operations impacted care or decision making by the providers.[13] Committee members should include the clinical leaders in the department representing the residents, attending physicians, and nursing. As the case is reviewed, copies of the patient record are analyzed to determine if there were any opportunities to improve.

During these discussions, it is common to hear some clinical discussions regarding standards of care or new studies cited in medical journals. It is also a time to discuss whether a policy or procedure would benefit from being updated, to standardize therapies or operations according to the current literature. If this has already been done, the opportunity to measure compliance presents.[14]

For larger organizational implications, others may be involved. For example, if the record being reviewed is of a neurosurgery patient, it may be presented to the neurosurgery quality assurance committee in addition to the ED quality assurance committee. For any unresolved follow-up, or for cases that did not meet the standard of care or failed to follow policies or procedures, the case may move forward to the institutional quality committee, consisting of leaders from all departments.

A more extensive discussion of quality assurance is found in Chapter 7.

---

**Case study 8.2. ED overcrowding**

Prior to 2009, emergency departments in the state of Massachusetts in the USA could request that the central ambulance dispatch center divert ambulances transporting new patients to the ED away from their facility if they felt that they were overcrowded. Healthcare policy makers had long felt

---

that this practice simply shifted the problem of overcrowding from one institution to another, and ambulance diversion was banned in 2009. The State Department of Public Health issued a mandate that all medical centers needed to develop an internal system for triggering a desired resource reallocation to decompress the ED. Medical centers in this state would no longer be able to go on diversion, unless there was an internal disaster that would shut down all internal medical services. Over the course of the year prior to implementation, departmental and institutional leaders within all of the affected hospitals met to determine how they would address the criteria and time frames outlined by the state.

A successfully written and implemented policy would be evident in the response to overcrowding in ED. Criteria were set not only regarding the expected turnaround time to move patients out of the overcrowded ED, but also establishing set expectations of the roles of different services. Table 8.4 shows an example of a "Code Help" policy and the response required, and Table 8.5 the department-specific roles.

This is an example of an organizational policy that resulted from a mandate by a regulatory body. It was a multidisciplinary and complex process. Leaders of the organization gathered key leaders from all departments to begin to draft a plan. After multiple drafts, tests, and evaluations, this plan was approved. The educational plan was rolled out to all frontline staff and physicians expected to take part in the process. The organization expects that when the regulatory body visits in the coming years, staff will be able to speak to the policy as well as demonstrate it in their practice.

## Leadership responsibility

Part of your role is to ensure the clinicians in your areas are following standards of care, clinical practice guidelines, and organizational policies. Auditing records to track compliance with regulatory standards is one method many organizations have used.[14] For teaching purposes, clinical case reviews offer opportunities to teach physicians-in-training or new nurses information that will assist them as they gain more clinical experience.

During any type of case review, leaders should think about the impact of the case on the department. Are there steps that could be taken to ensure that the potential for error is decreased? Would another similar physician come to similar conclusions in this particular case? Is there any opportunity to standardize practice through a policy or a guideline that will help ensure consistency in patient care? In addition to reviewing the individual case, leaders should also audit a sample of other similar cases in order to understand the scope of practice across the department.

## Conclusion

Policies and procedures play an intricate role in the foundations of care and standards of operations at a departmental as well as an organizational level. Differentiating between what is a policy and what is a procedure is the first important step. Every decision, from writing to implementation, requires leaders' attention to ensure that frontline physicians and nurses have the tools they need to make decisions in real time and operate within the accepted scope of practice while providing excellent patient care.

Assessment and reassessment of policies and procedures at departmental and organizational levels creates a foundation for care and a platform for informed judgment. As leaders, it is our job to look at our quality and safety programs and learn from the benefits of standardization.

Education of our frontline physicians and nurses will demonstrate the importance of clinical and operational consistency. Patients will have better outcomes and departments will run more smoothly. Leaders set the standard and motivate staff to work towards a more efficient system and higher quality of care. The influence of the partnership between physicians and nurses can make a positive difference in organizations. Through this partnership, we can build more efficient systems, continually improve patient-focused care models, and reflect this work in the formation of working policies and procedures that build excellence.

## Leadership tips

- Involve frontline staff in policy development, implementation, and evaluation.
- Develop a process for ongoing evaluation of policies and, as part of this process, ask the question "Do we need this policy?"
- Policies should be re-evaluated on a regular basis, and the dates for when it was written, approved, re-approved, and due for review should be tracked.
- Differentiate between a policy and a guideline. If the leaders are confused, the staff will be confused.

**Table 8.4** Example "Code Help" policy and the responses required (Source: Beth Israel Deaconess Medical Center)

| Medical center name |
|---|
| Policy manual |

**Title: "Code Help" – Emergency Department (ED) Saturation/Gridlock Response Plan**
Policy #: ADM-16
**Purpose**: To outline protocols for [medical center name inserted here] in responding as an institution to emergency department (ED) saturation.

**Policy statement/goals**

Surges in patient volume have been demonstrated to result in the boarding of patients in the ED, which in turn may limit the ED's capability and/or capacity to ensure ED patient care in an appropriate, effective, and safe environment. ED boarding of patients has been linked to increased adverse patient outcomes when compared to the boarding of patients in alternative inpatient treatment areas.

The Code Help plan is a three-tier response to optimize patient flow throughout the hospital and to address ED crowding. The main purpose of the policy is to re-deploy staff and resources within the medical center with the goal of expediting movement of all admitted patients out of the ED, in order to continue to provide the highest level of care to patients entering the medical center. This response is to be done in stages, when criteria for levels of ED saturation have been met.

**The goal of the Code Help plan**

- To respond to ED crowding and allow the ED to provide timely, appropriate care to the remaining patients in the department and to the patients presenting to the department
- To distribute throughout the medical center the burden of increasing volume so as to not overly strain a single unit or department

  - The movement of all admitted patient out of the ED to hallways in other departments will be the key method for immediate ED decompression
  - The goal of the Code Help activation is to move the patients from the ED within 30 minutes of activation
- To prevent adverse patient outcomes as a result of ED overcrowding

**Authority for activation**

- Initial activation for the plan will begin with the ED resource nurse and ED core attending, who will be alerted of triggers through the ED dashboard and send an automated page.
- If situation escalates to a Code Triage level, the administrator on call (AOC) will activate the emergency operations plan.

**Procedure(s) for activation**

- Guidelines for action should be followed when staffing and bed-space indicators approach or exceed specified levels. The three-tiered levels refer to degrees of saturation as defined by this institution (see Appendix A).
- The staffing, patient volume, and space indicators are the triggers for the level of response needed by the institution and include:

  i) no inpatient option exists
  ii) there is a lack of physical capacity and sufficient staffing available to provide care consistent with DPH, CMS, and Joint Commission standards
  iii) continuing to provide care to boarding patients interferes with the ability to provide timely, appropriate care to other ED patients

**Escalation to code triage (emergency operation plan activation)**

- If the activation of Code Help fails to relieve the burden *of admitted patients* on the emergency department after 2 hours or if the severity of the initial situation warrants, than the hospital's emergency operations plan (Code Triage) will be activated.

**Evaluation**

- After the Code Help plan has been activated it will be the responsibility of Patient Care Services (PCS) to review the event and elicit immediate feedback from areas and submit an after action report to approving committees. Each area involved should submit comments and feedback to PCS to apply continuous improvements.
- In the event this Code Help plan has not been activated in over 6 months the Emergency Management Program will coordinate a drill and after action process to encompass the scope of the policy.

**Table 8.4** (cont.)

| Medical center name Policy manual |
|---|

### Appendix A: Code Help levels
Vice President sponsor:
Approved by:
Medical executive committee:     Date
Requestor name:
Senior Vice President, PCS
Chairman, Emergency Medicine
Director, ED
Emergency management
Senior VP, Health Care Quality
Original date approved: 4/03
Next review date: 3/1/14
Revised: 8/03, 4/04, 6/05, 1/09, 10/10, 2/11
References:

### Definitions

| | |
|---|---|
| ED boarder | A boarder is a patient who remains in the ED > 2 hours after decision for admission is made. |
| Hallway bed | Temporary assessment of appropriate patients and/or as a temporary (< 2 hours) location for admitted patients transitioning to an inpatient unit. |
| Code help alert | A Code Help alert will be declared at any point when there is a ongoing burden on the emergency department. This is to include 10 or more patients in boarder status or a waiting room volume of 20 or more patients for over 2 hours or 54 or more patients in the evaluation stage of care in the ED for over 2 hours. |
| Code help activation | Code help will be declared at any point when there is a ongoing lack of inpatient capacity resulting in ED crowding. If the ED has 54 or more for 2 consecutive hours patients in the department and there are 10 or more patients in boarder status. |
| Code triage | A Code Help will be escalated to a code triage if after 2 hours Code Help activation fails to relieve the burden of admitted patients in the emergency department. |

**Table 8.5** Example of department-specific roles in a "Code Help" situation (Source: Beth Israel Deaconess Medical Center)

| Code Help level | Alert | Activation | Triage |
|---|---|---|---|
| ED triggers TBD | Any one of the following: 10 or more ED boarders or 20 or more patients in the ED waiting for 2 consecutive hours or 54 or more patients in the ED for over 2 hours | Activation will occur when there are: 10 or more ED boarders and 54 or more patients in the ED for 2 consecutive hours | A Code Triage will be declared if after 2 hours of activation status there remains an admitted patient burden on the emergency department |
| Communication | Director of throughput establishes bridge line within 45 minutes for initial meeting Email to all groups for situation report Hospital AOC alerted by Bed Facilitator | Email auto sent to all chiefs Page to chief medicine, surgery, ED regarding current status Open command center with key positions by decision of the IC | Open command center to coordinate operations |

**Table 8.5** (*cont.*)

| Code Help level | Alert | Activation | Triage |
|---|---|---|---|
| Admission facilitator | Prepares level 1 and 2 bed counts<br>At end of call reviews immediate next actions with plan to update in 2 h | All transfer through AF<br>Consult director of periop for review of OR case schedule<br>Hold transfers, elective cases<br>Consider alternative care settings (PACU etc.)<br>Utilize hallway spaces on inpatient 2 above on each floor (14 floors × 2 hall beds)<br>Notify case management to advance discharge time frame<br>Identify surge area for patient holding | Assume ICS role<br>Report to command center |
| Administrative clinical supervisors (west) | Reports to ED and rounds with resource to identify resource needs and facilities reallocation of staff to support the ED<br>Prepare to report out any concerns with impatient concerns/ staffing<br>Acts as liaison with floors to facilitate patients arriving when bed vacant<br>Directs floors to accept report on bed assignments regardless status of bed<br>Works with inpatient floors and communicates new vacant beds to ED resource<br>Communicates with East ACS for situational reports and resource needs | Works with AF and ED resource to identify ED patients that are hall appropriate<br>Communication to floor resource nurse to plan for patients to be sent to floors | Assume role in ICS as directed by Incident command |
| ED resource nurse | Prepares report on current departmental status and resource needs | Open dialogue with ACS/AF regarding ED status and resource needs<br>Fan-out list activated for staffing of unit over operational period | Assume ICS role and coordinates care of patients in the emergency department |
| ED RN AOC | Notification to hospital AOC for Code Help alert<br>Provide leadership support<br>Makes staffing operational decisions | | |
| ED MD AOC | Provide leadership support<br>Makes decision on transfers | Notified by ED core attending and will provide leadership | |
| Core attending | Report out on any known dispositions of patients to admit/ tele/ICU/obs<br>May choose after discussion with 33450 to forward all transfer request to the AF | All incoming transfers directed to AF | |
| Director of throughput | Assumes HICS role as designated<br>Alerts Case Management and medical leadership of capacity demands? | Contact director of case management to facilitate inpatient discharges (i.e. arrange patient transportation and work with sub- | Report to command center<br>Assume ICS role |

**Table 8.5** (cont.)

| Code Help level | Alert | Activation | Triage |
|---|---|---|---|
| Emergency management | Prepare to open command center<br>Assist with coordination of activities<br>Collect and document sit stat | acute facilities to create capacity for med/surg discharges<br>Contact Directors of Periop and Procedural Areas for alternative care settings<br>Consider elective Case Cancellations<br>Potential to activate command center<br>Coordinates conference call or meeting for key stake holders<br>Work on alternate care site<br>Activate planning section and activities | |
| Director of inpatient quality | Assists with assessment of planned / potential patient admissions and discharges<br>Contacts administrative hospitalist on call, medical directors as needed | Communicate with cobth reps coordinates with throughput director, incident commander (if command center activated), and aforementioned staff to deploy available contingencies in order to prevent Code Triage<br>Monitors safe hand-off of ED boarders to inpatient surge space. | |
| Transport supervisor | Prioritize ED admissions through call system<br>Additional stretchers brought to CC1 hold area tbd<br>Transport supervisor will report to ED | Code Help would supersede all Transport calls from call system. Transporters would be moved from East Campus to West Campus. | Transport supervisor would be in communication with incident commander to prioritized patient transports. |
| Material management manager on call | Ensure adequate supply of necessary equipment i.e. pumps<br>Responds to requests for additional items<br>Notifies ACS or command center of any potential supply issues | | Assume ICS role |
| Dietary manager | Call to ED resource tech to asses patient needs and adjust par stock for next 12 hours of needs | | Assume ICS role |
| EVS supervisor | Works with AF to prioritize work to beds with planned ED admissions<br>Report to Admitting<br>EVS staff in non-patient areas would be utilized to assist in Discharge Cleaning on patient floors. EVS Staff would identify location of all available beds for quick retrieval | EVS supervisor would be in communication with incident commander to prioritized discharges | EVS supervisor would be in communication with incident commander to prioritized discharges |
| Patient relations | Reports to ED and rounds through the department to speak with patients and families about current hospital status<br>Access to food/parking vouchers for patients and family members<br>If after hours or weekend hospital ACS will be available to the ED and is encouraged to round in the department | | |
| Inpatient floors | Activate fan-out list to determine ETA for additional staff | Activate staff from fan-out list | |

**Table 8.5** (cont.)

| Code Help level | Alert | Activation | Triage |
|---|---|---|---|
| | Communicate staffing status to staffing office<br>Make EVS aware of alert status for bed cleaning<br>Facilitate transport of patient from ED while assigned bed is being cleaned | Assess blocked beds on floor cohort as appropriate<br>NM/resource nurse will review all discharges with case management (during hours)<br>Identify appropriate patient in rooms that may be moved to hall<br>Refer to unit Code Help activation plan | |
| Specialty Care Sites Cath lab, Radiology Care unit, GI, WPC | Review planned admissions with af<br>Review current staffing for potential extended service hours | | |
| Nursing Directors | Receive notification and relays information to responsible areas to ensure all staff aware of current incident and to redeploy resources to facilitate d/c and admissions | Report to situation status to command center | Assume role in HICS structure |
| Medicine Directors | Expedite discharges / review potential admissions / transfers<br>Work with PCS to prepare for possible surge capacity space utilization | Review potential admissions and transfers for possible delay decision<br>Recruit Supplementary staff to expedite inpatient discharges and admissions<br>Work with PCS for managing patients in surge space (hallways) | Assume role in HICS structure |
| Case management | Director of CM and CM managers will receive Code Help page alert<br>Communicate Code Help to case management team<br>Director to ED and rounds with ED case manager to identify patients who can be discharged to alternative care settings (home with services, ECF, other facility)<br>Prepare to report out all definite patient discharges per nursing unit and pending discharges, to include barriers to discharge<br>Prepare to classify patients by unit using census:<br>Cannot discharge<br>OK to DC to ECF<br>Home with/without services)<br>Prepare for early discharges<br>Work with AF on all transfer requests, as necessary | Director of CM and CM Managers will receive Code Help Activation page<br>CM will review classification of patient disposition for all patients with NM/Resource Nurse (during hours)<br>Report definite discharges, expected time of discharges to command center (use classification system)<br>Report patients clinically ready with pending / actionable needs for discharge<br>Work with director of throughput, nursing, clinical teams to overcome barriers to discharge<br>Reach out to families/caregivers to facilitate discharges<br>Staff for extended hours coverage<br>Use taxi vouchers, chair car, ambulance (as necessary) for discharge transportation | Director of CM assumes role in command center in reporting all patient disposition classification.<br>Facilitation disposition classifications 2 & 3.<br>Staffing for extended CM hours<br>Use taxi vouchers, chair car, ambulance (as necessary) for discharge transportation |

**Table 8.5** (*cont.*)

| Code Help level | Alert | Activation | Triage |
|---|---|---|---|
| | Ensure taxi vouchers are available to all CMs<br>Prepare to extend CM staffing hours<br>Determine alternative care provider capacity (homecare, ECFs) (DCP Assistants)<br>Alert HC and ECF liaisons to be onsite for expedition of referrals and screens | | |
| Public safety | First officer on scene would contact police supervisor or designee. Supervisor would evaluate situation and make contact with command staff. | Try and restrict access to building and monitor situation.<br>Restrict outside traffic flow in the area.<br>Officer to respond to command center. | Assume ICS role<br>Work with the command center for any resource needs |
| Lab | Awareness to staff and lab mangers of situation | Work with command center to identify resource needs | Follow EOP |
| Radiology | Work with ED resource to prioritize studies | | |

# References

1. Howard PK, Steinmann RA, eds. *Emergency Nursing Principles and Practice*, 6th edn. St, Louis, MO: Mosby, 2010.

2. Paige JB. Solve the policy and procedure puzzle: bring together numerous departments to create one inclusive patient care model. *Nursing Management* 2003; **34** (3): 45–8.

3. Schyve PM. *Leadership in Healthcare Organizations: a Guide to Joint Commission Leadership Standards*. San Diego, CA: Governance Institute, 2009.

4. Hudson K. Policy and procedure management: a job that's never done. *Nursing Management* 2006; **37** (6): 34–8.

5. Kotter JP. What leaders really do. *Harvard Business Review* 1990; **68** (3): 103–11.

6. The Joint Commission. *History of the Joint Commission*. http://www.jointcommission.org/about_us/history.aspx (accessed January 2014).

7. Hudson K. From research to practice on the Magnet pathway. *Nursing Management* 2005: **36** (3): 33–7.

8. McLaughlin C, Kaluzny A. *Continuous Quality Improvement in Health Care: Theory, Implementation, and Applications*. Gaithersburg, MD: Aspen, 1999.

9. Institute of Medicine of the National Academies. *Advising the Nation / Improving Health*. Washington, DC: IOM, 2010.

10. Zavotsky KE. Developing an ED training program: how to "grow your own" ED nurses. *Journal of Emergency Nursing* 2000; **26**: 504–6.

11. Grimm JW. Effective leadership: making the difference. *Journal of Emergency Nursing* 2010; **36** (1): 74–7.

12. The Joint Commission. *Statement of Conditions: Compliance Document*, 2004. http://www.jointcommission.org/assets/1/18/0504_SOC.pdf (accessed January 2014).

13. Joint Commission on Accreditation of Healthcare Organizations. Appendix C in Performance Measurement report 1–15, 1998.

14. Graham N. *Quality Assurance in Hospitals*. Gaithersburg, MD: Aspen, 1990.

Chapter

# 9

# A framework for optimal emergency department risk management and patient safety

Carrie Tibbles and Jock Hoffman

## Key learning points

- Reducing the chances of a patient being injured in conjunction with an emergency department encounter is reliant upon the proper assignment of duties, the appropriate collection and analysis of data, and the informed development and implementation of interventions.
- Before implementing specific interventions to reduce the risk of patient injury, leaders need to determine if their emergency department's overall culture of risk and safety is capable of designing, adopting, and sustaining such efforts.
- Emergency departments that emphasize the importance of clear and effective communication have in place the most important component of risk management and patient safety.
- When a serious adverse event occurs, sincere sympathy and compassion expressed to the patient and/or family is often the most important response to help defuse a potentially volatile situation.

## Introduction

The single most important component of comprehensive risk management and patient safety in the emergency department (ED) is, quite simply, to practice and document good medicine.[1] Unfortunately, of course, medical errors do occur in the ED (as in other settings), and some lead to preventable injuries to patients. Effective management of

ED patient safety – reducing the risk of harm to patients during the course of examination, diagnosis, and treatment – is reliant upon several important factors (especially rapport, familiarity, and continuity) that are difficult to provide in an emergency care setting.

Improving patient safety and reducing adverse events in the ED can be challenging for a number of reasons. ED patients are typically treated by physicians and nurses who were not involved in their prior care and, most likely, will not be involved in their future care. These patients present with undifferentiated symptoms and may not be able to provide a comprehensive history. Time and production pressures force clinicians to perform patient assessments rapidly, often with incomplete information. The clinician is evaluating the patient at a moment in time when the underlying diagnosis may not yet be apparent. In the busy, unpredictable environment of the ED, communication between providers is often truncated, and physicians and nurses caring for the patient may have limited information available to them.

The most common medical error for ED patients is a missed or delayed diagnosis: being discharged without a completed workup, or with a diagnosis that misinterpreted symptoms, test results, or comorbidities.[2,3] Less common, but also troublesome, are injuries to ED patients caused during procedures performed in the ED, and by mismanagement of medication.[2]

Given the high-risk environment, ED leadership is challenged to understand not only the general risks inherent in emergency medicine, but also the particular patient safety challenges in the local setting. This chapter outlines the basic components of a risk

*Emergency Department Leadership and Management*, ed. Stephanie Kayden, *et al.* Published by Cambridge University Press.
© Cambridge University Press 2015.

management strategy, as well as some of the particular areas of vulnerability in emergency medicine.

## Optimizing an ED risk management and patient safety program

Effective ED risk management and proactive patient safety improvement depend upon a structure that facilitates both risk assessment and risk reduction. The proper assignment of duties, the appropriate collection and analysis of data, and the informed development and implementation of interventions are the foundation for reducing the chances of a patient being injured during an ED encounter.

### Responsibility

While the safety of ED patients is, essentially, everyone's responsibility, the responsibility for the department's risk management/patient safety program has to be clear to all staff (clinical and non-clinical) and, most importantly, to the individual expected to lead that effort. If the responsibility for risk management/patient safety is assigned informally, or listed at the bottom of someone's job description, then the program will lack the authority and respect necessary to effect change and fix problems.

Putting the risk management/patient safety responsibility in the hands of a clinician (or a team of clinicians) conveys the message that this is not simply an administrative function, that patient safety is a part of caring for patients. If the risk management/patient safety responsibility is assigned to a non-clinician, then having one or more clinical champions on board is essential. Whoever is responsible for risk management/patient safety in the ED, it is important that he or she is aligned with peers in other departments, or other EDs, and has the opportunity to share skills and experiences. Because he or she must address adverse events, errors, and potential hazards, the role of a risk management/patient safety officer can be isolating. The absence of peer support will exacerbate that isolation.

### Assessment

The starting point for an effective risk management/patient safety program should *not* be the last adverse event or the disgruntled patient/family in the ED this morning. Rather, existing and potential hazards should be assessed continuously through a variety of tactics, including executive walk-rounds, focus groups, third-party observation, and a thorough examination of indicator data.[4] Leadership should involve staff in identifying hazards and safety concerns.

### Data and reporting

ED leadership should establish a system to routinely review clinical care and important patient safety indicators to identify areas for improvement. Additionally, ED leaders need a reporting system for calling out adverse events/hazards and an environment that does not blame the individual who reported the error. Reporting should be encouraged and supported, or else staff will be reluctant to participate. When physicians and nurses see some evidence that the safety or risk-related information they report is put to good use, they then are motivated to continue or increase their participation as reporters.

Some data, such as adverse event reports, patient complaints, root cause analyses, and malpractice claims, provide direct insight to patient safety risks.[4] Other data, such as unexpected returns to the ED or patient satisfaction, will need to be examined to tease out indicators or trends that signal recurring or potential risk. A process for aligning and assessing data from a variety of sources – rather than each in isolation – will help direct the risk management/patient safety program to the most prominent areas in need of further investigation.

Contemporaneous reporting of adverse events is an essential source of data needed to understand the errors and potential risks impacting ED patients. It is important to have systems in place that enable ED clinicians and administrators to file reports which accentuate *what* happened over *who* was to blame. In addition to capturing the narrative of an adverse event or near miss, effective reporting systems provide required fields for entering information that helps analysts pinpoint both clinical and non-clinical factors.

### Investigation and analysis

Both individual events and aggregated data that raise serious concerns about ED patient safety necessitate further investigation before anyone begins to take action or institutes changes to procedures or protocols (except, of course, clear and present risks such as malfunctioning equipment, impaired caregivers, or undertrained staff assigned beyond their capabilities). Acting too quickly on preliminary data analyses or individual events or anecdotes may do more harm than good if the implemented changes are addressing a problem that no longer exists (or has already been resolved) or inadvertently create alternate hazards. A structured and in-depth investigation enables ED leaders to examine the root causes of adverse events and serves to confirm data analyses (for example, by cross-matching against a second or third data source). As with every stage in the process of understanding the current and potential risks to patient safety, taking the time to discuss findings, assumptions, and hypotheses with the physicians, nurses, and other ED staff working in this environment ensures that you have identified relevant problems to be addressed.

## Prioritization and resources

Determining where to focus finite risk management and patient safety resources – that is, which risks or hazards to tackle first – can be complicated by competing interests. Certainly, the problems that pose a significant risk and can be easily corrected deserve immediate attention. Leaders also need to determine if their ED is in need of broad interventions that supersede individual areas of risk. Does the department's culture of risk and safety need to be addressed before introducing any specific interventions? If so, then part of that process of culture adjustment may be to engage the entire ED staff in the task of setting risk management/patient safety goals and allocating remedial resources.[5] Let the data determine the appropriate blueprint to build a portfolio of interventions necessary to mitigate risk and improve patient safety. Early gains may prove helpful in building momentum and a positive ED culture change.

## Intervention and measurement

Organizations with a commitment to reducing risks to ED patients employ solid risk assessment and programmatic confirmation, based on well-designed reporting and data collection systems enriched by thoughtful analysis, investigation, and prioritization *before* introducing change. But if the changes that are introduced are misguided, unacceptable to the ED staff, or mismatched to the specific problem perceived to need attention, little will improve. In fact, botched attempts to implement patient safety improvements can undermine an otherwise well-designed and well-managed risk management/patient safety program.

The effectiveness of interventions implemented to reduce risks for ED patients ought to be measured, and that measurement ought to begin even before the interventions are introduced. An assessment that captures a snapshot of the key metrics for each targeted risk prior to implementation provides a benchmark for assessments done periodically after implementation. Without adequate metrics or credible benchmark data, assessing the value of any given intervention is essentially guesswork based on the staff's or leadership's intuition as to whether the intervention made a difference. While such input is valuable, it is also subject to bias and can be motivated by each individual's investment in the intervention process. Just as clear and consistent analysis of risk data will lead to a better understanding of which patient safety risks require intervention, those interventions need to be assessed with clear and consistent data in order to determine if they should be abandoned, continued, or adjusted.

## Reassessment

Staying on top of risks in the ED, knowing which problems are emerging (or persistently present), which have been addressed, what interventions are proving to be effective, and which are not, all requires commitment to a cyclical process of assessment, data collection and analysis, prioritization, intervention, and measurement. Periodic evaluation of both risks and interventions will help ED leaders stay on top of the most prevalent risks to ED patients and the most effective interventions to address them.

## Key risks for ED patients and physicians

As defined by their role, emergency medicine clinicians are asked to expose themselves to considerable risk of failing to satisfy their patients' basic needs. Emergency patients present with acute complaints to physicians and nurses often unfamiliar with the patient's medical history or any sense of their psychological, socioeconomic, or domestic backgrounds. Under those already challenging circumstances, the time-challenged clinicians are likely seeing these patients in moderate or extreme distress. The opportunity to progress through a comprehensive assessment is compromised; physicians may be left to fill in the information gaps with inadequate records, and with the patients' unreliable self-reporting of symptoms, prior treatment, drug allergies, test results, lifestyle factors, and so on. When an ED serves as a catchall for patients without access to a setting with more established physician–patient relationships, the ED providers are even more likely to experience difficult treatment encounters. ED leaders need understanding of the basic patient safety risks inherent in this environment to implement effective strategies, interventions, and training to reduce these risks both to providers and patients.

## Risk 1: The treating ED physicians have limited knowledge of the patient's background

Without a comprehensive understanding of the presenting patient's background, the treating physician faces an intellectual disadvantage and professional risk. Diagnoses and treatment (or stabilization) plans executed with incomplete knowledge about the patient – except, perhaps, in severe trauma cases – are tantamount to flying blind. Even the most acute needs of ED patients require physicians to make decisions based on a full complement of historic and contemporary data in support of the physical exam and the patient's testimony. Isolated reliance upon the notes of prior treating physicians – or worse, the patient's memory – runs the risk of biasing the diagnostic focus and obscuring contrary symptoms or test results.[6]

> **Risk reduction strategy 1**
>
> Enhance or devise systems to provide ED physicians with adequate knowledge of the patient's background and relevant prior medical records.

## Risk 2: The patient's diagnosis cannot be confirmed during the ED visit

ED patients often present with a constellation of symptoms that may or may not be amenable to a definitive diagnosis during the ED visit. In each case, the ED physician performs a workup to evaluate potential life-threatening or serious causes of the symptoms as well as other likely possibilities. After sufficient diagnostic testing, a definitive diagnosis may not be obtainable. In this circumstance,

a sicker patient may need to be admitted for further evaluation and observation. A patient who is appropriate for discharge from the ED needs explicit and clear discharge instructions describing steps to take if he or she becomes sicker or develops new symptoms, as well as a clear follow-up plan with his or her primary doctor or the relevant specialist.

> **Risk reduction strategy 2**
>
> Ensure that all complaints are followed to an appropriate conclusion even in the absence of a clear diagnosis, which may include hospital-based observation, explicit discharge instructions for the patient (and family members), or scheduled post-discharge follow-up by the ED staff or other physician. Establish a protocol for contacting the primary caregiver for patients seen in the ED – especially for patients instructed to follow up with their primary physicians.

## Risk 3: The patient is discharged with incomplete or inadequate discharge instructions, or without full comprehension of the instructions

An adequate discharge process – not just providing written instructions, but ensuring that the patient or family member understands them and can carry them out – is an essential component of every patient's ED visit.[7] This includes providing the patient with specific instructions (what to do and when) in the event of any recurrence, change, or worsening of symptoms, drug reactions, or exacerbation of comorbidities. An inadequate discharge process can undo any good the patient receives during his or her ED visit if he or she is left exposed to the risk of injury (including death) after leaving the ED. If the staff determines that a patient cannot adequately carry out the discharge instructions (or does not have appropriate support in the home) then an alternative to home discharge needs to be found.

> **Risk reduction strategy 3**
>
> All ED staff should be trained for preparing and delivering discharge instructions, and any written instructions should be tested for the appropriate language, reading, and health literacy levels.

# Risk 4: Changes in the patient's condition during his/her stay in the ED are not addressed

Busy physicians and nurses are focused on caring for multiple patients simultaneously, and often the patient receives the most comprehensive assessment at the initial encounter. Subsequently, providers move on to other tasks and may fail to recognize and account for changes in the patient's clinical status or critical new information. For example, failing to recognize neurological changes in a patient waiting to have a broken wrist set and immobilized may result in the patient being discharged home with no appreciation for the minor stroke that led to the wrist-breaking fall.

### Risk reduction strategy 4

Enhance or devise systems to ensure that the patient's status is periodically reassessed during his or her ED stay, including vital signs and appropriate physical and neurological markers. Significant changes should trigger the same degree of attention as the initial presentation.

### Case study 9.1

An 83-year-old woman presented to the ED after her daughter noticed her voice sounded strange and her speech was unclear on a telephone call. Upon arrival, the patient was noted to have a mild facial droop and some garbled speech. Initially, it was not clear when the symptoms had begun. The patient was triaged to the waiting room. Three hours later, when examined, it was noted that the patient had significant and progressing right-sided weakness and that her symptoms had started within three hours of the ED presentation – within the window for thrombolytic therapy, which the patient had missed. The patient had a prolonged hospital course and a persistent inability to walk.

- Developing standardized protocols and treatment algorithms for high-risk chief complaints is an effective and important risk reduction strategy. This includes the rapid triage of these patients.
- ED leaders must be intentional about ensuring the competency and education of each staff member to perform his or her role. Ongoing professional development is essential to maintaining high-quality care.

# Risk 5: The patient's care is transferred to another provider during a change of shift, or the patient is discharged before the results of ordered tests are received or pending issues resolved

Without a protocol in place for closing the loop on test results that are received after the patient has left the ED or has been signed over to another physician, key information can be lost, putting patients and providers at risk of bad outcomes.[8] Physicians who order tests for ED patients need to have a plan for receiving and communicating those results that may be received after the patient's ED stay or after the providers have left the shift. Patients who are discharged before all test results have been received in the ED must be given clear instruction on how those results will eventually be communicated, and to whom (to the patient directly or to the patient's primary caregiver). At shift transitions, is it essential to communicate any pending tests or issues to the physician assuming responsibility for the patient.

### Risk reduction strategy 5

Enhance or establish protocols for closing the loop on tests ordered in the ED to ensure that all results are reconciled with the ordering physician, the patient, and subsequent caregivers (if appropriate).

### Case study 9.2

A 72-year-old man presented with fever and chills and mild shortness of breath progressing over several days. He had a white blood cell count of 18, and signs of mild dehydration. He was given intravenous fluids; his chest x-ray was normal. Feeling better after the intravenous fluid, he was discharged home. Blood cultures were sent. The next day two of the blood cultures grew Gram-positive cocci. The patient's telephone number was not accurate on the record, and he was reached only after four days. At that time, he returned to the ED with worsening shortness of breath and was found to have acute bacterial endocarditis that eventually required a mitral valve replacement.

- A system to follow up pending tests sent from the ED should be established to ensure the timely and proper follow-up of these results, particularly if they are abnormal.

## Risk 6: Following discharge, the patient suffers an unexpected outcome unbeknownst to the ED staff

Tracking adverse outcomes of discharged patients is a challenge for ED leaders. Such events are relatively rare, and thus routine tracking is generally not practical. On the other hand, ED leaders who are uninformed after a recent patient suffered an outcome that was unexpected or preventable have no opportunity to determine if any part of the ED visit was mishandled, and then to factor that occurrence in to the ongoing patient safety assessment and improvement process. Where possible, leaders may consider small-scale tracking projects with a specific subset of patients (for example, patients with a complaint of chest pain discharged home with a gastrointestinal diagnosis), or coordinating with a third party that records certain conditions (stroke, myocardial infarction) to see if any of those patients had been seen in the ED prior to their change of condition.

**Risk reduction strategy 6**

Consider opportunities to identify occurrences of unexpected/adverse outcomes for patients recently seen in your ED.

**Case study 9.3**

A 45-year-old woman presented with epigastric pain since that morning. The patient was primarily Spanish-speaking, but could speak some minimal English (the primary language of the ED staff). She was noted to be tachycardic and given some intravenous fluid. A basic chemistry panel and complete blood count and liver function tests were normal. After the change in shift, she was discharged home with a prescription for an antacid. Her heart rate was 120 beats per minute upon discharge. An ECG was not performed. The patient died of a cardiac arrest later that day; subsequent autopsy revealed a large myocardial infarction.

- Persistently abnormal vital signs can be a sign of a potentially serious condition that has been missed, or that the patient is sicker than initially appreciated. A persistently abnormal vital sign must be addressed.
- An interpreter should be used routinely with every patient that does not speak the primary language of the providers, as critical information can be lost during communication.
- The missed diagnosis of myocardial ischemia remains an important area of ED adverse events, and the possibility should be carefully considered in patients with potential symptoms.

## Communication as a key to managing ED risk and patient safety

EDs with robust systems, recruitment, and training programs that emphasize the importance of clear and effective communication (both spoken and written) have in place the most important component of risk management and patient safety.[9–11] While the importance of expressing and comprehending clinical facts and emotional responses pervades all aspects of a patient's ED visit, the following are the key points leadership should focus on as part of its commitment to exemplary communication practices:

(1) **Communication among providers** that enables multiple clinicians sharing responsibility for a single patient to keep abreast of all critical patient information breaks down barriers to a timely diagnosis and initiation of treatment.

(2) **Communication between clinicians and patients** that aligns the patient's status, the physician's assessment, their mutual expectations, and the ongoing plan for diagnosis and treatment reduces the opportunity for wrong turns along the course of treatment or unanticipated decisions.

(3) **Communication between the radiology department or the laboratory and the ED** needs to ensure timely, standardized, and reliable transfer of test orders and results. This includes the need for a system to ensure that findings incidental to the reason for the test being ordered are communicated to the ordering physician and to the patient and his or her primary physician.[12]

(4) **Communication from ED physicians to specialty consultants** needs to be precise about the reason for the consult and convey whatever information the ED has gathered about the patient's history, current complaint, symptoms,

and test results. The communication from the specialist back to the ED clinicians should, first and foremost, respond to the primary reason for the consult request, but should also convey any observations or findings that will inform the patient's immediate treatment or any subsequent care.

(5) **Communication between the ED and the patient's primary physician** should serve to enable the patient to receive subsequent care informed by the reason for the ED visit, any findings or diagnosis stemming from the ED visit, and any newly prescribed medications or follow-up recommendations generated from the ED. If possible, the primary physician should be encouraged and enabled (that is, provided with contact information) to communicate directly with the ED physician who saw his or her patient.

(6) **Documentation of ED care** poses challenges in a practice settings where (a) the pace and intensity of each patient interaction complicates contemporaneous record keeping, and (b) the reliance by subsequent providers on the record of the patient's ED visit is often minimal. Nevertheless, medical record documentation is the primary evidence of what took place while the patient was under the ED's care and it should reflect accurately and without extraneous commentary the patient's complaint and presentation, the results of his or her examination, and the diagnosis and discharge plan. While ED notes may not always be accessible by subsequent (non-ED) providers, they should be comprehensive enough to account for all aspects of the patient's ED visit.

## Reactive strategies following an adverse event

The role of ED leaders in being prepared to react to an unfortunate adverse event is as important as their role in proactive risk management and patient safety. An inadvertently injured ED patient – already vulnerable upon arrival at the ED – must remain the primary focus of attention in the aftermath of a medical error. The following advice for responding to an adverse event is adopted from materials originally prepared by the Risk Management Foundation of the Harvard Medical Institutions.[13]

When a serious adverse event occurs, sincere sympathy and compassion expressed to the patient and/or family is often the most important response to help defuse a potentially volatile situation. Rather than taking a defensive stance against accusations of substandard care, the healthcare team should refrain from castigation or infighting and immediately begin the following positive measures:

- take care of the patient
- contact institutional resources
- disclose as immediately as possible
- do not speculate about causation
- convey compassion for the patient's pain and suffering
- take responsibility (for what needs to follow)
- assign accountability for follow-up
- preserve evidence
- report the incident

## Ongoing assessment and staff training

As is true in all professions, physicians learn from their mistakes. In the ongoing process of assessing patient safety risks in the ED, teaching from case examples from your very own setting is an incredibly powerful technique. When paired with routine data collection and analysis, local examples help capture your staff's attention, raise awareness of tangible risks, and garner their investment in devising solutions to the underlying problems. That degree of participation is vital to sustaining a successful patient safety/risk assessment and improvement program. Relevant case examples from other EDs also provide exceptional learning opportunities (and are often recognized as similar to past local events).

## Summary

The best formula for a strong risk management and patient safety program in the ED is having a well-trained staff of physicians and nurses practicing good medicine. When their leadership, training, and systems are focused on continuously identifying and addressing risks, those clinicians are supported by a safety net that enables them to focus their energy and attention on delivering excellent patient care.

# References

1. Smith HW. Legal responsibility for medical malpractice IV. Malpractice claims in the United States and a proposed formula for testing their legal sufficiency. *Journal of the American Medical Association* 1941; **116**(24): 2670–9.

2. Kachalia A, Gandhi TK, Puopolo AL, *et al*. Missed and delayed diagnoses in the emergency department: a study of closed claim malpractice claims from 4 liability insurers. *Annals of Emergency Medicine*. 2006; **49**: 196–205.

3. Campbell S, Croskerry P, Bond WF. Profiles in patient safety: a "perfect storm" in the emergency department. *Academic Emergency Medicine*. 2007; **14**: 743–9.

4. Studdert DM, Mello MM, Gawande AA, *et al*. Claims, errors, and compensation payments in medical malpractice litigation. *New England Journal of Medicine* 2006; **354**: 2024–33.

5. Patterson PD, Huang DT, Fairbanks RJ, *et al*. Variation in emergency medical services workplace safety culture. *Prehospital Emergency Care* 2010; **14**: 448–60.

6. Stiell A, Forster AJ, Stiell IG, van Walraven C. Prevalence of information gaps in the emergency department and the effect on patient outcomes. *CMAJ* 2003; **169**: 1023–8.

7. Thomas EJ, Burstin HR, O'Neil AC, Orav EJ, Brennan TA. Patient non-compliance with medical advice after the emergency department visit. *Annals of Emergency Medicine*. 1996; **27**(1): 49–55.

8. Roy CL, Poon EG, Karson AS, *et al*. Patient safety concerns arising from test results that return after hospital discharge. *Annals of Internal Medicine* 2005; **143**: 121–8.

9. Morey JC, Simon R, Jay GD, *et al*. Error reduction and performance improvement in the emergency department through formal teamwork training: evaluation results of the MedTeams project. *Health Service Research* 2002; **37**: 1553–81.

10. Salas E, DiazGranados D, Weaver SJ, King H. Does team training work? Principles for health care. *Academic Emergency Medicine* 2008; **15**: 1002–9.

11. Frankel A, Gardner R, Maynard L, Kelly A. Using the communication and teamwork skills (CATS) assessment to measure health care team performance. *Joint Commission Journal on Quality and Patient Safety* 2007: **33**: 549–58.

12. Laxmisan A, Hakimzada F, Sayan OR, *et al*. The multitasking clinician: decision-making and cognitive demand during and after team handoffs in the emergency care. *International Journal of Medical Informatics* 2007; **76**: 801–11.

13. Truog RD, Browning DM, Johnson JA, Gallagher TA. *Talking with Patients and Families about Medical Error: a Guide for Education and Practice*. Baltimore, MD: Johns Hopkins University Press, 2011.

# Further reading

Biros MH, Adams JG, Wears RL. Errors in emergency medicine: a call to action. *Academic Emergency Medicine* 2000; **7**: 1173–4.

Brown TW, McCarthy ML, Kelen GD, Levy F. An epidemiologic study of closed emergency department malpractice claims in a national database of physician malpractice insurers. *Academic Emergency Medicine* 2010; **17**: 553–60.

Elshove-Bolk J, Simons M, Cremers J, van Vugt A, Burg M. A description of emergency department-related malpractice claims in The Netherlands: closed claims study 1993–2001. *European Journal of Emergency Medicine* 2004; **11**: 247–50.

Fordyce J, Blank FS, Pekow P, *et al*. Errors in a busy emergency department. *Annals of Emergency Medicine* 2003; **42**: 324–33.

Hurwitz B. Learning from primary care malpractice: past, present and future. *Quality and Safety in Health Care* 2004; **13**: 90–1.

Karcz A, Holbrook J, Auerbach BS, *et al*. Preventability of malpractice claims in emergency medicine: a closed claims study. *Annals of Emergency Medicine* 1990; **19**: 865–73.

Chapter

# 10

# Emergency department staff development

Thomas Fleischmann

## Key learning points

- Well-trained and dedicated physician and nursing staff are essential to providing high-quality and efficient medical care in an emergency department (ED).
- Emergency care delivery in the ED differs significantly from physician and nursing activities in other medical disciplines that take place in other parts of the hospital, and thus requires specific training in an ED.
- Finding, forming, leading, monitoring, and developing the medical and nursing staff is one of the most important tasks for the leader of an ED.

After studying this chapter the reader will be able to:

- address the need for trained medical and nursing staff in an ED
- define the core competencies of physicians and nurses in an ED
- specify the impact of communicating a clear vision of an ED, as well as setting goals and expectations
- formulate ideas for finding physicians and nurses for an ED
- discuss strategies for training and supervising medical and nursing staff in an ED

## Introduction

Many countries around the world have recognized emergency medicine as a specialty or a supraspecialty, while others have yet to do so. Regardless of the status of emergency medicine as a specialty, the need for high-quality, efficient emergency medical care remains the same everywhere in the world. The institutional resources necessary for providing high-quality emergency care include a well-designed clinical area that supports the operational model for emergency care delivery, well-defined policies and procedures, relevant equipment and medical supplies, rapid access to diagnostic studies and therapeutic resources. However, the most important resource, by far, is a dedicated emergency physician and nursing staff with the necessary knowledge, skills, and competencies and an appropriate attitude.

Working in an ED is very different from working in other fields of medicine. It requires specific knowledge, skills, and competencies. In addition, a unique style of medical decision making and action is necessary in order to simultaneously manage multiple patients of varying acuity and underlying conditions, often with limited data and clinical information. Working clinically in the ED differs from working in an outpatient clinic, inpatient ward, operating room, or intensive care unit, although it shares some characteristics with each of these settings. Delivering high-quality, efficient emergency care can only be learned and taught in the ED, and it must be continuously practiced there.[1,2]

Relatively speaking, it is less difficult to recruit emergency physicians and nurses in a country where emergency medicine and emergency nursing are recognized specialties and accredited training programs produce adequate numbers of qualified personnel to meet the staffing needs of hospital EDs within the country. Under these circumstances, the required competencies are typically well defined and taught by locally accredited postgraduate medical education institutions. Applicants for clinical positions in the ED who have graduated from accredited training programs will generally have a certain minimum level of defined expertise, which simplifies the process of reviewing applications and selecting candidates.

*Emergency Department Leadership and Management*, ed. Stephanie Kayden, *et al.* Published by Cambridge University Press.
© Cambridge University Press 2015.

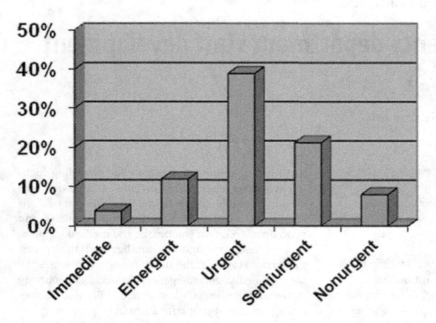

**Figure 10.1** Triage acuity among patients presenting to US emergency departments (2008). Source: Centers for Disease Control and Prevention (www.cdc.gov/nchs/data/ahcd/nhamcs_emergency/nhamcsed2008.pdf).

However, in countries where emergency medicine has not yet been recognized as a specialty and standardized clinical training programs have yet to be established, finding adequate numbers of doctors and nurses who are both dedicated to, and capable of, providing high-quality emergency care can prove to be more challenging. Under these circumstances, the ED leader still has the responsibility to build a skilled clinical team capable of providing the best possible clinical care. Accomplishing this requires time and effort by the ED leadership team, who must work closely with individual physicians and nurses to identify gaps in knowledge and skills, supplement these with relevant educational and training activities, and implement sufficient policies, procedures and clinical pathways to ensure the delivery of standardized, evidence-based care. Continuing medical education for both emergency physician and nursing personnel is essential for staying current with evidence-based emergency medicine practice standards and maintaining a high standard of care. In all cases, including countries where emergency medicine is a recognized specialty, ED leaders need to monitor the ongoing continuing medical education (CME) activities of emergency physician and nursing staff in their department. And finally, quality assurance mechanisms including routine audit of selected patient cases are necessary to ensure that care meets the established standards.

## Characteristics of a good ED team
### The role of the emergency department

The role of the hospital-based ED has evolved over the past several decades to become the primary portal of entry to the hospital for patients with acute illness or injury. Under this model, patients may be referred to the ED by their primary care or other physician, arrive at the ED by ambulance, or seek care in the ED based on their own concerns about an illness or injury. As a result, the patient population presenting to the ED includes a wide range of levels of severity and complaints, most of which do not have a definitive diagnosis on arrival. Data from the US National Hospital Ambulatory Medical Care Survey (NHAMCS) shows the distribution of triage acuities among over 123 million patients presenting to the nearly 5000 US hospital EDs in 2008 (Fig. 10.1).[3]

Approximately 13.4% of ED patient visits described in the NHAMCS data resulted in hospital admission. At one university teaching hospital in Boston, Massachusetts, over the course of 12 months in 2009, over 1200 different ICD-9 codes were encountered among patients admitted to hospital from the ED, and over 2000 different ICD-9 codes were encountered overall among patients presenting to the ED (personal communication, Philip Anderson, Department of Emergency Medicine, Beth Israel Deaconess Medical Center, Boston, MA, USA, 2011).

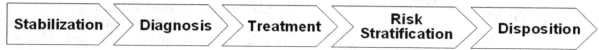

**Figure 10.2** Phases of emergency department care. Source: Missions in Emergency Medicine.[5]

In order to meet the emergency care needs of this diverse patient population, the ED needs to be organized and function as a high-volume acute diagnostic and treatment center with the appropriate space, equipment, supplies, and personnel to rapidly stabilize and evaluate patients arriving to the department. The practice of delivering ED care can be broken down into five steps (Fig. 10.2).[4]

## Unique characteristics of ED patient management

There are a number of characteristics of ED patient management, which uniquely define this area of clinical practice and illustrate many of the inherent challenges. The first of these is that patients arriving at the ED tend to present with symptoms, as opposed to a diagnosis.[1,5] Furthermore, patients with common conditions may present with uncommon signs and symptoms, and patients with unusual conditions may present with common signs and symptoms: thus the cautionary saying about ED patients, "Atypical is typical."[4] As a result, ED providers need to always consider a broad differential diagnosis when approaching the initial evaluation and avoid the temptation to arrive at a diagnosis too soon. However, it is often difficult or impossible within the time frame of the ED encounter to obtain all of the clinical data that one might ideally want in order to establish a definitive diagnosis in every case. Yet despite the sometimes inadequate datasets, effective ED providers must still act decisively to stabilize and manage patients, even when the definitive diagnosis is uncertain.

Because of the uncertainties that arise, ED providers necessarily have to take a diagnostic approach of ruling out potential threats to life, limb, and organ, rather than simply focusing on the most likely cause of the patient's condition. Discharging a patient from the ED with an unrecognized time-sensitive condition can result in morbidity, mortality, and disability that could have been prevented and often cannot be undone.

Unlike most other healthcare settings, patients present to the ED in an unscheduled fashion with variable acuity and complexity of care needs. We never know if the next patient to arrive will be unstable and require immediate attention, or how extensive a workup will be required. As a result, the ED nearly always has multiple patients with a variety of problems at different stages in their workup and treatment. In order to ensure that patients with time-sensitive problems are rapidly identified and stabilized, while at the same time ensuring effective overall patient flow through the ED, providers need to manage multiple patients in parallel, moving from one patient to the next to monitor their progress through the management phases outlined above. This requires specific competencies to avoid errors or delays.

## Standardization of knowledge and skills

Achieving standardized healthcare outcomes within a given domain or specialty (such as surgery or anesthesia) is generally viewed as being dependent upon standardized knowledge and skills among the providers in that domain or specialty.[6] The scope of work and workplace environmental characteristics in the modern ED constitutes a unique domain that similarly requires a specific set of knowledge, skills, and decision-making abilities in order for providers to perform at a consistently high level.

Given the increasing similarities in the epidemiology of medical emergencies around the world,[7] it is not surprising that curricula for postgraduate physician specialty training in emergency medicine bear remarkable similarity regardless of where in the world they have been developed.[8,9]

The European Curriculum for Emergency Medicine, for example, contains the following sections:[9]

- core competencies of the European emergency physician
- system-based core knowledge
- common presenting symptoms
- special aspects of emergency medicine
- core clinical procedures and skills

**101**

# Core competencies

The European Curriculum for Emergency Medicine identifies a range of necessary competencies for the emergency physician in addition to medical knowledge. These include:[9]

- patient care
- communication
- collaboration and interpersonal skills
- professionalism
- ethical and legal issues
- organizational planning
- service management skills
- education and research in emergency medicine

The importance of such non-technical skills has been recognized for their association with improved safety in the ED.[10] Perhaps the most important competency of all among team members in an ED is the ability to communicate effectively with many different types of people. ED providers need to communicate extensively with patients, relatives, doctors and staff from other departments, administration, emergency medical services, primary care physicians, and amongst themselves, to name only a few. The need for effective and empathetic communication is important not only for physicians but for all members of the ED team.[11]

# Knowledge

The knowledge base necessary for the practice of emergency medicine is broad, encompassing the range of conditions associated with all types of acute illness and injury, and has been well described in international curricula.[8,9] Knowledge areas are typically grouped according to symptoms as well as organ systems. System-based knowledge is usually subdivided following the medical specialties, which are themselves oriented by organ systems, functions, or age. The symptom-based approach is uniquely characteristic of emergency medicine, because of the undifferentiated nature of most patient presentations to the ED, and is reflected in the organization of most emergency medicine textbooks, which include chapters focused on symptom-based presentations.[12,13]

# Skills

There is also common agreement on what procedural skills an emergency physician and emergency nurse should possess. The skills required by an emergency physician are well described and include those necessary to resuscitate and stabilize unstable patients, as well as diagnostic procedures and therapeutic interventions commonly needed by patients presenting to the ED.[8,9] There is greater variety in the descriptions of emergency nursing skill sets used in different countries, which may be due to the fact that some countries have adopted the concept of mid-level providers in the ED, for example physician assistants and nurse practitioners, while other countries have not.[14–16] One example of a knowledge and skill set description for emergency nurses in a country without a recognized physician specialty in emergency medicine is that from Switzerland.[17]

# Attitudes

In order to perform at a high level in the sometimes chaotic environment of the ED, providers need to adopt professional behaviors and attitudes that allow them to provide care that is both compassionate and effective.

Patients presenting to the ED typically are in pain or experiencing other symptoms that are distressing to them; they are confused, uncertain, or afraid about the nature of the underlying diagnosis causing their symptoms; they may be the victims of assault or other trauma that has been inflicted upon them. There are innumerable reasons why patients in the ED may feel irritable, unhappy, or angry. ED providers need to have the capacity to empathize with the stressful circumstances of patients in the ED and strive to provide compassionate care even when patients are difficult or ungrateful. Our job is to bring order to inherently chaotic situations, and a friendly compassionate attitude towards patients is essential for providing reassurance in the face of uncertainty and stress. Keeping the balance between too much and too little empathy is sometimes a challenge even for experienced providers in an ED.[18]

ED providers also need to take a sense of ownership for the patient during the period where the patient is in the ED and advocate strongly for them. This means taking responsibility for ensuring that the initial stabilization, diagnostic evaluation, and initiation of treatment is carried out appropriately and in a timely fashion, even if this requires the involvement of other specialists. This can be particularly challenging because of the undifferentiated nature of the conditions with which many patients present to the ED. The ED providers need to advocate for their patients to ensure they receive appropriate care even when the definitive diagnosis is uncertain, and to ensure that care is appropriately prioritized when patients have multiple medical or surgical problems at the same time.

ED providers need to think broadly and avoid the temptation of premature diagnostic anchoring as they approach the stabilization, diagnostic evaluation, and treatment of their patients. This can be challenging for all ED providers, but especially in the case where the ED provider has a background in a specialty area other than emergency medicine, which is often the case in countries where emergency medicine is not yet a recognized specialty. Under these circumstances, ED providers need to be able to think and act outside the comfort zone of their primary specialty. This requires the ability to recognize the limits of one's own knowledge and skill set, and to know when to get assistance in a clinical situation. It also requires a commitment to continual self-improvement and acquisition of new knowledge and skills to meet identified needs.

The European Curriculum for Emergency Medicine articulates the following about the professional behaviors and attitudes of emergency physicians:[9]

> The general professional behaviour and attributes of emergency physicians must not be adversely influenced by working in stressful circumstances and with a diverse patient population. They must learn to identify their educational needs and to work within their own limitations. They must be able to self-motivate even at times of stress or discomfort. They must recognise their own as well as system errors and value participation in the peer review process.

ED providers also need to have the capacity for self-reflection and recognition of their own potential for personal biases, which can include racial or social-status bias.[19] Biases can have a detrimental influence even on otherwise skilled caregivers, and can be hard to detect at times. A good way to protect from biases

is to have team members from diverse backgrounds, who trust each other and are united by a common mission.

And finally, the practice of emergency medicine is invariably a team-oriented operation, uniting many people from different professional and social backgrounds, who need to be willing and able to work closely as a team in order to perform at a high level.

# Building and maintaining the ED clinical team

The process of building and maintaining an excellent clinical team of ED providers dedicated to deliver high-quality emergency care can be subdivided into the following five steps: finding, forming, leading, monitoring, developing (Table 10.1). These five steps are the same for all members of the ED, regardless of whether they are doctors, nurses, or other personnel.

## Finding a good ED team

Medical emergencies happen in every country of the world, and these patients are cared for by the providers that work within the local emergency care system. Sometimes the providers working in the ED are there not entirely of their own free will; it may be an unpopular part of their training, or they may have to work in the ED as an obligatory component of their job in the hospital. These doctors and nurses may do a good job in the ED, but they may not feel a sense of commitment to this type of work. Not infrequently they may try to avoid the work in the ED or terminate it as soon as possible. This is an unfortunate reality that ED leaders in many countries have to live with.

But even in countries where emergency medicine and emergency nursing are not yet recognized as independent specialties, there are however still doctors, nurses, and other staff who feel attracted to this job. Sometimes they may suffer from a lack of appreciation by colleagues and the public of their

**Table 10.1** The five steps of building and maintaining an ED clinical team

| Finding | Recruitment |
| --- | --- |
| Forming | Orientation, supplemental education and training |
| Leading | Strategic vision, planning, setting goals/expectations, protecting, role modeling |
| Monitoring | Quality assurance, performance, satisfaction, CME, risk management |
| Developing | Diversification, specialization, designing future trends |

work in the ED. Some providers working in an ED may actually regret having to leave the ED in order to advance in their professional career. Others may even accept a delay in career advancement in order to remain working in the ED. In fact, this is the way in which the specialty of emergency medicine developed several decades ago in a number of countries, by individuals making this career choice.[20]

These providers, who choose to work in the ED, are often intrinsically motivated on a high level. And, once again, they are already present in every country of the world. They are the perfect core team members to start an ED staff. Thus it makes sense to look first at applicants who are already working in an ED to find physicians and nurses with a high level of motivation and experience, who are interested in working in a well-organized and high-performing ED. Applicants with foreign experience in countries with highly developed EDs may also prove to be useful.

Classified advertisements in emergency medicine journals, newsletters, and other print media, as well as internet websites, and even social media, can all be useful strategies for seeking applicants for ED positions.

The leader of an ED may increase his or her visibility and the desirability of the department as a workplace if he or she is an active speaker at medical conferences or is the author of books or journal articles related to emergency medicine.

Another approach is to publicize the fact that you are opening a newly designed ED in which there will be professional leadership, training and support for professional staff development, and commitment to high performance. The professional vision and personal attitude of the ED leader can be a significant factor in attracting motivated and talented team members. Therefore it is fundamental that the ED leader develops and articulates a clear vision for what his or her ideal ED operation looks like, as well as a clear and realistic vision for how this will be achieved. Successful leaders must be able to inspire their teams, and this begins with having a compelling vision that all members of the team can relate to.

If conditions in one's regional labor market are favorable, and the ED leader has developed a compelling vision and advertised well, there will ideally be an excess number of applicants relative to openings that need to be filled. It then becomes prudent and necessary to define selection criteria and an interview and selection process. In terms of selection criteria, first

and foremost is the ability to work as a team member within a team structure, as this is central to the success of the ED. Having an open mind and flexibility, as well as resilience to working under stressful situations, is important given the changing and varied nature of the work in the ED. For providers who have a prior background in a single specialty outside of emergency medicine, this need for open-mindedness extends to the preparedness and ability to work in an interdisciplinary fashion, across specialty boundaries. In this regard, work experience in multiple specialty areas, ideally including both medical and surgical specialties, is particularly desirable. And lastly, prior experience in an ED setting is highly desirable characteristic of a suitable candidate.

> **Case study 10.1**
>
> The Northwest Hospital is a mid-sized community hospital. The annual volume of ED patients has risen steadily over the past few years. The ED patient volume now exceeds the capacity of the emergency care area of the hospital. Until now, the nurses working in the ED were employed primarily in the ICU and were called to the emergency care area on an as-needed basis when patients arrived. There were no doctors assigned to the ED. The nurses had to decide which doctor to call from one of the inpatient departments when an unannounced patient arrived at the hospital. The doctors often refused to come, telling the nurse to call someone else or find a doctor of another specialty. This led to long waiting times, even for patients in pain or with hemodynamic instability, to multiple encounters with different doctors, and to unclear, unpredictable, and sometimes even unsafe care. Patients and nurses were increasingly unhappy. After several serious complaints by patients and unfavorable reports in the local media, the hospital leaders decided to establish an ED and to employ a doctor well known for his competency and skills in organizing an ED. His preconditions for accepting the position were that the ED be established as an independent department and that he be able to hire his own clinical team that would work exclusively in the ED. Both conditions were granted.
>
> After the arrival of the newly appointed ED director, the hospital leaders launched a large media campaign, announcing the planned improvements in emergency care delivery. The campaign also mentioned that they were seeking doctors and nurses interested in working exclusively in a modern and professionally organized

ED. This attracted widespread attention by the media and resulted in a wave of applications from both doctors and nurses who wanted to work in a high-performing ED, including many who were willing to move into the area only to work in this ED. The number of the applications significantly outnumbered the open posts.

This is a true story.

## Forming a good ED team

Once a team of doctors and nurses dedicated to working in the ED is found, the ED leader needs to unite all of the members of the ED team around a compelling vision of the idealized future state of the ED. This vision needs to incorporate the elements of efficient, effective, and empathic emergency care, but also must be accompanied by a clear and realistic plan for how this will be achieved.

In countries where there are no postgraduate specialty training opportunities in emergency medicine for doctors and nurses, it will be necessary to provide additional, supplemental education and training in order to achieve a high level of clinical competency among the ED providers. The starting point for determining what additional education and training is required should ideally be a description of the scope of care that is to be provided in the ED, which in turn will define the scope of practice of the doctors and nurses that are responsible for providing this care. One example of such a scope of care document is the "Model of the clinical practice of emergency medicine,"[21] which describes in detail the range of conditions, stratified by acuity, that emergency physicians in the USA are expected to be able to manage. This document also details the types of clinical tasks, procedural skills, and administrative and other non-clinical competencies that are essential to the successful practice of emergency medicine. This document, which is periodically updated every few years by relevant professional organizations, serves as a basis for developing the educational and training curricula for emergency medicine postgraduate specialty training programs as well as the board certification examinations that emergency medicine specialty trainees complete following completion of their training programs.

The description of the scope of ED care may very well differ from country to country, and even by type of hospital within a given country. The important practical point is that whatever the actual intended scope of care that will be delivered in the ED, it should be explicitly defined with sufficient clarity and detail so that the ED practitioners know what is expected of them and so that they can, over time, become experts within this domain. If the boundaries of the ED scope of care are not agreed upon and made explicit, then it will be extremely difficult for the ED providers to ever become experts, or for care delivery to ever become standardized, as the desired scope of practice is ill-defined.

Once the scope of practice and corresponding knowledge and skill sets have been defined for the ED providers, it then becomes possible to carry out an individual gap analysis for each provider, which will define the knowledge and skill areas that need to be supplemented with additional education and training.

Identifying the necessary resources to support the ongoing professional education and training of healthcare providers can be challenging. In many cases it will be necessary for the ED and the hospital to provide resources to cover the costs associated with professional staff development, especially if there is a shortage of qualified personnel in the local labor market and these educational opportunities are viewed as an important incentive for attracting applicants. Resources are needed to cover both the costs associated with the educational programming itself, and the cost of replacement staff to cover the clinical duties of the staff who are away attending educational programming, as it may be difficult or impossible to ask staff to work a full clinical load and attend mandatory educational programming in their free time or vacation.

The reality is that in most healthcare systems the available resources to support ongoing professional education and training for healthcare providers are limited. In many healthcare systems, resources for continuing professional education of care providers, and in some cases also research, may be funded from the same pool of resources as actual clinical care delivery, and thus these activities compete for the same resources.[22] Resources allocated for continuing professional development of providers must be viewed as a strategic investment in the emergency care delivery system that is justified by a future return on investment that can be measured in terms of improved quality, reduced complication and error rates, and improvements in productivity.

In countries where emergency medicine is not a recognized specialty, and where there are no formal postgraduate specialty training programs, there may be courses for doctors and nurses in emergency medicine that are organized locally, regionally, or internationally that staff can attend. Such training courses and seminars are often publicized on the websites of emergency medicine professional organizations. If appropriate training resources are lacking in one's local region, developing and running local training programs can be accomplished more easily by working together with other local or regional ED leaders with similar training needs.

In addition to didactic education and training course, there are other useful strategies and tools that can be employed. Bedside teaching involves formal supervision of junior providers by senior providers in real time in the ED, whereby junior providers briefly present their cases to a senior provider present in the ED and discuss management plans. Bedside training in the ED is one of the most effective and efficient ways to train both doctors and nurses on the job.[23] Regular and frequent rounding in the ED, where the clinical team gathers and reviews the status and management plans for patients in the department, either at the bedside or in a central location, is an effective, evidence-based practice, assuring quality of care and patient safety, as well as promoting standardized practice and adherence to departmental policies.[24]

Simulation-based training, using either high-fidelity simulation centers or in-situ methods, is becoming an increasingly valuable educational strategy in emergency medicine. Learning and practicing common high-stakes procedural skills or clinical management and decision making in a simulated environment allows emergency medicine practitioners the opportunity to develop and expand their expertise without subjecting live patients to potential risk or harm. Simulation also provides opportunities to train in performing lifesaving procedures that are rarely performed in real life, but nonetheless require expertise to perform successfully, such as cricothyroidotomy and pediatric cardiac arrest resuscitation.

It is equally true, for nurses as well as for physicians, that the ability to perform at a high clinical level in the ED requires that the individual possess the specific knowledge and skill set associated with carrying out the clinical tasks and patient management duties that comprise the scope of care delivered in the ED. However, comprehensive training in ED nursing competencies is typically limited or absent in the nursing school curricula in most countries, or in

the training that nurses receive in other areas of clinical nursing practice. Therefore, it is often necessary to establish a competency-based training program within the ED to augment nursing competencies for newly hired nurses, as well as maintaining competencies for all members of the ED nursing staff.[15,25]

Lastly, whenever possible, less experienced providers should always be scheduled to work clinically in the ED together with more experienced providers, in order to ensure that many of the educational opportunities described above can take place and to ensure patient safety. Having only team members in the early stages of their careers at the same time in the ED can create unsafe conditions.

## Leading a good ED team

Leading a high-performing ED team is a demanding and never-ending task for the ED leader and his or her leadership team. A clear vision of the idealized ED has to be defined, deployed, and defended on a daily basis. This requires the continuous attention, presence, empathy, and fortitude of the ED leader. Setting clear goals and defining expectations are central parts of the strategy for leading and developing any team.

Establishing a culture of communication and mutual respect is highly dependent upon the personality and example of the department leader. He or she is the primary role model not only for clinical care but also for the communication and interpersonal dynamics within the department. The way in which staff members communicate and interact with each other is likely to reflect the way in which they communicate and interact with patients and their families. Therefore, establishing a respectful and friendly tone among staff is likely to have a positive impact on the way staff interact with patients and their families.

The circumstances and conditions under which the ED operates are likely to be in a state of continual change. This includes the clinical practice of emergency medicine, the resources available within the ED and the hospital, including the ED team members and other personnel, and even the legal, organizational, and financial framework of emergency care delivery. The ED leader must assume a skeptical stance and view any changes as having the potential to negatively impact the ED and its operations. The ED leader must therefore continuously monitor internal and external circumstances and conditions that have the potential to impact the department, and must address these openly and decisively.

Creating an environment that promotes safety and reduces the frequency of errors requires trust among ED team members, such that any member of the team feels empowered to call a time-out if they suspect a problem that could lead to an adverse event. The hierarchical nature of relationships within the clinical team can sometimes result in subordinate team members being reluctant to call out potential problems that they observe, because they may feel it is not their place to interrupt or question a senior team member. All team members, even the most junior or subordinate, must be encouraged to voice concerns about potential errors in patient care or to ask for help when needed. This approach to error reduction is borrowed from the crew resource management (CRM) model pioneered in the aviation industry and is highly relevant to ED operations.

The ED leader also needs to create working conditions that are conducive to high performance and staff satisfaction. Excessively long or frequent shifts can lead to lapses and mistakes due to exhaustion, as well as low morale and potential burnout.[26]

## Monitoring a good ED team

The ED leader needs to monitor how the team is doing over time, both in terms of outcomes and performance, and also in terms of motivation and readiness to perform at a high level. Outcomes and performance should be monitored systematically by a quality assurance team that tracks locally and regionally mandated quality markers, as well as performing case audits of selected cases. Quality assurance mechanisms are discussed in more detail elsewhere in this book (see Chapter 7). In addition to tracking performance metrics, the ED leader and his or her leadership team also need to participate in and supervise clinical care in the ED in order to have first-hand knowledge and experience with departmental operations and care delivery. Working clinically in the ED, including nights and weekends when patient volumes may be higher and hospital resources less available, gives the ED leader enormous credibility, both with the ED staff and with other hospital departments, when talking about challenges facing the ED.

In addition to having the necessary knowledge and skills to carry out the scope of care in the ED, as discussed above, personnel also need to be motivated and engaged to perform at a high level. Staff who are dissatisfied with their job are less likely to be motivated to perform well, and therefore one of the most important goals of the ED leader is to assure the satisfaction of providers. There are many control levers to influence team satisfaction. Examples are choosing the right people for the team, communicating goals and policies and defending them, enhancing decent behavior, and controlling diversions. A very important issue is to limit the workload of the team members, to distribute the exposure equally, and to detect an impending burnout problem early. These efforts translate directly into patient safety and staff satisfaction at the same time. An exhausted and hostile group is much more prone to errors than a trusting team working in a controlled environment.[26]

Striving to improve staff satisfaction is also likely to have a positive impact on the satisfaction of patients and their families. Comparing complaints of patients and of nurses in the ED shows significant similarities.[27] Both groups express dissatisfaction with long waiting times, delayed and infrequent attendance to pain, and lack of communication in the ED. Short waiting times, early pain control, and clear communication seem to please both patients and nurses.

---

**Case study 10.2**

Some weeks after his start as director of the Northwest Hospital ED, the newly appointed ED director called for a staff meeting. He asked the team members to describe their vision of a perfectly functioning ED. The staff came up with a number of goals that they all agreed on including: that all personnel would treat each other with respect, trust, and empathy; that provider–patient interactions would also be this way; that the scope of ED care would be clearly defined, including the procedures and responsibilities of all providers; that the workload would be controlled and equitably divided; and lastly that comprehensible quality, performance, and risk management metrics would be established.

One of the team members then asked what was preventing this from happening. The team came to the agreement that this was how they wanted their ED to function. They decided to adopt a "code of conduct" describing the accepted interpersonal behavior and style of communication, and to immediately address deviations. They established a taskforce to explicitly describe the tasks and procedures that constitute the scope of care delivered in the ED, thereby creating a manual for daily use and for the orientation of new team members. In the future they planned to define and monitor quality, performance, and risk management metrics.

Following this, the team morale improved and remained high, even under pressure. The rate at which providers called in sick dropped and stayed low. Patient complaints fell to an all-time low. The changes that had taken place in the ED attracted the attention of employees in other departments in the hospital, and job applications for positions in the ED started to flow in. The number of patients seeking care in the ED rose steadily.

This again is a true story.

## Developing a good ED team

Once the initial challenges of establishing a new department and ED team have been overcome, new challenges are likely to present themselves over time as the physician and nursing staff discover their own aspirations and seek further professional development and career advancement. This may manifest itself in staff members moving on to accept leadership positions in other EDs, which the ED leader should welcome as a marker of success in helping to build the specialty of emergency medicine, but it may also be reflected in staff seeking to pursue special interests and acquire further expertise and qualifications in particular aspects of emergency medicine. These may be areas of medical subspecialization such as pediatric emergency medicine or toxicology, particular skills such as emergency ultrasound, or a particular interest in medical education and teaching. Providing opportunities for committed staff to acquire new skills and bring them back to the department can be a strategy for building the depth of expertise within the team and disseminating this across the team through ongoing CME within the team.

Foresighted ED leaders also need to play a role in envisioning and advocating for the future development of emergency care delivery and emergency medicine as a profession within one's own region and country. Active participation in regional and national emergency medicine organizations by all ED leaders is an essential step towards developing a strong collective voice for addressing healthcare policy and decision makers on issues affecting emergency medicine.

## Summary

Building a dedicated team of full-time physician and nursing staff based in the ED is crucial to the success of a high-performing ED.

Finding suitable team members may prove to be more challenging in countries where emergency medicine is not yet recognized as a specialty. However, healthcare providers who are dedicated and motivated to work in emergency care delivery can be found in all countries.

Starting with providers who already work in an ED is often a natural starting point, as these individuals often welcome the vision of a well-designed and supportive ED.

When starting from scratch, the dedication of the team members may be more important than extensive experience, but structured training, instruction, and supervision must follow soon after. Explicitly defining the local ED scope of care to be delivered provides a basis from which physician and nursing providers' scope of practice can then be described. The knowledge and skill set necessary for delivering this scope of practice can then be determined, and gap analysis can be used to determine educational and training goals for individual providers. Established curricula for emergency medicine training are available internationally and provide valuable references for developing local education.

Leading a good ED team first depends on a clear and well-communicated vision, enhanced by comprehensible and achievable goals and expectations. Good role modeling by the ED team leader is essential.

After the ED team is established, formed, and united by a vision, then quality assurance, performance, and risk management issues have to be addressed. Monitoring and maintaining patient and provider satisfaction is of fundamental importance.

Continuous medical education and improvement by all team members is a hallmark of an advanced ED team. Job specification and diversification among both doctors and nurses may follow, and advance emergency medicine further.

Anticipating and even designing future trends in emergency medicine may be a rewarding mission to which foresighted emergency care providers can aspire.

# References

1. O'Connell E, Kleinschmidt K. Adult learners in the emergency department. In RL Rogers, ed., *Practical Teaching in Emergency Medicine*. Chicester: Wiley-Blackwell, 2009; 3–15.

2. Fleischmann T. Core competencies in emergency medicine. In T Fleischmann, ed., *Clinical Emergency Medicine*. Munich: Elsevier, 2012; 15–27 [German].

3. Centers for Disease Control and Prevention. National Hospital Ambulatory Medical Care Survey: 2008 Emergency Department Summary. http:// www.cdc.gov/nchs/data/ahcd/ nhamcs_emergency/ nhamcsed2008.pdf (accessed March 19, 2012).

4. Fleischmann T. Missions in emergency medicine. In T Fleischmann, ed., *Clinical Emergency Medicine*. Munich: Elsevier, 2012; 8–11 [German].

5. Fleischmann T. The biology of an emergency. In T Fleischmann, ed., *Clinical Emergency Medicine*. Munich: Elsevier, 2012; 11–13 [German].

6. Timmermans S, Berg M. *The Gold Standard: the Challenge of Evidence-Based Medicine and Standardization in Healthcare*. Philadelphia, PA: Temple University Press, 2003.

7. Anderson P, Petrino R, Halpern P, Tintinalli J. The globalization of emergency medicine and its importance for public health. *Bulletin of the World Health Organization* 2006; **84**: 835–9.

8. Perina D, Beeson M, Char D, *et al.* The 2007 model of the clinical practice of emergency medicine: the 2009 update.

*Annals of Emergency Medicine* 2011; **57**: e1–15.

9. UEMS Multidisciplinary Joint Committee on Emergency Medicine, European Society for Emergency Medicine. European Curriculum for Emergency Medicine. http://www.eusem.org/ cms/assets/1/pdf/european_ curriculum_for_em-aug09-djw. pdf (accessed March 19, 2012).

10. Flowerdew L, Brown R, Vincent C, Woloshynowych M. Identifying nontechnical skills associated with safety in the emergency department: a scoping review of the literature. *Annals of Emergency Medicine* 2012; **59**: 386–94.

11. Woloshynowych M, Davis R, Brown R, Vincent C. Communication patterns in a UK emergency department. *Annals of Emergency Medicine* 2007; **50**: 407–13.

12. Multiple authors. Section Two. Cardinal presentations. In J Marx, R Hockberger, R Walls, *et al.*, eds., *Rosen's Emergency Medicine*. Philadelphia, PA: Mosby Elsevier, 2010; 83–240.

13. Multiple authors. Common emergency presentations. In T Fleischmann, ed., *Clinical Emergency Medicine*. Munich: Elsevier, 2012; 29–170 [German].

14. O'Hara S. The nursing perspective and role in planning a simulation modeling: historical, experimental, and future applications of complex adaptive system thinking. In J Shiver, D Eitel, eds., *Optimizing Emergency Department Throughput*. New York, NY, Taylor & Francis, 2010; 67–107.

15. Stewig-Nitschke A. Prerequisites for nurses in an emergency department. In W von Eiff, M Brachmann, T Fleischmann, *et al.*, eds., *Management of an Emergency Department*. Stuttgart:

Kohlhammer, 2011; 363–75 [German].

16. Swiss Joint Venture for Nurses in Emergency Departments. www.notfallpflege. ch (accessed March 19, 2012) [German].

17. Swiss Joint Venture for Nurses in Emergency Departments. Curriculum for Emergency Department Nursing. http://www. notfallpflege.ch/rlpd.pdf (accessed March 19, 2012) [German].

18. Van Groenou A, Bakes K. Art, chaos, ethics and science (ACES): a doctoring curriculum for emergency medicine. *Annals of Emergency Medicine* 2006; **48**: 532–7.

19. Bernstein E, Bernstein J, James T. Multiculturalism and care delivery. In J Marx, R Hockberger, R Walls, *et al.*, eds., *Rosen's Emergency Medicine*. Philadelphia, PA: Mosby Elsevier, 2010; 2540–6.

20. Zink B. *Anyone, Anything, Anytime: a History of Emergency Medicine*. Philadelphia, PA: Mosby Elsevier, 2005.

21. Perina DG, Brunett CP, Caro DA, *et al.* The 2011 model of the clinical practice of emergency medicine. *Academic Emergency Medicine* 2012; **19**: e19–40.

22. Bohrn M, Kramer D. Teaching and patient care in emergency medicine. In R Rogers, ed., *Practical Teaching in Emergency Medicine*. Chichester: Wiley-Blackwell, 2009; 24–32.

23. Rodgers K. Bedside teaching in the emergency department. In R Rogers, ed., *Practical Teaching in Emergency Medicine*. Chicester: Wiley-Blackwell, 2009; 35–47.

24. Baker S. Hourly Rounding with individualized patient care in the ED. In S Baker, *Excellence in the Emergency Department*.

Gulf Breeze, FL: Studer, 2009; 1127–43.

25. Becker D. Emergency nurses training: subspecializing nurses in an ED. In M Moecke, C Lackner, T Kloss, eds., *The ED-Book*. Berlin: Medizinisch-Wissenschaftliche

Verlagsgesellschaft, 2011; 371–81 [German].

26. Wachter R. Basic principles of patient safety. In R Wachter, *Understanding Patient Safety*. New York, NY: McGraw-Hill, 2008; 17–26.

27. Fleischmann T. Stakeholder satisfaction in the ED. In M Moecke, C Lackner, T Kloss, eds., *The ED-Book*. Berlin, Medizinisch-Wissenschaftliche Verlagsgesellschaft, 2011; 216–21 [German].

# Costs in emergency departments

Matthias Brachmann

## Key learning points

- Understand why costs are of increasing importance.
- Review cost types and typical cost distributions in emergency departments.
- Learn how to measure costs and how to apply this knowledge to make useful and efficient decisions.
- Understand new ways to improve the budget balance and how to allocate fixed costs in different ways.

## Introduction

The pressure to improve the efficiency of service provision in hospitals is increasing globally for many reasons. National health systems are faced with increasingly tight fiscal restrictions. As life expectancy continues to rise, so too does the risk of multiple morbidities – and, with it, the demand for the provision of relevant services. This latter development is also driven by ongoing medical and technical progress. Increasingly expensive medical–technical innovations are being introduced into the daily functioning of hospitals at a rapid rate. At the same time, these innovations are embedded into workflow and administrative mechanisms that have hardly changed since the 1950s.[1] As part of efforts to solve the problem of increasing costs and the lack of efficiency-enhancing innovations, governments increasingly introduce measures to enhance competition and/or cost regulation programs. Internationally, these changes in incentives have been associated with a reduction both in the capacities of hospitals and in patients' average length of stay.[2] Figure 11.1 depicts the rise in healthcare expenditure and the simultaneous decline in healthcare capacity,

as well as the decrease in length of hospital stay for selected countries. Given the slight increase in the total number of patients treated, hospitals today must deal with more patients in fewer beds and within markedly reduced time frames.

Expenditures related to inpatient hospitalization account for a substantial percentage of overall healthcare expenditures in many countries, ranging from 22.5% to 49.5% among OECD countries in 2008.[2] However, when expenditures related to emergency department (ED) care are disaggregated from other healthcare expenditures, they account for a relatively smaller percentage of overall healthcare expenditures. For example, in the USA, the country with the world's highest level of expenditure on health care as a percentage of GDP, and which is also regarded by many observers as having a resource-intensive emergency care delivery system, expenditure on ED services amounted to only 4% of overall healthcare expenditure in 2009 (Fig. 11.2).[3]

Despite the modest proportion of healthcare expenditure consumed by ED services, the ED plays an increasingly important gateway function in many healthcare systems. One-third to one-half of all inpatients in an acute-care hospital enter the hospital by way of the ED. However, it is not uncommon that certain ED operating costs are included in the operating budgets for inpatient wards, other inpatient care units, and ancillary services.[4,5] As a result, it can be difficult in many healthcare systems to determine what the actual costs of ED care delivery are with a high degree of certainty. The true costs of ED care can be even more elusive, because of the often arbitrary methods by which overhead and support costs are allocated across departments, based on metrics such as the size of direct costs, number of patients seen, numbers of procedures, length of stay, and so on,

*Emergency Department Leadership and Management*, ed. Stephanie Kayden, *et al.* Published by Cambridge University Press.
© Cambridge University Press 2015.

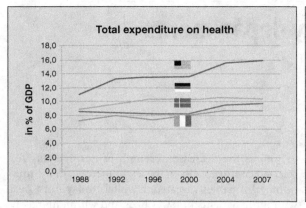
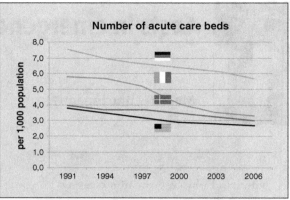
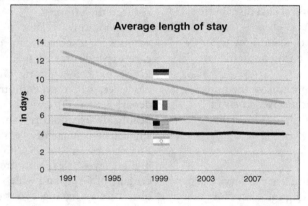

**Figure 11.1** Healthcare costs are on the rise, whereas capacities decline. Total expenditure on health in USA, Germany, Denmark, Italy; number of acute care beds in Germany, Italy, Denmark, USA; average length of stay in Germany, France, USA, Israel. Source: OECD health data.[2]

rather than the actual utilization of support services.[6] This can create a misleading picture of the true efficiency of individual departments. Furthermore, costs with no relationship whatsoever to ED operations may be hidden in the ED's budget when it is not under the direct control of the ED leader. It was recounted by a participant in a recent International Emergency Department Leadership Institute (IEDLI) course that soon after taking on a position as new head of an ED, he began probing into the costs that were being allocated to his ED only to discover, much to his surprise, that the costs for the personal care of the hospital CEO were included in the ED budget.

Despite the difficulties that can be associated with understanding the true costs associated with operating one's ED, it is essential that the ED leader understand the departmental costs to the best of his or her ability. Improving the efficiency of resource allocation is one of the primary aims of management, and it can only be reached through excellent

organization.[7,8] To make useful, effective, and efficient decisions and to put available resources to optimal use, the ED leader needs a maximum of transparency concerning the conditions and consequences of his or her actions.[9] Without cost transparency, the degree to which economic efficiency can be achieved is limited. In other words, "to contain costs, emergency department managers need to know their costs and use cost accounting."[4]

## Types of costs

To understand the cost framework of an ED, one needs to distinguish between two types of costs: *short-term* (or *variable*) and *long-term* (or *fixed*) costs. This distinction is important because of the resulting management implications: for example, fixed costs are relatively difficult to reduce in the short term. Together, variable and fixed costs add up to the total costs of the ED.

## Overall US Healthcare Expenditures, by service,
### Medical Expenditure Panel Survey, 2009

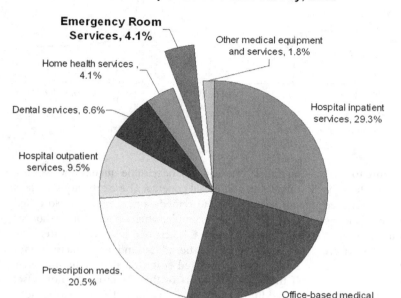

**Figure 11.2** Total healthcare expenditures by category, USA, 2009. Source: AHRQ Medical Expenditure Panel Survey.[3]

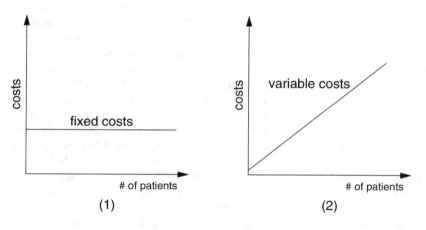

**Figure 11.3** (1) Fixed costs remain constant, while (2) variable costs increase proportionally with the number of patients

Fixed costs comprise all costs that accrue independently of the number of patients treated. They are borne by the total number of patients treated. Accordingly, the more patients that are treated in the ED during a given time period (for example, one year), the lower the share of fixed costs that each individual patient must bear. Examples of fixed costs include the rent, electricity and heat for the building that the department is located in, personnel costs, and the costs for purchasing medical equipment.

Variable costs are those that are directly related to the number of patients treated. They include all costs

that are incurred during the process of caring for individual patients. As variable costs accrue on a per-case basis, they can usually be allocated directly to the treated patient. Examples of variable costs include dressing materials (gauze), drugs, and standard forms. Figure 11.3 provides an overview of the two cost types.

Above, we noted that fixed costs are also referred to as long-term costs, while variable costs are referred to as short-term costs. This is because fixed costs are relatively difficult to modify in the short term. For example, it is not feasible to dynamically change

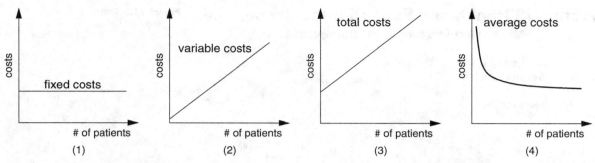

**Figure 11.4** (1) Fixed costs and (2) variable costs together make up (3) the total costs. (4) Average costs are calculated by dividing the total costs by the number of patients.

the size of the floor plans of an ED in response to daily fluctuations in patient flows. Likewise, while it is important to align staffing numbers with anticipated patient volumes, one cannot hire and fire personnel on a daily basis in response to fluctuations in patient volume. While personnel costs for full-time staff are relatively difficult to modify in the short term, this can in some cases be partly offset by strategies such as per-diem hiring, whereby some personnel are hired on a part-time, as-needed basis, and their utilization can then be dialed up and down in response to shorter-term fluctuations in departmental activity.

Hospital overhead costs including, for example, general administrative and management costs, marketing and human resources costs, as well as ancillary and support services that are not directly allocated to an individual patient's care, must also be included in the total costs of the ED.

Dividing the total annual costs of the ED by the total number of patients treated there that year returns the average cost per patient for that year.

Average costs are relevant in establishing whether or not the average revenue per patient is sufficient to cover the average costs. The average cost per patient decreases with every additional patient treated – rapidly at first, and then asymptotically approaching the variable cost per patient, as can be seen in Figure 11.4. This is due to the fact that each additional patient treated reduces the proportion of the fixed costs that is borne by each patient.

Within this cost framework, it follows that health systems that reimburse hospitals on a "per treated patient" basis provide strong incentives for treating as many patients as possible. From an economic standpoint, it is therefore desirable for an ED to increase the number of patients treated. But the problem of capacity limitations of scarce resources (for example, CT scanners) can lead to undesirable queues and waiting times with additional patients. These capacity shortfalls can be expensive to remedy and may lead to so-called *step-up costs*. For example, when an additional resource such as a second CT scanner or another attending physician needs to be added and its capacity is not fully utilized, the fixed costs for all patients increase. If the additional costs of this resource are not offset by additional revenue generated from treating additional patients, then the ED leader needs very convincing arguments to justify the resulting higher cost structure. To fully consider step-up costs in making resource decisions, the ED leader has to thoroughly understand the capacity of his or her fixed resources.

However, it is not sufficient to refer only to average costs when calculating the additional costs incurred by an additional patient. After all, average costs include the ED's fixed costs, which would accrue regardless of whether that additional patient were treated or not. Since treating the additional patient would have no effect on the department's fixed costs with the exception of the above-described step-up costs, each additional patient needs only to cover those costs that are incurred in his/her treatment. The variable costs incurred by the treatment of one additional patient are referred to as *marginal costs*.

If the marginal cost of treating one additional patient is less than the average cost of all patients already treated, then treatment of this additional patient will lower the average cost of all patients treated. This phenomenon is referred to as *fixed cost degression* and underlies what in economics is referred to as *economies of scale*.

For EDs, the economies of scale mainly stem from the reduction of average fixed costs per patient and increases in patient volume, which lowers the variance of resource demand. The added utility of improved planning given increases in patient volumes applies for small departments but is negligible for EDs of average or greater size: if the daily number of patients treated is sufficiently large (around 100 patients per day or more), then daily fluctuations can be anticipated reasonably well and the workload of the department can be planned with a sufficiently high level of confidence. The effects of fixed cost degression (the fact that additional patients treated will lower the share of fixed costs borne by each patient) also diminish with increasing patient numbers. This applies particularly to EDs that are already operating at the limits of their capacities. In such cases, there are hardly any more economies of scale to be realized, as Bamezai et al. show.[10] In this sense, increasing the size or capacity of an ED is only of limited benefit. Reaching a capacity limit where further step-up costs would be needed to continue operation, as well as having reached a daily number of patients which allow for better planning with low variances, the ED will have found its optimal size. There are no studies or other publications so far determining the optimal size for EDs from an economic and operational perspective. The ideal size will depend on hospital size, existing capacity, and resource utilization. Looking at the evolution of existing EDs in different countries in Europe and North America would suggest an upper size limit of around 60 000 patients a year for tertiary care centers as being desirable.

## Cost distribution within EDs

The provision of emergency care, as with other types of health care, is personnel-intensive, as evidenced by the fact that personnel costs represent the largest single item in the cost structure of EDs and make up 60–85% of total costs.[10] Other cost items include equipment, such as medical equipment, office equipment, computers, software; supplies, such as pharmaceuticals, blood products, other therapeutic products, medicals aids; and rent and utility costs for the facility space required, or care delivery and other related non-clinical activities (administration, education, research, etc.). This distribution of costs tends to be similar across different countries. One example of such a cost distribution across categories is shown in Figure 11.5.

One of the maxims frequently voiced in connection with reorganization efforts and cost reduction measures is that one must focus on the largest cost items first. Personnel costs are therefore a common initial target of cost-cutting initiatives. However, a qualified and motivated staff is crucially important for the success of the ED, so any consideration of cutting personnel needs to be done carefully. If the quality of services provided is to remain constant, then any reductions in personnel (given constant or increasing patient inflows) must be accompanied by improvements in workflow and efficiency; otherwise, personnel reductions will lead to increased waiting times, error rates, and overcrowding, resulting in declines in patient satisfaction. None of these effects is desirable for successful ED management.

A problem with allocation and reimbursement of ED costs occurs in healthcare systems in some countries when the costs for some care that is provided in the ED are allocated to the ED, while the reimbursement for that care is allocated to another hospital department. For example, patients seen in the ED will have an initial evaluation which may include taking

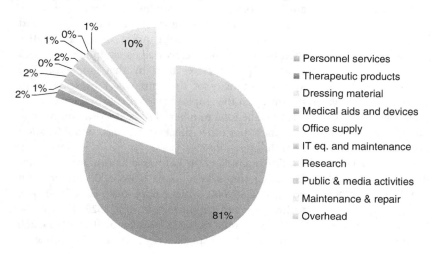

**Figure 11.5** Cost distribution of a typical European emergency department. Source: Project data of the author.

- Personnel services
- Therapeutic products
- Dressing material
- Medical aids and devices
- Office supply
- IT eq. and maintenance
- Research
- Public & media activities
- Maintenance & repair
- Overhead

vital signs, performing a focused history and physical exam, obtaining an ECG or other bedside testing, obtaining initial diagnostic imaging and blood tests, initiating therapeutic interventions, and so on. For patients in the ED who are subsequently admitted to a hospital inpatient service, the ED portion of the patient's care may represent a significant portion of the overall care provided for the patient during the hospital stay. In many countries that have only recently adopted the emergency medicine-based model of ED care, inpatient hospital departments receive the same diagnosis-related group (DRG)-based reimbursement for patients admitted to their service, regardless of whether that patient was admitted on an elective basis, directly to their department, or on an acute basis, via the ED; while the ED receives only a flat, non-DRG-based reimbursement for all patients seen in the ED, regardless of whether they are admitted or not, and regardless of the level of complexity of the care that is provided in the ED. Under this cost allocation and reimbursement model, the ED accrues costs that it is never reimbursed for, which negatively impacts its balance sheet.

ED leaders should strive for a fair allocation to the ED of hospital revenues received for care provided, which is proportional to care delivered in the ED. Depending on the local reimbursement system and on possible ways of reallocating resources within the hospital, the ED may be able to receive a portion of inpatient department reimbursements to cover the costs of the ED care provided to patients admitted to those inpatient departments. If reallocation of revenues is not feasible within the institution, the ED may alternatively consider billing the other departments for delivering these services as a way of reallocating its costs.

## Measuring costs

The types of costs described in the preceding sections provide a solid basis for understanding the overall aggregate cost framework at the level of the ED itself. However, in order to make cost-efficient ED management decisions related to process improvements or investments in additional resources, it is often necessary to determine cost structures at the level of specific medical conditions, patient groups, or other categories.

In the case of variable costs, this allocation process is generally straightforward, as variable costs can

usually be linked directly to specific patients' treatments. In fixed budget systems, however, even this step may pose a challenge, since cost accounting may not reflect this level of detail. In countries with free-floating currencies, converted sample costs from foreign EDs can be used to approximate these costs.

The allocation of fixed costs, however, is often more difficult. One approach may be to distribute the fixed costs according to estimates of their actual use within the facility. For example, an elderly patient with multiple medical and orthopedic issues who occupies a treatment room for four hours would be allocated a proportionally greater percentage of the department's rental costs than a patient with a simple complaint who occupies a treatment room for half an hour.

Special care must be taken in measuring and allocating personnel costs at the patient level. Although EDs do require a certain minimum level of staffing in order to safeguard the desired access to and availability of high-quality emergency care 24/7, one cannot therefore say that simply because the staff would have been on duty anyway their associated costs cannot be allocated to the individual patient. One still needs to understand the contribution of personnel costs to the overall cost of treating a patient in order to identify cost drivers with a potential for optimization efforts, as well as being able to align decisions about increasing staffing levels with the economic implications.

Personnel costs are best allocated according to the *capacity cost rate* of each occupational group.[6] Capacity cost rates are calculated by dividing the average annual expenses attributable to the employee by the available capacity of that individual. Average annual expenses for an employee include total salary and benefits and a prorated share of costs associated with employee supervision, office or other facilities used by that employee, as well as equipment, IT, and other support services used by that employee. The available capacity of the employee represents all of the time that the employee is available for actual work, which is the total number of days at work, minus time for lunch and other breaks, meetings, and education or training sessions.

For example, if an ED nurse has an annual salary including fringe benefits of US$65 000, supervision costs of US$9000, office space costs of US$10 800, technology and support costs of US$2560, then the total costs would be US$87 360 annually, or US$7280 monthly. The available capacity of the nurse is

365 days/year – 104 weekend days – 20 vacation days – 12 holidays – 5 sick days = 224 working days/year = 18.7 days/month. Starting with 7.5 hours/day – 0.5 hours for scheduled breaks – 1 hour for meetings, training, education = 6 hours/day. The nurse's availability for patient care is therefore 112 hours/month (6 hours/day × 18.7 days). The nurse's capacity cost rate is therefore US$7280 for 112 hours = US$65/hour, or US$1.08 per minute.[6]

If such values are calculated for each of the department's personnel groups, then personnel costs can be allocated to patient treatments in proportion to the time spent with patients for each process step. If, for example, a nurse spends on average 20 minutes with a chest pain patient, then the nursing cost for this patient group is: 20 minutes × US$1.08 = US$21.67 per patient. Adding up the total time spent on an average chest pain patient by each professional group and multiplied by the minute cost of each profession provides the total labor cost caused by an average patient with chest pain.

As mentioned earlier, hospital overhead costs must be taken into account when assessing the economic profitability of an ED. Strategies for allocating hospital overhead costs to individual departments may vary by institution and may be based on metrics such as departmental size as measured by square feet (or meters), total clinical revenues, numbers of patients seen, or other metrics.

The method of allocating overhead costs can have a major impact on the financial performance of the ED. For example, if the allocation is based on the number of patients treated, the ED will end up with a relatively higher share of overhead costs due to its high patient volume relative to other hospital departments. Unfairly allocated overhead costs can greatly influence a department's perceived financial performance such that a highly efficient and productive department can appear to be suffering financial losses simply because of inaccurate cost accounting.

This is why it is essential for ED leaders to understand the methodology by which overhead costs are allocated to their department. Using an innovative approach, Robert Kaplan and Michael E. Porter show how fixed overhead hospital costs can be more accurately allocated to the patient level using time-dependent activity-based costing.[6] Without going into further detail here, this method can provide administration as well as department leaders with a calculation which better reflects the share of overhead costs for each department.

These cost analyses are interesting not only for budget plans and general assessments of profitability. They can also be a basis for investment decisions in the ED. After all, economic implications must be taken into account when considering investing in equipment and/or changing processes within the ED.

Several financial models have been developed to assess whether or not a specific investment is profitable. All these models are based on the effects that the investment or process redesign in question is expected to have on the costs and the revenues of the department. Due to differences in the emergency care reimbursement modalities of different countries, we cannot present detailed calculation models such as the *net present value* model in this chapter, but will instead focus on the more general *cost–benefit analysis*. For cost–benefit analysis, the expected benefit of a measure (an investment or process redesign) is offset against that measure's expected cost. Here, the term *benefit* extends beyond purely monetary factors. Rather, benefits encompass all advantages realized by the measure, including parameters such as patient satisfaction and increased motivation of staff. Even though both of these variables are difficult to express in monetary terms, they play a key role in ensuring the long-term success of an ED.

On a critical note, most cost–benefit analyses have a problem of accuracy: their quality always depends on how accurately the costs and benefits have been estimated. Also, the findings of such analyses will always depend strongly on the factors taken into consideration. For illustrative purposes, the following case study on point-of-care testing (POCT) provides an indication of how complex such analyses quickly become.

> **Case study 11.1. Cost–benefit analysis of point-of-care testing (POCT)**
>
> The use of point-of-care diagnostics in emergency care can have potential medical, as well as financial, advantages: savings in diagnostic costs, streamlining the diagnostic processes, and improving overall workflow management – which together can theoretically reduce a patient's overall length of stay (LOS) in the ED. As part of a German study undertaken across three hospitals, a cost–benefit analysis was carried out for a POCT panel for patients with shortness of breath (troponin, D-dimer, CK-MB,

**Table 11.1** Process costs with and without POCT

| Description | Process cost with POCT | Process cost without POCT |
| --- | --- | --- |
| Labor costs: nursing care (7 Min) | €3.36 | €3.36 |
| With POCT: labor costs nursing care and S.O.B. panel | €20.50 | |
| With POCT: lab values | €2.90 | |
| Without POCT: lab values incl. troponin | | €12.00 |
| Labor costs: nursing care (8 min) | €3.84 | €3.84 |
| Labor costs: physician (14 min) | €11.20 | €11.20 |
| Cost of general materials (syringes, tubes, etc.) | €0.95 | €0.95 |
| ECG | €0.55 | €0.55 |
| Administration of O2 | €0.02 | €0.02 |
| With POCT: further diagnostics (chest x-ray, echo, etc.) | €7.70 | |
| Without POCT: further diagnostics (thorax x-ray, re-requisition for D-dimer, echo, etc.) | | €16.26 |
| Labor cost: physician (10 min) | €8.00 | €8.00 |
| Labor cost: nursing care (15 min) | €7.20 | €7.20 |
| ECG | €0.55 | €0.55 |
| Troponin (lab) | €9.10 | €9.10 |
| Total cost | €75.87 | €73.03 |

Source: Brachmann, 2011.[11]

BNP, and myoglobin).[11] The process-related costs of treating patients with shortness of breath were first measured without POCT. Costs were then measured for the same processes, with the difference that bedside POCT was used. All costs were measured comprehensively and allocated completely.

For example, hidden costs such as administrative and maintenance costs of the laboratories were taken into account, as well as additional personnel expenditures arising from operating the POCT system. The findings are summarized in Table 11.1.

Comparison of the costs related to ED processes showed that use of the POCT panel incurs additional ED costs of €2.84 per patient, despite the fact that bedside testing and early test results reduced the amount of further diagnostics that were required. A narrow interpretation of this data is that POCT costs more than it saves on additional diagnostics. However, it was found that the introduction of POCT also resulted in an average decrease in ED LOS of 45 minutes.

This reduction in LOS increased the ED's capacity to care for additional patients; the number of walk-outs who left a hospital without any examination by a physician was reduced, and both patient and employee satisfaction levels were increased. Together, these effects have a cumulative impact on the performance and attractiveness of the ED, which in turn increases the department's reputation and attracts more patients. In assessing whether or not to introduce POCT for patients with shortness of breath, €2.84 of added costs must be weighed against an average reduction in ED LOS of 45 minutes and the associated tangible and intangible benefits that this brings.

## Summary

The economic pressures on EDs to improve their efficiency can be expected to increase further in future. To be successful in the long run, EDs must therefore continue to work on optimizing their processes and on creating the transparency that is necessary for making economically sensible decisions. Along with optimizing the revenue side of activities, this also means ensuring full knowledge of the cost structure of the department.

The distinction between fixed and variable costs provides the ED leadership with a fundamental orientation: in the shorter term, variable costs are more amenable to cost containment, while fixed costs can only be influenced in the longer run. This is not to say, however, that fixed costs may be neglected. Even though they cannot be reduced from one day to the next, it is in the long-term interest of an ED to find ways to reduce the fixed costs.

From this chapter, it should be clear that in order to make useful, effective, and efficient decisions and to put available resources to optimal use, the ED leader needs a maximum of transparency concerning the conditions and consequences of his or her actions. This requires that hospital management supports the head of the department accordingly and provides him or her with access to the relevant data, including detailed revenues as well as costs. The way fixed costs are allocated to the different departments also is of great importance to fully appraise the department's performance. After all, it would seem only reasonable that an ED director, who is typically responsible for a greater number of patient contacts in the ED every year than is admitted to all of the inpatient hospital departments combined, can be entrusted with data on the ED's cost structure. Only with access to the relevant data can the ED management properly assess the economic consequences of its decisions.

Of course, basing decisions solely on cost deliberations would be negligent. This could be shown in the example of point-of-care testing. Instead, non-monetary factors must also be taken into consideration. In the end, efforts towards improving efficiency and reducing costs must never be made at the expense of compromising the quality of services or risking patient satisfaction.

# References

1. Plsek P. Complexity and the adoption of innovation in health care. In *Accelerating Quality Improvement in Health Care Strategies to Speed the Diffusion of Evidence-Based Innovations*. Washington, DC: National Institute for Health Care Management, 2003.

2. Organization for Economic Cooperation and Development. *Health Data 2011*. Paris: OECD, 2011.

3. Agency for Healthcare Research and Quality. *Medical Expenditure Panel Survey (MEPS)*. AHRQ, 2009.

4. Welsh F. Cost containment in emergency departments. *Healthcare Financial Management* 1995; **49**: 42–3, 45–6, 48.

5. Van de Leuv JH. *Management of Emergency Services*. Philadephia, PA: Lippincott Williams & Wilkins, 1987; 416.

6. Kaplan RS, Porter ME. How to solve the cost crisis in health care. *Harvard Business Review* 2011; **89**: 46–52, 54, 56–61.

7. Robinson JC. Hospital tiers in health insurance: balancing consumer choice with financial incentives. *Health Affairs (Millwood)* 2003; Suppl Web Exclusives: W3-135–146.

8. Carter P, Jackson N. Management, myth, and metatheory: from scarcity to postscarcity. *International Studies of Management and Organization* 1987; **17**: 64–89.

9. Georgopoulos BS. Organization structure and the performance of hospital emergency services. *Annals of Emergency Medicine* 1985; **14**: 677–84.

10. Bamezai A, Melnick G, Nawathe A. The cost of an emergency department visit and its relationship to emergency department volume. *Annals of Emergency Medicine* 2005; **45**: 483–90.

11. Brachmann M. Prozessoptimierung durch Point-of-Care-Testung In W von Eiff, C Dodt, M Brachmann, *et al.*, eds., *Management der Notaufnahme*. Berlin: Kohlhammer, 2011: 321–6.

# Further reading

## Costs in general
Mankiw G. *Principles of Economics*. Cincinatti, OH: South-West College Publishers, 2010.

## Advanced economies of scale
Krugman PR. Scale economies, product differentiation and the pattern of trade. *American Economic Review* 1980; **70**: 950–9.

Frisch R. *Theory of Production*. Dordrecht: D. Reidel, 1965.

## Cost accounting
Colin D. *Cost and Management Accounting: an Introduction*. London: Thomson, 2006.

## Cost–benefit analysis
Folland S, Goodman AC, Stano M. *The Economics of Heath and Health Care*, 5th edn. Upper Saddle River, NJ: Pearson Prentice Hall, 2007.

# Human resource management

# 12

Mary Leupold

## Key learning points

- The importance of marketing an organization for prospective employees.
- Understanding the employment laws that govern the industry.
- The need for continual monitoring of staff satisfaction.
- How to create and implement a comprehensive performance review program.
- How to mediate when faced with a disruptive employee.

## Introduction

It is 4 o'clock in the afternoon and somewhere a parent is concerned about a child's fever not breaking; a car accident with multiple injuries just took place; a local factory is being evacuated for hazardous fumes – and all of these people are headed to your trauma center. While you may identify with this as a routine day in the life of an emergency department (ED), one facet that will dictate the level of care these patients receive will center upon your ability to build a successful ED team. This team will need to work as a cohesive group in order to provide the highest attainable standard of health care for patients, no matter what continent you practice on.

## How to create, develop, and enhance your workforce

If you are looking to create or enhance the emergency services in your organization, it is necessary to first review your existing structure. To assist you with this, your first hire should be a chief administrative officer (CAO). While the title may vary depending on the organization, this position provides internal and external coordination, management, and oversight of all administrative activities related to the development and implementation of the mission and instructional goals of the organization.[1] Filling this role with an experienced person whose personality and work ethic complements your ideals is crucial to building a strong practice.

Together, you will need to complete a comprehensive assessment of the current operational structure. One key element of the assessment will be the staffing plan. Your ability to successfully hire qualified staff will be critical to providing quality patient care. Finding the right people to complement one another will bring about a positive environment for both patients and existing staff. Fundamentally, your process for recruitment through hiring, if designed correctly, will amount to a successful physician hire.

Figure 12.1 may be helpful when drafting your departmental hiring practices. This illustrates the various areas requiring consideration before you can have a successful physician hire.

## The marketing message

Before you can move forward on your staffing plan, it is necessary to develop a clear message that promotes your department's assets for the recruitment process. Take the time to identify favorable attributes that exist within your organization and use this as the foundation of your marketing plan. This message allows applicants to assess their eagerness to know more about your organization and potentially develop a desire to want to come and work there.

Talented physicians know they have a choice in where they work, and you will therefore need to allocate time and money toward marketing your department. How do you make your department

*Emergency Department Leadership and Management*, ed. Stephanie Kayden, *et al.* Published by Cambridge University Press.
© Cambridge University Press 2015.

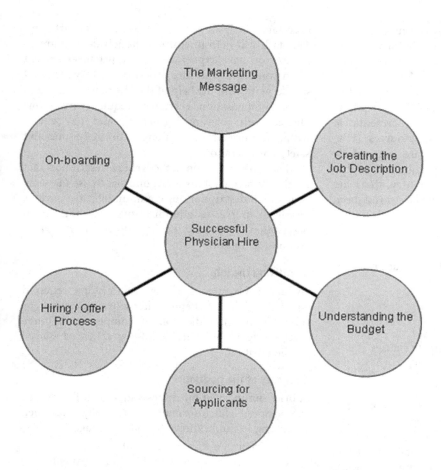

**Figure 12.1** The components of successful physician hire. The process starts at 12:00 (the marketing message) and proceeds clockwise around the circle.

stand out among the competition? When creating your marketing message you should consider your existing organization's mission statement or vision and tie it into your department's message. Think about what your department is known for. How do your employees, and possibly your patients, rank your organization as compared to the competition? Do they remark on your dedication to customer service? Are you recognized for certain types of patient care? Applicants today have access to more information than ever before. It is not uncommon for candidates to have researched your organization and department before they even consider interviewing for a position in your department.

Increased globalization has allowed workers the opportunity to find work in other countries. Today, for a well-trained and experienced emergency physician, increased opportunities exist where they once did not. Keep in mind that there may be immigration laws that you need to be familiar with. Physicians

looking for the opportunity to experience life in a different part of the world are more apt to be successful in this endeavor. There are many things that can attract a physician to relocate. Sometimes marriage or extended family obligations contribute, the location may capture one's attention, or in other cases the pay and benefits may be the deciding factor. Other physicians may find working in a developing country, or providing humanitarian assistance in the wake of disasters or other catastrophic events, to be a fulfilling experience. These and other experiences can offer the employee a range of opportunities that, together with providing patient care, constitute a compelling professional position.

## Know the law

How does one tackle the issue of maintaining one's knowledge of industry and government regulations? A skilled employment lawyer can assist you in working through numerous issues you may encounter in the employee/employer work relationship. The experienced attorney will have a method to stay abreast of the current changes in legislation and keep you informed. Not every employment matter requires the advice of an employment lawyer. Many issues can be worked through with a representative from your organization's human resources (HR) department. However, those that are particularly challenging may require legal expertise. While it is impossible to list regulations by country, there are some topics that are referenced in law throughout the world:

- labor/trade union
- dispute resolution
- behavior – harassment and discrimination
- benefits
- workplace health and safety
- immigration
- termination
- loyalty, trade secrets, non-compete clauses
- taxation, wages and salaries
- privacy

Although typically it is your HR or legal department that will most likely negotiate the legal fee arrangement with any outside employment lawyer that you use, it is important for you to understand the details of this arrangement to avoid any misunderstandings concerning billing hours, fees, and other costs that you might occur.

While avoiding costly litigation is not always possible, there are some things you can do to minimize your exposure. Treating all employees consistently, having effective communication, and documenting interactions as required will aid in creating a positive work environment. It is important to react to and defuse behaviors that might interfere with the functioning of the workplace. In other words, lead by example. If you work to create a positive and cohesive work environment for your team, their ability to address issues and formulate solutions will pay off with increased productivity.

## Job analysis

Before you can set out to attract qualified employees you must understand each skill set needed for your staffing plan. Although creating a list of roles, duties, and responsibilities is not that exciting, it is a necessary analysis for a functioning department. This task will help in crafting the job description to ensure you have expressed the competencies needed when you begin your hire process. You or your CAO should work with the help of the HR representative to assess compensation, recruiting requirements, compliance with relevant legislation, and pay equity within the organization, along with ergonomic and safety considerations.

The job description is the written description that details the actual job. It is not unusual to use the same general job description for common job titles such as physician, nurse, or administrative assistant. A job description is usually broken down into various sections, as follows.

### Identifying the job

Include a job title, reporting relationships, required work schedule (weekends, alternative schedules, or telecommuting), indication of compensation grade level, along with other identifying criteria required by the position.

### Summary of the position

A brief summary of the duties and responsibilities for the position. This information is typically used when recruiting in publications. Sample language:

- physician in a full-service, acute-care community hospital with 45 000 ED patient visits annually
- 24-hour single attending MD coverage
- proven skills to assess, evaluate, diagnose, and provide initial treatment to patients of all ages and cultures
- trained in core emergency medicine procedures preferred

### Details of duties and job responsibilities

In this section you will want to list both the essential and non-essential job responsibilities. You may want to consider a bullet format for easier reading by the prospective candidate, such as:

- airway techniques
- anesthesia
- cardiac procedures
- diagnostic procedures
- genitourinary techniques
- head and neck
- hemodynamic techniques

- thoracic procedures
- other techniques as required

### Skills and education requirements

Outlining core skills, required certifications, licensure, and educational requirements for the position will allow candidates to determine whether they meet these requirements. Depending on the job, it may be prudent to include physical requirements such as an ability to lift a specific weight.

## Review and authorization

Depending on your organization and its approval criteria, you may need both departmental and HR authorization prior to a position being approved.

## The recruitment budget

When you set out to create your budget, you may need to set aside funds for recruitment activity if your HR department does not cover this expense. Recruitment costs can vary by position. If you find the need to recruit beyond the local market, decisions on use of recruitment firms, medical journals, and other media sources will require financial resources. If you are recruiting for positions in leadership areas, you may want to cover travel expenses. Your organization may have special negotiated pricing with local hotels. Another area to be aware of is the potential request for relocation assistance. This can come in the form of low-interest housing loans, moving expenses, or temporary housing. Since tax regulations can vary by country, it is recommended that you consult with your finance department or tax attorney.

## Looking for applicants

Now that you have identified the marketing message, job analysis, and recruitment budget you can finally begin to create a candidate pool. Knowing where to search for applicants can mean the difference between a lengthy vacancy and timely hire. There is no single way to find applicants; over time you will discover what options result in the greatest return on investment. One of the most powerful and least costly strategies is word of mouth. Let your current organization and team spread your message. When that is not enough, other options to consider include both internal and external routes.

### Internal pipelines

Looking within your organization may be an option for enticing recruits. Consider sponsoring a residency or training program that will provide access to a well-trained candidate pool. Promoting from within can pay off in numerous ways, including increased employee satisfaction, upfront knowledge of the candidate's work ethic, and heightened interest from potential future candidates on the training program.

### External recruitment

When you do not have the option to look within, you may find yourself looking beyond even your community for qualified individuals. Knowing your organization's strengths and weaknesses will help define the routine sources you may need to use. Types of external opportunities can include:

- Recruitment firms
  - use the resources of a larger candidate pool
  - screen candidates prior to interview process for realistic matches
- Media at the local, national, and/or international level
  - examples of international publications
    - *Annals of Emergency Medicine*
    - *Internal and Emergency Medicine*
  - examples of US publications
    - *New England Journal of Medicine*
    - *JAMA*
- Aligning with an educational, military, or training institution
  - for difficult-to-fill positions consider working with a local or international academic institution to sponsor a fellowship training program to enhance your talent pool
  - consider local military branches that have trained emergency medical professionals
  - align with an international partner to attract talent to your region of the world
- Internet marketing/job posting
  - consider various internet candidate pools to reach a larger market of candidates
  - posting on the organization's website
  - posting with local or international medical schools

You have received notice that one of your senior physicians is leaving to take on a new role outside your organization. This termination will result in numerous uncovered shifts that now must be absorbed by existing staff. In an effort to expedite the hiring process you forgo placing advertisements in local and national journals and opt to select from CVs you have kept on file. Following your screening of CVs and a phone interview, you inform the staff that Dr. Y will be starting in three weeks. Three months into the employment you are surprised to hear from your senior staff less than favorable comments concerning his interactions with staff and patients. On paper this candidate looked promising, and he interviewed well over the phone. You wonder what you could have done differently to avoid this.

# Hiring practices

Hiring practices vary throughout the world. It is important to have policies at the organizational level that support these practices. You can use your job description to identify general qualities and skills that you will look for from a qualified candidate. You have marketed your position in a variety of internal and/or external locations. Now it is time to decide on how to screen, interview, and select a candidate for the position.

It may be beneficial for you and your CAO to designate a group of people to participate in a search committee. While you may not need this with all positions, professional staff hiring brings a need for this type of committee. Consider selecting three senior physicians with expertise in the areas of clinical, teaching, and research. Responsibilities of the group will include applicant screening, interviews, and follow-up assessments.

You should inquire whether your HR department offers training to support the hiring process. Committee members may benefit from the regulatory, diversity, and formal hiring guidance. This training supports consistency throughout the organization. Beth Israel Deaconess Medical Center, located in Boston, Massachusetts, USA, has adapted an interviewing skills workshop for all managers fittingly called "Does a fish know it's swimming?"[2] Managers are required to participate in this course. The premise is that if you have a standardized practice for

applicant flow review, interviewing, offers, and new hire orientation, each applicant will be treated in like fashion without consideration of gender, race, or other defining aspects.

It helps for a search committee to have an agreed-upon procedure to follow throughout the recruitment process. A suggested process includes the four steps of CV screening, interviewing, debriefing, and offering the position.

## Step 1: CV screening

When completing an initial CV screening, focus on required education level, hospital of training, and any previous experience. Assessing experience will vary depending on the duties of the position. For example, a research position will have additional weight given to first or senior authorship on papers and other publications, as well as past and future potential for grant funding. In contrast, a purely clinical position will value hands-on emergency medicine training and clinical experience. Finally, if you are hiring for a management position, previous experience in management positions will be an indicator of a potential match.

## Step 2: interviews

Phone interviews are useful if candidates are not local or if you want to expand on elements of the presented CV before committing to a formal interview. On-site interviews will narrow down the candidate pool. Typically the department chief will take part in this process when the field of candidates is narrowed down.

If you have candidates coming from outside your area, prepare a welcome packet with reference material on a variety of subjects such as shopping, schools, theater, arts, and sporting events. If you offer the candidate a position in your organization this extra material may help him or her to decide on whether to accept your offer. Another successful part of the interviewing process is to provide your candidates with an itinerary ahead of time so that they have an idea of what to expect and how to prepare. Providing this information in advance will present your organization in a positive light. A sample itinerary is shown in Table 12.1.

Prepare for your interview. Asking the same types of questions of each applicant will provide you with

**Table 12.1** Sample itinerary for the interview process

| Itinerary item | Value to applicant | Value to employer |
|---|---|---|
| Interview schedule with time, location, directions, name and job title of each person who will be interviewing the candidate | Positive impression of the company and shows the process is taken seriously | Assesses applicant's ability to prepare for interviews; create "best foot forward" image |
| Tour of facility or work unit | Allows applicant to assess a typical day | Allows for assessment and feedback on relating past experience to your facility |
| Impromptu introductions to other workers | Starts to formulate the work culture fit | Assesses ability to interact with various subsets of employees |

**Table 12.2** Sample areas for questioning during an interview

| Area | Sample questions |
|---|---|
| Service quality | Explain a time when you had to deal with an extremely emotional patient or family member and how you handled the situation. What was the outcome? How did you resolve a major conflict with a patient? |
| Cultural competency | You will encounter employees or patients that are different from you, be it in culture, belief, or mental or physical abilities. Describe a situation where you encountered a patient different from you and what approach you took in caring for them. Work situations require us to interact with some people we dislike. Describe a situation like this that you have encountered, and explain how you handled it. |
| Collaboration and teamwork | Tell me about a situation when you encountered conflicting priorities with a co-worker. What did you do to work out an agreement? When contacting your co-workers for references, how would they describe you as a team player? |
| Initiative | Give an example of a time when you sought to improve the way work is done in your department? What are the most important contributions or improvements you have made to your practice, community, or hospital? |
| Communication | Describe a time when you had to communicate something unpleasant or a mistake made to your direct report. How did you handle the situation? How do you avoid communication mishaps at your place of work? Tell me about a time when you did not communicate effectively, and what you did to fix the problem. |

comparisons. During the interview consider the following process:

- Welcome the candidate
  - outline what the interview will entail
- Areas of questioning and examples (Table 12.2)
- Close the interview
  - recap the position and the organization
  - invite questions
  - tour the facility

## Step 3: debrief

The committee members should be prepared to discuss their observations concerning the candidate's competencies with respect to the job. Were there any concerns about the candidate? Will he or she be a good fit? When you are done answering these questions you may want to assess your responses. Were your comments driven by any personal biases? Did you draw positive or negative conclusions because of them? It is important to give a candidate the opportunity to be assessed on the same merits as all other applicants. As you narrow down the pool of candidates, you will want to check references prior to presenting final candidates to the department chief. The chief will then interview, and a final decision will be made. A job offer will need to be prepared. The committee is feeling good about the process and decision, but what if the candidate does not accept? It is important during the process to keep a watchful eye on the candidate's continued interest in the job. For those just finishing their postgraduate specialty training, it may be prudent to ask where else they have interest in working.

## Step 4: the offer

Offers of employment are handled in a variety of ways. You may want to check with your HR department for established procedures. An example of this may be first making a verbal offer then following up with a written formal offer and contract, typically called an employment agreement. While it is not required, you may wish to request a written acceptance. Your offer should outline any items that are conditions of employment, such as licensure, credentialing, and other pre-employment requirements. The offer should instruct the candidate to review the employment agreement with their counsel, then to sign and return. Consider creating a template for an employment agreement for your professional staff. This will provide consistency among employment offers and offer a baseline of expectations. It is important that the wording in this document explicitly states that it replaces any other verbal or written offers previously discussed.

It is important that you support your organization's pre-employment requirements and ensure that they are completed prior to the start date. This is another task that is easily delegated to your CAO. These can include but are not limited to the following:

- A pre-employment health screen is routinely required for healthcare workers. Typically these screens will assess immunization and other precautionary measures to protect both patients and staff.
- Background screens can be considered intrusive, but it can be in the organization's best interest to know whether your prospective hire has been convicted of a crime or some other offense.

Understanding the laws that apply to your organization with respect to protecting patients and other staff will assist in determining the need for these reviews. There are a number of firms that can provide both domestic and international reviews.

- Not all organizations require drug and alcohol testing prior to employment. Your HR department can work with you if you feel this is necessary.
- Credentialing is another important aspect of hiring physicians and other medical professionals. A prescribed format for obtaining documents and confirming authenticity should be a standard part of your hiring practice. Your organization may have a department that handles these verifications. Regardless who is responsible, the ideal way to gather this information is to ask the new hire to complete a credentialing packet that will be used to ascertain the legitimacy of the candidate's history. Items to consider reviewing are:

  o education and certificates received (make sure that you request contact information, dates of attendance, and other vital information)
  o license and any other mandated requirements for treating, prescribing, and caring for patients
  o if malpractice insurance is a requirement, request a history to better understand any possible prior claims on the provider
  o references are important from former supervisors and colleagues to better understand work behavior and knowledge of the specialty
  o employment history will highlight any breaks in employment history

You should plan to work with the prospective hire to ensure a successful and timely start date. Tracking of your desired timeline is prudent.

## New hire process

Having a formal hiring process for your new employee will aid in a successful orientation to your organization. A part of this process will include payroll, benefits, general orientation information, training requirements; even a map of your institution is helpful to someone new to your facility. With all the effort put into hiring quality staff, it is important that the new hire process helps to bring about a welcoming environment, job satisfaction, and retention.

## Staff satisfaction and retention

Having spent a significant amount of time and money to recruit excellent employees to work for you and your organization, the one thing you do not want to happen is for the new hire to leave your organization because you were not able to keep him or her satisfied. It is important to spend time developing strategies on how to support and retain your employees. Retaining qualified, dedicated, and satisfied employees requires that you get to know them well and respond to their needs. This will ensure that your employees are highly satisfied, committed, and loyal both to your department and to the organization as a whole.

When setting out to create this structured program, make sure to include those within the department and organization who can sell the message. The first few weeks should focus on making your new employee feel part of the team. Welcoming your new staff member and his or her family into your community will get you off to the right start. This includes simple things such as providing an extensive tour of your facility so that the new employee is able to get around easily (if yours is a large facility you may want to consider a map). Another thoughtful gesture would be to consider how your new employee will be getting to work (car, public transportation, bicycle). If your organization is in a location where parking is not easily accessible, something as simple as arranging for temporary parking for the first week will go a long way.

Making sure your new employee has the right tools to successfully get the job done is essential. In the first few weeks you should be prepared to have someone in your organization adequately train your new employee on the computer systems as well as the phone systems. Provide a list of important phone numbers to avoid lengthy searches. This may sound insignificant, but to a new employee it is critical. Meeting key players in your organization who can help answer clinical and operational questions in the beginning will be helpful. Making sure your new employee has an assigned "go-to" person or role model in the organization can positively influence your new employee in the long run. The bottom line is that you need to make sure each employee has

what he or she needs to get settled in the new position and ultimately perform the job successfully.

Make sure you follow up at various intervals within the first year to assess the new hire's progress. This dual feedback will benefit both the employee and the orientation program. Remember to include in your orientation any other training requirements such as employee compliance, fire safety, or organization-specific training. The more you empower each new employee with the required expectations, the greater will be that person's successful transition to your organization.

Your HR department will most likely want to meet with your new employee prior to his or her start date, but at the very least it should be done within the first few days. Some laws may require your new employee to complete paperwork for work authorization in a timely manner. Another important reason for your new employee to meet with someone in the HR department early is to assist him or her with choosing benefits. Benefits and compensation can be viewed as a form of motivation that is used to attract and retain your workforce.

The benefits and compensation package you offer is usually very important to your employees and their families. Understanding mandatory benefits, costs, tax structure, and any labor union requirements is of great importance. One must identify programs that enhance the quality of life for people. You will need to understand the needs of health insurance, life and disability insurance, and saving for retirement. Access to these programs and how they are funded will vary. Understanding what government benefits are available will help to tailor your organization's package. Knowing whether certain regulations require or prevent offering certain benefits is essential. Working with your HR department to design a comprehensive program will enhance your leverage for attracting talented personnel and improving the morale of existing staff. How you value your workers will have an impact on patient satisfaction.

When considering what to offer, your program will have to conform to your budget. Knowing what mandatory programs you are required to offer will start to scope out your program. Do you need to offer traditional welfare, retirement, and/or accident and sick leave programs? Consider identifying what brings the greatest value. If your culture puts greater emphasis on caring for your elders, retirement income replacement programs may be top on your list.

Other aspects of the job that add to the physician's satisfaction will include the patients and case mix at your hospital, the culture of the company, including rapport among colleagues, and other administrative or academic advancements provided. The more a new employee feels like a part of your organization and community, the more likely it is that he or she will be committed to the success of your organization.

## Evaluation of performance

The relationship between an employee and an employer can be complex. While both the employee and the employer have an expectation of a cohesive work environment, often this can be marred by internal and external issues that disrupt business objectives. Learning to navigate, diffuse, and eliminate sources of tension may not be as easy as you think. If labor laws apply they can be complex. It is important that you, your CAO, and/or HR representative have a clear understanding of any company-defined dispute resolution programs that may come from labor contracts or government regulations.

## Creating a code of conduct

Consider using a code of conduct as one way to drive your desired work ethics and behavior. A document that everyone agrees to abide by is a method to ensure your workforce understands what is considered acceptable conduct.[3] A code of conduct can contain the following:

- Statement of commitment, e.g., "We are committed to helping all employees, staff physicians, and contractors act in a way that preserves the trust and respect of those whom we serve and with whom we deal"[3]
- Definition of core values that guide actions in the workplace: core values may include integrity, community, excellence, service, compassion, and respect
- Statement on confidentiality and protecting patient privacy
- Statement on quality and standards for professional practice
- Statement on legal responsibilities
- Statement on payments, discounts, and gifts
- Statement on billing and claims

- Statement on false claims
- Statement on conflict of interest
- Statement on responsible use of assets
- Statement on treatment and work environment practices
- Statement on HR policies and treatment of others
- Information concerning voluntary reporting: stress confidentiality and no-retaliation rules
- Certification and impact of violation of the code of conduct policy

## Creating an evaluation process

Employees in general tend to need validation of their work performance. Employers can provide this by creating an evaluation process. This can be used for a number of positive outcomes. Consider the poor performer who requires counseling, the average employee who meets expectations, and the employee who exceeds expectations. Every employee can benefit from performance feedback. Creating a formal review process that outlines expectations will enhance the desired effects for both new and existing employees.

Feedback for a new employee in intervals of 3, 6, and 12 months, and yearly thereafter, increases the effectiveness of the employee's ability to transition into his or her job duties. Annual reviews can highlight the past year's successes. It is also important to identify areas of improvement or goals for future development and potential compensation adjustments. Items discussed at these meetings will differ depending on position (e.g., physician vs. nurse).

Standard expectations in a review can include:

- ability to collaborate and work with the team
- respect for privacy and confidentiality of both patients and other employees
- attendance and punctuality
- responsibility and follow-through on assignments
- patient/customer service excellence
- quality of work
- specific job competencies (assessing procedure outcomes, number of admits, and patient satisfaction)

While we strive to create an environment that allows employees to exceed expectations, this does not always happen when it comes to employee interactions. It is important for management to address, defuse, and educate staff when issues arise. Having a well-established corrective action process will allow you to be consistent in dealing with similar issues. We are all human. At some point you will come across a performance issue for which management will need to investigate the root causes. This assessment should determine if this is systemic to the department or specific to the individual. If departmental, you may want to consider bringing in someone from HR's occupational development team or an outside consultant to help work through the issues. If it is determined that the individual is the problem, you need to go further in your assessment to identify what further action needs to be taken.

## Creating a fitness-for-duty policy for health-related issues

Evaluate the need for a fitness-for-duty policy. The purpose of this type of policy is to ensure that clinicians receive timely and appropriate attention when issues arise concerning their own health, such as chronic, acute, or mental problems, and/or substance abuse. Assess whether you have the resources for an on-site clinician health services program or need to outsource this service. This policy works best if there is a two-tiered approach, giving both the clinician a self-referral option and the chief a process to follow in case of a potentially harmful situation.

### Self-referral

The self-referral option allows individuals to confidentially discuss any personal or work-related issue they may be experiencing before it escalates into a larger issue.

Creating this confidential self-referral program allows the clinician to request and expeditiously receive the opportunity to discuss health concerns, seek assistance with problem solving, and receive recommendations for ongoing treatment if needed. The fact that the program is cost-neutral to the clinician eliminates the financial deterrent to obtaining help. It is recommended that the number of sessions be capped, as this should be used as assessment rather than ongoing treatment, and it does not become part of the medical record. It is important to remember that chiefs will not receive any feedback or confirmation of these visits before, during, or after, unless it is requested by the clinician seeking the assistance or it is determined that the impairment has the potential to impact the quality and safety of the clinical practice

of the clinician. In fact, you may not even be aware that one of your clinicians is taking advantage of the program.

> **Case study 12.2**
>
> A clinician recently experienced a traumatic event in his personal life. The clinician is now feeling overwhelmed and preoccupied at work and is struggling to keep it from interfering with patient care. Particularly difficult is providing care for patients who present with a similar condition. The clinician remembers receiving information from HR regarding a program that provides a safe place to discuss concerns, assist with problem solving, and make recommendations for ongoing treatment, if indicated. Reaching out to Clinician Health Services (CHS), arrangements were made to meet with one of the psychologists that same day. The clinician was reminded when scheduling that up to three confidential psychiatric consultations would be provided with no out-of-pocket cost, and that information would not be shared with others unless permission was granted or in extreme circumstances, such as threat of harm to self or others. Together with the psychologist, a treatment program was suggested to continue forward progress in working through these issues while at the same time continuing employment and effectively caring for the patients.

### Chief referral

It would be easier if you could always count on clinicians being able to recognize their own personal issues, but this is not always the case. Over time it is inevitable that you will encounter an employee who may exhibit conduct or behavior that indicates the possibility of mental health or substance abuse issues. The chief must move in quickly to minimize any harm to patients and staff by initiating an investigation. This may include a meeting, or a mandatory requirement to present to your on-site employee occupational health services. It is always important to remind the clinician of the clinician health services program. These types of events will illustrate how important it is to have a well-thought-out assessment tool.

It is important to foster an environment where employees, both clinical and non-clinical, feel comfortable bringing concerns to your attention, whether it relates to professional conduct, patient care, or patient and/or personal safety. Having a pre-designed process will allow you to treat all concerns consistently from one employee to the next. It will be important to determine if the individual is not fit to perform some or all of his or her work functions and if necessary to remove him or her from service until cleared to return to work. Depending on the individual situation, a formal return-to-work plan may be needed for a successful re-entry to the workplace. Given the delicate nature of such matters, chiefs should not be the sole decision maker when it comes to a return-to-work plan. Your policy should include a senior-level independent panel to review anonymously the situation and action plan, with the expectation that they may accept, amend, or deny it. Having a panel should help to defuse any concerns of biased treatment between employee and chief.

## Expanding your policy for non-health-related issues

Having a disruptive employee or an employee whose conduct is inappropriate can result in loss of productivity, decrease in patient satisfaction, and poor morale among other employees. Understanding your institution's tolerance for these types of behaviors is the first step in arming yourself to identify, defuse, and resolve the situation. While a fit-for-duty policy helps to assess health-related situations, having a formally adopted set of rules to which clinicians and management must adhere for patient care and job conduct will eliminate the guesswork should an incident occur. Earlier we discussed the need for a code of conduct, which can be included with what some institutions call "medical staff bylaws." These bylaws outline expectations with respect to patient care and privileges. This is a document that should be presented during your orientation process, along with subsequent updates to reinforce the importance of proper patient care and conduct.

How do you define a disruptive employee? Factors that can contribute to these elements of dissatisfaction can include items that relate to:

- attendance and/or tardiness
- on-the-job conduct
- hygiene or choice of inappropriate clothing
- use of profanity and tone when speaking
- aggressive or threatening behavior
- insubordination or violation of company rules

While there are many other variations, how you handle any form of misconduct must be addressed in a consistent manner. Much as when patient presenting to the ED with a medical problem, you must complete an initial assessment on the circumstances leading up to the behavior. Typically you can break down an issue into one of three classifications:

- level 1: minor issue that can be addressed internally within the department
- level 2: serious issue that requires peer/independent review
- level 3: critical issue that requires immediate action by governing board

### Level 1: minor infraction

Disruptive behaviors such as those involving attendance, attitude, and department dynamics usually can be handled informally through a discussion with the chief or another senior member of the department. Different people may exhibit similar behaviors, yet the issues leading up to the event(s) can vary dramatically. The ability to differentiate minor departmental issues from those that are more serious in nature will result in your ability to address the issue in a timely fashion.

---

**Case study 12.3**

You have two employees who are both having issues interacting with colleagues, patients, and visitors. They differ in age, demographics, and family life. Over the past three months both have exhibited unusual behavior that is disrupting workflow and staff morale. As chief, you know you need to speak with both employees regarding these issues. The first employee is recently widowed and a parent of small children who is trying to manage work while adapting to the loss of a spouse. The other employee is single and has a laid-back attitude with respect to authority and work in general. Do you treat them the same, in a similar way, or vastly differently?

Consistency in how you handle any employment situation is best. The way in which you handle the situation not only adds to the credibility of department rules, it emphasizes your recognition of the importance of the contribution of each member of the team to the overall functioning of the department. That said, it is important to understand and assess each situation individually.

Meeting with the employee is the first step in investigating the circumstances surrounding recent

---

complaints or behaviors. It is hard to imagine that the team would not feel empathy for the newly widowed employee; however, the impact on the rest of the staff must also be taken into consideration. While the behavior must be corrected, you may find your discussion centering on ways to assist the employee. Offering a leave of absence, schedule modifications, and access to the clinician assistance program may prove beneficial. Subsequent follow-up with the employee should be scheduled as needed.

Your meeting with the second employee does not reveal options for easily mitigating the behavior. In fact, the employee does not recognize the behavior as problematic. In this instance further intervention may be needed. You suggest that the employee consider attending a class in behavior modification or dealing with difficult encounters. The individual does not follow through with these suggestions, and while the behavior tempers it does continue. Complaints from other staff and patients continue and you are now faced with a second meeting, where you mandate enrollment in the class.

While the first example does not require the need for an independent disciplinary review, it is important to document the department-level investigation. If the behavior continues, or if there is a pattern of recurrence, you may find the need to take more aggressive action. In the case of the second employee, the individual did not improve, and the situation required initiating the disciplinary action process under level 2: serious infraction.

## Level 2: serious infraction

The initiation of a disciplinary process should include a series of events that result in determination of the clinician's ongoing employment. Whether it is clinically related or professional conduct inconsistent with, or harmful to, patient care and safety, the chief of the department should formally request a disciplinary review, citing the evidence supporting the need for disciplinary action. While your process will be unique to your institution, you may consider the creation of an independent investigative committee made up of three or four individuals, which should include peer members and other senior-level personnel familiar with the details of the investigation. This committee should have a set timeline and report back to senior leadership with recommendations for remediation.

When a recommendation for disciplinary action occurs it is important to allow the clinician the ability to appeal the decision. Your process should include having an appeal process with a pre-described governing board. Setting a maximum timeline for each stage of the appeal will keep the process moving and result in a timely resolution. The outcome of this appeal process will result in upholding, modifying, or overturning the findings and the disciplinary action.

In the case of the employee who has had repeated complaints concerning behavior and fails to follow up on the department-suggested behavior modification class, the independent peer review could result in the recommendation for an unpaid suspension until there is documentation that a behavior modification class has been completed. A return-to-work plan should include scheduled check-ins to reinforce improvement initiatives. If the employee cannot improve, it may be best to start discussions for moving into a more suitable work environment. If there is an employment agreement, it may be best to exercise the "termination without cause" notification even though you may be at a "termination for cause" point. This should allow for an easier passage of the termination process.

## Level 3: critical infraction

If the nature of the action or behavior is critical enough, it may require an automatic removal of clinical privileges and employment. These types of events usually include the revocation of a license to practice medicine or a violation of physician standards of care. In certain cases the employee may be able to rectify the condition causing the suspension. It is the responsibility of the clinician to request a re-evaluation and reinstatement. In certain conditions the governing board may reinstate a physician, but in most cases a plan for continued correction or monitoring will need to be implemented to ensure ongoing adherence to the rules. This is especially important if a clinician is returning from a substance addiction. Given the circumstances, an appeal process similar to that used in level 2 should be implemented; however, the clinician should not be allowed to return to patient care until the outcome is determined. The situation will dictate if this is a paid or unpaid administrative leave. If the critical situation is health-related, the employee should be encouraged to follow up with the clinician health services program and the HR department for care and determination of eligibility for sick/disability pay.

It is important to remember that while clinicians are trained to take care of others they may neglect to take care of themselves. The role of management is to recognize and respond to situations that impact their employees' personal well-being. Having resources that can help the clinician work through personal issues will make him or her a better physician and create a positive work environment.

### Case study 12.4

You receive a call from your manager on call that a clinician is acting out of the norm and is exhibiting behaviors that resemble being under the influence of an unknown substance. You are familiar with the clinician and instruct the manager to arrange for coverage, to remove the clinician from service, to call security if the situation warrants, and to tell the employee to present to the chief. The chief must assess the situation for concern for professional conduct or personal and/or patient safety. In the chief's professional opinion there is a concern for professional conduct, personal and patient safety, and the clinician is referred for a "fitness to serve" evaluation. The chief or her designee informs HR to place the employee on administrative leave and works to enact an independent investigative committee. The committee evaluates the findings of the fitness-to-serve evaluation, which supports that there is concern for personal and patient safety. The employee is then referred for clinical care. After two months of care it is determined that the employee may be able to return to the workplace, but the treating clinician recommends a return-to-work plan. The plan is presented to the independent investigative committee for evaluation. The committee must decide whether the employee can return to work based on the plan, or whether the original offense violated policy and requires termination of employment.

## Conclusion

This chapter is intended as a starting point for some of the more important aspects to consider in your quest to create or enhance your ED. These human resources concepts will help you establish the foundation of running the "people" part of your department. It is important to develop an administrative working relationship with your HR and legal departments. Knowing when to involve these professionals can directly impact your employment outcomes.

## References

1. Chief administrative officer: job duties, requirements and career information. *Education Portal. com.* http://education-portal.com/articles/Chief_Administrative_Officer_Job_Duties_ Requirements_and_Career_Information.html (accessed November 15, 2010).

2. Interview with G. Shillin, Chief Administrative Officer, Emergency Medicine, November 4, 2010 (M. Leupold, interviewer).

3. Interview with A. Jarvey, Director, Professional Staff Affairs/Regulatory Compliance, Health Care Quality, Beth Israel Deaconess Medical Center, April 14 and 28, 2010 (M. Leupold, interviewer).

Chapter

# 13

# Project management

Lee A. Wallis, Leana S. Wen, and Sebastian N. Walker

## Key learning points

- Project management is a structured, repeatable approach to planning and guiding a project from initiation to completion.
- Applying the fundamentals of a robust project management methodology to emergency medicine projects maximizes efficiency and impact.
- Every project has three main components: scope, timeline, and cost. Any change to one element invariably alters the others.
- The four steps of the project management cycle are initiation, planning, executing/controlling, and closing.

## Introduction

Co-authored by two emergency medicine (EM) physicians and a project manager, this chapter explains the fundamentals of project management as applied to EM. We start with the framework of delineating what a project manager would require to start planning a project, and work through the four-step cycle of project management methodology. Examples of three EM-specific projects are provided along the way to illustrate the practicalities of each step as they apply to our field. Project management is a critical skill used daily by EM leaders, and our objective is that by the end of the chapter readers will be able to incorporate the key aspects of project management into maximizing the impact and efficiency of their next project.

Running an organization as complex and multifaceted as an emergency department (ED) requires the simultaneous management of multiple projects. All emergency physician and nurse leaders and administrators who have planned and executed a project have had experience in project management. We have an intuitive understanding of what is required to manage a project, yet few of us have the business and administrative training to clearly define all the steps involved. In the same way that advanced cardiac life support and advanced trauma life support provide time-tested algorithms for standard complaints, project management methodology is an algorithm that ensures all key components of planning and executing a project are addressed.

## The basics of project management

### What is a project?

It may seem obvious what a project is; we have all worked on projects. Generally, projects may be thought of like art: we don't know how to define it, but we know it when we see it. Certainly if a project is put in front of us, we would recognize it for what it is. The definition of a project is quite broad. It can be considered as *any undertaking that requires a defined list of actions by one or more parties*. Based on such a definition, a project can run the gamut from running a simple lemonade stand to sending a man to the moon. The reader will see that many of the activities he or she has undertaken will be considered projects.

### What is project management?

*Project management* is a structured, repeatable approach to planning and guiding a project from initiation to completion. There are four key stages to project management:

- initiation
- planning
- execution/controlling
- closing

*Emergency Department Leadership and Management*, ed. Stephanie Kayden, *et al.* Published by Cambridge University Press.
© Cambridge University Press 2015.

By definition, there are critical components in each of these four key stages. A *project manager* is the person who takes primary responsibility for the entire project and directs all four key stages.

## Why use project management for a project?

Other than the simplest of projects, most projects run the risk of going over time and budget without a robust project management plan. The most common reasons for the failure include:

- lack of ownership and poorly defined roles and responsibilities
- inaccurate initial budgeting
- poorly defined scope
- failure of project control
- inadequate management of risk

By following a standard set of time-tested guidelines and checklists one can increase the likelihood that all aspects of the project are thought of ahead of time, and that all contingencies can be addressed.

## The project management triangle

The *project management triangle* forms the basis for understanding the concept of project management (Fig. 13.1). All projects are carried out with three constraints: scope, cost, and timeline. Represented graphically, this amounts to a triangle where each side of the triangle represents a constraint. The sides of the triangle are defined as follows:

- scope: what must be delivered by the project
- cost: the budget for the project
- timeline: the time available to complete the project

If any of these often-competing constraints are altered, it affects the other sides of the triangle and thus impacts the quality. For example, if the budget is decreased unexpectedly, the quality will suffer. To maintain the same quality, a corresponding change – in this case, in scope – would have to occur. Similarly, if the timeline is suddenly altered so that the project must be delivered within a shorter-than-anticipated period, the scope or the budget will have to be adjusted.

## Project scenarios

In this chapter, we will give three examples of ED-specific projects for which you are the project manager. We will apply the fundamentals of the project management methodology to define what needs to be done for each of the three projects. We also give examples of common pitfalls and what could be done to address them. Tables 13.1–13.3 show a sample approach using project management methodology. Here are the scenarios:

(1) **Implementing a central-line checklist** to prevent blood-borne infections in an academic teaching hospital (Table 13.1). You are the medical director of the ED. Your department chair has asked that you implement a standardized checklist for the insertion of every central line, to reduce the rate of blood-borne infections. You are told that this checklist needs to be followed 100% of the time by all physicians, attendings, and residents, within the next two months. Part of this checklist involves getting nurses and nursing assistants to assist with placement of central lines, a level of participation that has not been required or expected in the past.

(2) **Expanding the capacity of the ED** from a small 10-bed urgent care operation to a 20-bed acute care operation capable of handling major traumas and resuscitations (Table 13.2). You were just hired as chair of the ED to oversee its conversion from a small 10-bed urgent care operation that is open 16 hours a day and can only handle the walking well (Emergency Severity Index [ESI] 3–5), to a 20-bed acute care operation with 24/7 service. The plan for construction has already begun, and the 20-bed unit is slated to open in one year. The new ED has two trauma and resuscitation bays; another goal is to handle major traumas and resuscitations.

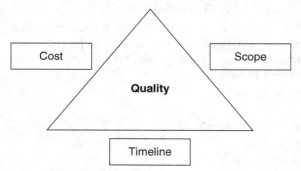

**Figure 13.1** The project management triangle, showing the three constraints of scope, cost, and timeline.

**Table 13.1** A sample project management outline as applied to the central-line checklist scenario

| Initiation | |
|---|---|
| Success of project | 100% compliance by all ED attendings and residents within 2 months. |
| Deliverables | Demonstrated completion of checklists every time central lines are placed. |
| **Planning** | |
| Project plan (team, who does what, timeline) | Team would consist of chair of the department, director of the residency, nurse manager, nurse assistant manager, and an ED administrative person. The project manager would delegate training of attendings and of residents to the chair and residency director, respectively, who would make sure that in 1 month that all 15 faculty and 10 residents have been trained in the usage of the checklist. The nurse manager and nurse assistant manager would need to familiarize their corresponding staff with the necessity of their participation and create buy-in within the same month. Then, in the month following, the ED administrative person would be in charge of documenting compliance in using the checklist. The compliance statistics would be compiled by the administrator or his/her designee, and non-compliance would be addressed by the project manager so that by the 2-month deadline, the department can fulfill the 100% compliance rate. |
| Resource plan (people, materials) | People include all attendings, residents, nurses, nurse assistants, administrative assistants including those will measure compliance. There may also be technical support required to assist with computerized training module or having a poster up to remind people of the checklist. Other materials are what is required by the checklist, for example, an ultrasound machine, sterile drapes, etc that are different from what was previously required. |
| Financial plan | Budget for training module or poster creation, administrative assistant time, any additional nurse and assistants who may need to be hired to implement this project. |
| Quality plan (how to assure quality, measure quality) | Quality is addressed in the front-end by ensuring buy-in from key stakeholder representatives (also members of the project team). Equipment needs to be functional to ensure that it is possible to do lines in sterile fashion. Documentation of quality needs to be through appointed observers, initially every day for every line, then spot checks to ensure there continues to be 100% compliance. |
| Communications plan (internal, external) | Internal to team: weekly group meetings and progress reports to the project manager. Other communication includes frequency of oral, email communications to residents, attendings, nurses, and other stakeholders. |
| Risk plan | Anticipated risks in this example primarily pertain to failure of buy-in and failure of 100% compliance. These can be addressed through both positive and negative incentives. Other things like increased staffing and increased education can be implemented to ameliorate such risks. Technical failure to implement the central line checklist should also be taken into account, i.e., what happens if ultrasound fails or other components of checklist fail. |

| Execution and controlling | |
|---|---|
| Change management | Anticipating changes such as decreased budget, change in scope (only non-emergent lines), or timeline (hospital accreditation committee coming in 1 month; what to do if timeline is pushed up). |
| Quality management | Anticipating for what happens if quality is not up to par: if only 20% of residents are compliant after a month, additional education and/or incentives need to be implemented. |
| Communications management | Continued education during weekly conferences for residents and during staff meetings for faculty. |
| Risk management | As above in the risk plan. |
| **Closing** | |
| Checking against scope | Was there 100% compliance by the second month? Is the compliance continuing to be 100% at random spot-checks later? |
| Accounting | Detailed budget accounting to the chair. |
| Publication | Can include internal publications to the department, hospital, and medical school; or publications and presentations of lessons learned to EM journals and conferences. |

**Table 13.2** A sample project management outline as applied to the ED redesign scenario

| Initiation | |
|---|---|
| Success of project | ED restructured as requested as 24/7, 20-bed acute care ED. |
| Deliverables | Full-capacity, functioning 20-bed ED that is staffed accordingly and has patient-care volume; ability to handle traumas and resuscitations as evidenced by statistics. |
| **Planning** | |
| Project plan (team, who does what, timeline) | This is a very complex multi-year project requiring multiple stakeholders. An initial project plan can be as follows. The team would consist of hospital administrator, IT expert, building/facilities manager, nurse manager, other staff manager, patient relations liaison, EMS liaison, and heads of major inpatient services (ICU, medicine, surgery). The building manager will be in charge of ensuring construction takes place as requested by the deadline, to budget, and that the new ED has all the requested capabilities. The hospital administrator and IT expert would create modeling scenarios to figure out patient flow and how much new staffing is required. The nurse manager and other staff recruiter would start the process of recruiting and making schedules. Redesign is also a chance to make the ED more patient-friendly, and the patient liaison person can assemble committees to see what other aspects of this new ED could have to improve service and patient satisfaction. The EMS liaison would spread the word to local crews that this new ED can accept higher acuity around the clock and ensure that patient flow accompanies the increased capacity. Heads of major inpatient departments need to provide buy-in to support increased volume and they will assist with enhanced procedures for admission, consults, etc. A timeline would be constructed for all of these duties, and a second follow-up plan would be devised well ahead of the 2-year roll-out of the new ED. |

| | |
|---|---|
| Resource plan (people, materials) | People include all ED attendings, attendings from other services, existing and new nurses and assistants, EMS, patient liaison, publicity, etc. Materials include the things needed to build a new ED, i.e., Actual building materials, medical supplies. It may also include new electronic documentation and charting methods, new patient tracking board, new laboratory or diagnostic test possibilities, and/or new ways to streamline ED flow. |
| Financial plan | There would need to be an extensive budget not just for the construction of the new ED space but also for increased staffing and all the accompanying changes in the redesign. |
| Quality plan (how to assure quality, measure quality) | Quality would be addressed in the front-end by making sure that all tasks in the construction are done to budget and on time. Sufficient buy-in from the outset by all involved will prevent further problems along the line. Measurement of quality is when the new ED can be rolled out, how many visits, what is length of stay, what is patient satisfaction, what is acuity of patients, and how this measures according to initial expectations of quality. |
| Communications plan (internal, external) | Internal to team: weekly group meetings and progress reports to the project manager by each component team. External: communication with other hospital departments, EMS groups, patient groups, and the media. |
| Risk plan | Anticipated risks run the gamut from inability to finish construction on time to lack of anticipation of staffing needs to not having enough patients to not having enough capacity to handle patients. Many of these should be addressed by the early planning and meticulous modeling, but much of the risks should be dealt with in a comprehensive plan for what happens if patient acuity exceeds capacity (i.e., is there divert plan), if staffing needs change, if there are significant issues with disposition and length of stay (i.e., if there is significant pushback from medical or surgery service to admit patients). |
| **Execution and controlling** | |
| Change management | Any alteration to budget, timeline, scope – which in this case is any change to almost any parameter – would require a change to the project management triangle. |
| Quality management | Anticipating for problems with quality along the way (i.e., if enough nurses cannot be hired) and when fully implemented (i.e., if patient volume overwhelms ED). |
| Communications management | Close management internally and close watch externally to ensure PR is appropriate and timely |
| Risk management | As above in risk plan |
| **Closing** | |
| Checking against scope | Did ED open on time? Is it functioning as initially proposed in terms of numbers of patients, acuity, length of stay, flow, and other metrics? |
| Accounting | Detailed budget accounting to the hospital and any internal or external donors. |
| Publication | Can include internal publications to the department and the hospital; or publications and presentations of lessons learned to EM journals and conferences and publications aimed at hospital/ED redesign. |

**Table 13.3** A sample project management outline as applied to the disaster relief scenario

| | |
|---|---|
| **Initiation** | |
| Success of project | Sending 5 physicians and 2 nurses to assist with disaster relief within 1 week of disaster. |
| Deliverables | Helping a significant number (say 50 patients/day) in their efforts; aiding with establishment of temporary medical clinic that can be sustained after these initial providers leave. |
| **Planning** | |
| Project plan (team, who does what, timeline) | The team would consist of the 7 providers who are heading to the disaster site. It should also involve an administrator who can help to coordinate finances and trip details and communications as well as a physician located in the home hospital. Ideally the team would consist of multiple people trained in disaster relief who have coordinated similar relief efforts in the past. Team assignments would include having one person in charge of trip logistics (where to stay, when to go, where is safe, how much water to bring); medical equipment; coordinating the clinic operations on the ground; liaising with other volunteer clinicians; fundraising and coordinating with the government and NGO and IGO relief efforts. Because this is a disaster situation with a limited timeline, the program would be condensed. Say the decision is made to leave in a week's time. Within the week, each person would have specific tasks assigned, i.e. in three days, to ensure there is a safe place to stay, in four days to select the location of the temporary clinic. Daily meetings would probably need to be assembled so as to get everyone on the same page and to have continuing reassessments of the rapidly changing plan. Continuing planning once the project gets underway is also necessary to deal with changes. |
| Resource plan (people, materials) | People who are able to leave as well as people who are assisting the relief efforts at the home hospital. This also includes stakeholders who may assist, i.e. potential fundraisers, availability of help by the home and host government, NGOs, IGOs, etc. Materials include food, water, and shelter for the workers as well as key supplies that they will bring to supply the temporary clinic. |
| Financial plan | The budget would include for all the resources above and travel and safety. There should be sufficient resources budgeted for contingencies, should they arise. |
| Quality plan (how to assure quality, measure quality) | In this project, quality assurance is difficult because of the many unknowns including the conditions at the disaster site. On the front end, quality can be addressed by making sure the right people go, the equipment is working and appropriate, and safety is assured. Quality in terms of number of patients treated and continuity is more difficulty to control, and would have to be an ongoing assessment process. |
| Communications plan (internal, external) | Initially there would be constant internal meetings. During the project, stakeholder meetings would be frequent; plans would have to be adjusted to allow for more NGO input, for example. There would be plan for PR and external communication as well to establish ongoing funding and commitment. |
| Risk plan | This is a risky project by the very nature of the work. Risks that may be encountered include personal risk to the workers (repeat disaster, lack of water, food, and shelter, and threat to personal safety); lack of ability to deliver care; and any unexpected obstacles, including those erected by the government or other groups. These risks can be anticipated to some extent, and certainly things like personal safety and a method to evacuate need to be considered, and buy-in could be obtained from the beginning, but as this is a dynamic process, the risk plan in particular will need to be constantly modified. |

| Execution and controlling | |
|---|---|
| Change management | There should be preparations made for potential changes in budget (one funder pulls out) to change in scope (two clinics will be more effective than one) to even change in timing (it might take more than one week to make preparations for departure). |
| Quality management | This scenario, more so than the other two, carries greater likelihood of inconsistent quality. Not only should there be mechanisms in place to improve quality, the quality metrics themselves may need to be adjusted, i.e. if it is not reasonable to treat 50 patients/day, or if it is found that a sustainable clinic is not in the best interest of the community. |
| Communications management | Communication between those on the ground and those back in the host country needs to exist on a fixed schedule. |
| Risk management | As above in risk plan: dynamic changes need to be anticipated |
| **Closing** | |
| Checking against scope | How many patients treated? Was this what was expected? Is the clinic functioning even after physicians left? |
| Accounting | Detailed budget accounting to the department and other funders |
| Publication | Can include internal publications to the department, hospital, and medical school; publications and presentations of lessons learned to EM journals and conferences and publications aimed at international medicine audiences. |

(3) **Initiating a humanitarian disaster relief program** for a disaster that has occurred in a neighboring country (Table 13.3). A natural disaster has just occurred in a neighboring country. You are one of five emergency physicians and two emergency nurses in your department who wish to donate their time for one month to assist with this disaster. Your chair has given all of you protected time to go. Your job is to coordinate a response plan to make the most use of these physicians' time and expertise, in the context of assisting local needs.

## Project management methodology

There are four steps involved in basic project management methodology: initiation, planning, execution/controlling, and closing. This section will describe each component and how it applies to each of our three scenario projects.

## Initiation

For every project, it is important to begin by establishing the *project charter*. This is a one-page summary that provides the big-picture, high-level plan for what the project is. It defines what constitutes success

of the project, delineates the deliverables, and outlines the preliminary scope. In our scenarios, the brief paragraph would be expanded to explain each of the above. For example, in the central-line example, success of the project would be 100% compliance with the central-line checklist in two months' time by all resident and attending physicians. The deliverables would include demonstrated completion of the checklist every time. The scope would be all central lines performed in the ED.

## Planning

Planning for a project is the most time-consuming and difficult part of the process, and should be undertaken with great care. There are six parts to the planning process, which should be done in conjunction with each other: project, resource, financial, quality, communication, and risk.

### The project plan

The project plan is the core of the planning process. It should include a detailed scope, the activity definition for each specific task that needs to be done, and a timeline for when these tasks should take place. At this point, the project team should be appointed so that a work breakdown structure for who is going to be doing what specific task can be created. In the case of the central-line checklist, those who are part of the team could be chair of the department, director of the residency, nurse manager, nurse assistant manager, and an ED administrative person. The project manager would delegate training of attendings and of residents to the chair and residency director, respectively, who would make sure that in one month that all 15 faculty and 10 residents have been trained in the usage of the checklist. The nurse manager and nurse assistant manager would need to familiarize their corresponding staff with the necessity of their participation and create buy-in within the same month. Then, in the month following, the ED administrative person would be in charge of documenting the compliance of using the central line checklist. The compliance statistics would be compiled, and non-compliance would be addressed by the project manager so that by the two-month deadline the department can fulfill the 100% compliance rate.

### The resource plan

The resource plan is an accounting of all the resources available and required. It includes a documentation of all the stakeholders involved and all people/organizational resources. It should also include all materials needed. In the case of the disaster relief program, for example, the resource plan should include an accounting of all individuals involved including allies at non-governmental organizations (NGOs) and intergovernmental organizations (IGOs), as well as materials needed such as tents, water, medical supplies, medicines, ground transportation, and so on.

### The financial plan

The financial plan is the detailed budget for the project. All administrators are used to creating budgets; this is no different from any other detailed budget you are used to preparing.

### The quality plan

The quality plan is put in place to ensure that there is good quality in the final product. This includes both pre-emptive planning (such as making sure a physician with mass casualty planning experience is on the disaster relief trip) and quality control measures (such as an external validation for quality and success of the mission).

### The communication plan

The communication plan covers how the project manager engages with the project team and outside stakeholders. In the example of the ED redesign, the project manager may propose weekly internal meetings with the key team members: the physician clinical director, the nurse manager, and the ED administrator. There would be monthly activity reports issued by each team member to the project manager, and a bimonthly accounting and summary back from the manager to the team. There should also be a communications plan with others involved in the project: for example, a plan for engaging other stakeholders such as heads of other clinical departments so they know of higher acuity coming their way and increased rate of admission, EMS services so they know to send more critically ill patients to this new ED, the public and media so they are aware of the increased capacity of the hospital, and so on.

### The risk plan

The risk plan is a comprehensive process that aims to identify, prevent, and manage risks. It includes all anticipated and possible risks and provides alternative plans and contingencies. EM physicians are trained in anticipating and managing risk, and in the project management setting this is no different. In the case of disaster relief, the risks are numerous, including unexpected equipment failure, threats to personal safety, resistance from the government, etc. Plans should be in place to maximize the chance of equipment working, ensure safety of volunteers, and develop connections with those in the positions of power to facilitate the project. Should these plans fall through, a "plan B" could include borrowing equipment from other volunteer agencies and finding safe transport back.

## Execution and controlling

Once the project has been mapped out, the six aspects of the plan can be executed. The project manager's role in the execution is to oversee the implementation of the project plan and to manage the project team. Along the way, careful control and monitoring should be applied so that problems are immediately detected and corrective action applied. Hence, execution and controlling are done simultaneously.

A key component in this process is the concept of *change management*. Change management needs to occur any time there is a change to the project management triangle: whenever there is an alteration to the cost, timeline, or scope. If the ED capacity needs to increase to 25 beds instead of 20 beds, the scope is changed, and the cost and timeline would likewise need adjustment. If three of the five physicians who agreed to go on the disaster relief operation pull out, or if a major donor withdraws, then that would also require some readjustment on what can be delivered. Change management encompasses the range of responses necessary to any alterations, deliberate or unplanned, in the project. It allows for a consistent, standardized method for identifying and applying corrective actions to any sides of the project management triangle.

Related to change management is the management of other aspects of the plan: quality, communications, and risk. *Quality management* refers to the constant assessment to measure against performance expectations. The goal of the project should be kept in mind, and adjustments made if it appears that the quality is not up to par. For example, if only 20% of residents are compliant with the central-line checklist after the first month, a more intensive education campaign accompanied by possible punitive actions would need to be enforced to assure quality. *Communication management* is the monitoring and control of information flow to internal and external sources. It includes a continuing reassessment of buy-in by stakeholders and corresponding adjustments to the communications plan. Similarly, *risk management* is continuing risk monitoring and control and, if necessary, improvements to the initial risk plan.

## Closing

The final part of a project is to perform the project closure. This involves not only double-checking against the initial detailed project scope, but also producing final documentation, including final accounts, ongoing operations information, and communication to the key stakeholders in the form of summary reviews. A "lessons learned" presentation can be given by the doctors who participated in the disaster relief effort. That team, as well as the teams that incorporated the central-line checklists and expanded ED capacity, can publish their work in EM and other publications.

## Common pitfalls

Tables 13.1–13.3 illustrate the four steps of the project management cycle as applied to each of the three scenarios. Below are common pitfalls that we have observed in EM projects. We provide advice on how to pre-empt and address each of these pitfalls.

### Pitfall 1: the project is over budget

You find out that the teaching modules for preventing central-line infection require programming expertise that costs $150/hour. The trainers that you hired are now estimating that it will cost double the number of hours and want to charge for overtime. What do you do?

Underestimating the budget is a frequent problem in project management. There are often pressures from administration to come up with the tightest possible budget from the start. Unfortunately, this results in budgets that have little leeway for extra costs. It is advisable to include a contingency of between 5% and 20% for unforeseen budget costs.

It goes without saying that the best way to prevent going over budget is pre-emptive: for example, to carefully research costs, obtain quotes from a number of reliable vendors, and use conservative estimates when possible. What if it is too late and you are now faced with a project that is over budget? The project management triangle is clear: unless you can raise additional funding somehow, you will need to change the scope or the timeline. Perhaps fewer people will be educated, or over a longer time period. Perhaps the module could be cut for length to allow trainers to work on budget. If there is no money for the computerized training, perhaps another form of training will need to be carried out. Emergency physicians who are used to working in resource-limited settings will be able to think creatively about how to raise money at the last minute, and also to work with what they have. The best strategy, though, is always pre-emptive.

### Pitfall 2: time has run out

It is the day that you are due to open your new acute care 24/7 unit. Most of the equipment has not yet arrived. The unit has no phones. Only half the rooms are fully equipped; the rest do not have a stretcher.

But the unit is advertised to open, and all your new staff will show up in a few hours.

This situation should never happen. One way to manage time is to set three dates: the goal date, the realistic date, and the absolute deadline. Make arrangements with your vendors and whoever you anticipate to have the most time limitations to have everything be done by the goal date. Depending on the project, this would include utilities and equipment companies that take time to source your needs, and major national and international organizations that require time for political buy-in. The rollout of the project should ideally be the realistic date. If for whatever reason it still does not happen, make sure that there are steps in place to implement the project by the absolute deadline.

If all the planning took place as intended, and for whatever reason time has still run out, it is time to put your thinking cap on again. Can the staff work with their cell phones only? Can they improvise other areas in the department if only half of the new bays can be used? Can some of the staff be deployed to try to get the equipment from the warehouse themselves? Getting the support of everyone involved will help to salvage the situation.

## Pitfall 3: there is confusion about outcomes

You thought that the purpose of your trip to the country in the middle of a natural disaster was to assist those most in need. Now you are back, and your department chair is asking you what contacts you have established for him and where your publications are. How can you justify the investment that the department placed in you in terms of time and resources?

The very first step of the project management cycle is to establish the project charter. The major objectives should be clearly delineated and agreed upon by the major parties involved. This prevents confusion later. It is particularly important to define the scope of the particular project. Perhaps, from your perspective, the publicity and contacts could be an ideal outcome or a goal for the future, but it is not the specific goal. That should be clearly defined ahead of time.

In the event that it is too late and the project has already been executed, there is still time to redefine the objectives. You probably still have the option to make contacts and publish on your experiences. If that is very important to your chair, establish that as a new goal and make it happen. If there is no way it is possible for this project, this could be a good segue to ask for another project – one that you will define the scope and timeline for at the outset.

## Pitfall 4: there is confusion about responsibilities

You have asked one of your colleagues to look up price estimates for tents and food and another to make contact with three major NGOs. Your budget is due today, and your first colleague says he never agreed to look up price estimates. You call an NGO and they say that they have never heard from your other colleague. Why are people so unreliable?

How many times has the above scenario happened to you? As a leader and project manager, your challenge is to delegate responsibility and hold people accountable to their duties. This is much easier said than done, but there are concrete steps to making this happen. From your experiences, you know a lot about these management skills already. One tip is to hold people accountable in a public forum. When you have conference calls or meetings, set the agenda ahead of time and make it clear that this is where responsibilities will be divided. At the end of the meeting, have a verbal accounting of who needs to be doing what. Then send out minutes over email so that there is a written record of what was agreed. That way, if there is ever any question of why someone did not do something, you will have a record of it – and there will be others who will help you hold the individual responsible.

Ultimately, pitfalls in project management are all about pre-empting and then managing risk. We emergency physicians should be particularly good at both, as our minds are tuned to figuring out contingencies, worst-case scenarios, and alternative plans. The same skills we use at the bedside can be applied to our projects.

## Summary

As emergency physicians, nurses, and administrators we manage multiple projects in our daily work. Project management is an essential tool that provides a standard framework for planning, executing, and monitoring our projects. Understanding and applying the key principles and techniques of project management will allow EM practitioners and leaders to maximize impact and efficiency in future projects.

## Further reading

The concepts referenced in this chapter are industry-standard practice for project management. Some references for further reading:

Association for Project Management. http://www.apm.org.uk (accessed January 2014). Membership allows access to a broad range of templates and project management literature.

Berkun S. *The Art of Project Management*. Sebastopol, CA: O'Reilly, 2005.

Kerzner HR. *Project Management: a Systems Approach to Planning, Scheduling, and Controlling*, 11th edn. Hoboken, NJ: Wiley, 2013.

Project Management Institute. *A Guide to the Project Management Body of Knowledge (PMBOK® Guide)*, 5th edn. Newtown Square, PA: PMI, 2013. Available through the PMI website: http://www.pmi.org.

**Chapter**

# 14

# How higher patient, employee, and physician satisfaction leads to better outcomes of care

Christina Dempsey, Deirdre Mylod, and Richard B. Siegrist, Jr.

## Key learning points

- Gain an understanding of how patient, employee, and physician satisfaction are highly correlated with clinical outcomes, operational metrics, and financial performance.
- Find out how patient and staff satisfaction are critical to healthcare quality and patient safety, how good communication reduces patient anxiety and stress, and how patients accurately perceive problems of care quality.
- Learn about emergency department processes that lead to more satisfied patients, including triage, staffing, and scheduling practices, as well as how improving processes in the rest of the hospital can streamline emergency department operations.

## Introduction

Over the past quarter-century, the realization that patients are good judges of the quality of care they receive in hospitals and other care settings has begun to slowly take root around the world. In the United States, measuring patient attitudes through ever more sophisticated surveys is now a routine part of running most healthcare organizations, and it is now effectively mandated by the federal government. Patients are not surveyed just to find out if the food is bad or the nurses are nice; a wealth of academic research has traced close correlations between patient satisfaction and clinical outcomes.[1–4]

The World Health Organization has developed measures of patient experience intended to capture the "responsiveness" of the health system, specifically the manner and environment in which people are treated when they seek health care.[5] In Europe, Asia, South America, and Australia, hospitals have sought data on the patient experience, part of a growing movement to improve the quality of care, enhance patient safety, and lower the cost of services.

The USA has led the way in the movement toward "transparency," where information on quality of care and evaluations of the patient experience of care are becoming readily available to help patients choose where to get treatment for medical conditions. Surveys now allow organizations to drill down to the department and individual clinician level. Emergency department (ED) surveys and reports are now seen as one of the most important department-level measures to track, and with good reason: roughly half of all non-obstetric hospital admissions in the USA come through the ED, which has become most hospitals' front door. How patients are greeted, how long they must wait to see a physician or triage nurse, the competence of the caregivers – all are of primary importance to maintaining a hospital's reputation.

In the USA, the movement toward transparency has been fostered in large part by the federal government, which has now embarked on a large-scale effort to link a portion of hospital payment under the Medicare program – which provides health coverage to more than 44 million people, mostly senior citizens – to the quality of care provided. Thirty percent of the complex formula for determining how much hospitals receive under this program is based on patient satisfaction measures.

Of course, there are obvious differences in reimbursement, staffing, provider incentives, culture, and resource availability between EDs in the USA and in other countries. And yet the trend towards value-based purchasing by the government and other payers is not unique to the United States, suggesting that the USA is only a bellwether for the future for healthcare payment elsewhere.

---

*Emergency Department Leadership and Management*, ed. Stephanie Kayden, *et al.* Published by Cambridge University Press.
© Cambridge University Press 2015.

In the ED, long waits for care – a factor of perception as much as actual wait times – are ingredients of patient stress, which leads to negative outcomes.[6] Long waits for care prompt some less-emergent patients to leave the ED without being seen by a physician. And logjams in the ED also impact the rest of the hospital. Patients boarded in ED hallways may result in lower-quality care and outcomes.[6–8]

Evaluations of patient satisfaction that began in the 1980s fairly quickly expanded to measuring the satisfaction of the people who work in hospitals and other care settings. With retention of quality physicians and nurses becoming a continuing problem for many institutions, the idea was to identify and address the issues that affected the ability to hire and keep top performers on the job. It turned out that there are strong, positive correlations between patient satisfaction and employee satisfaction.[9] In fact, without satisfied caregivers, it is highly unlikely you will find satisfied patients.[9]

## Using data to drive transformational change

Valid patient satisfaction surveys for the ED provide a wealth of structured data in the form of numerical ratings and unstructured data in the form of patient comments. Proper analysis of both types of information enables an organization to identify areas that need improvement, undertake root cause analyses to gain a deeper understanding of the issues, and design interventions that can lead to transformational change.

There are several critical issues that need to be addressed to ensure the proper use of patient satisfaction data. First, the sample size should be sufficient to draw reasonable conclusions from the data, rather than responding to anecdotes that may not have broad applicability. A sample will be representative of the overall population if all members of the population have an equal (random) chance of being surveyed. Sampling error is the difference between a survey's results and the results if every patient in the population were to respond. For proportional-level data (percentage of patients indicating they are satisfied) needed sample size can be determined based on the size of the population and the desired level of precision. For data where mean scores are used, needed sample size is determined based on estimates of sampling error using historic data for EDs. For example, a commonly used ED survey within the USA recommends a range of 127–145 survey responses as a minimum number of returns to assess the experience as a whole.[10] For subunits of analysis it is recommended that at least 30 and preferably 50 survey responses be used. These sample sizes are based on estimated confidence intervals and ensure a minimum of error has been achieved for the ED as a whole on a quarterly basis.

Second, the data analysis should focus on trends over time and not on individual data points that may simply be aberrations or an indication of natural fluctuation by time of the year or day of the week. Special attention should be paid to individual questions that correlate highly with the patient's overall perception of the care experience in the ED.[6] Those questions can form a list of areas on which to focus improvement efforts that reap the largest possible reward in terms of higher patient satisfaction. Table 14.1 reflects the combined priorities of more than 1.5 million patients at nearly 1900 US hospitals in 2010, as identified by analyses of ED patient satisfaction survey reports.

Third, appropriate benchmarking to EDs of similar size in terms of annual patient volume and type, such as urban academic medical centers, puts an

**Table 14.1** National emergency department priority index[6]

| Survey item | Mean | Correlation | Priority rank |
| --- | --- | --- | --- |
| How well you were kept informed about delays | 71.3 | 0.726 | 1 |
| How well was your pain controlled | 77.9 | 0.722 | 2 |
| Degree to which staff cared about you as a person | 82.0 | 0.795 | 3 |
| Overall rating of care received during your visit | 83.0 | 0.897 | 4 |
| Nurses' concern to keep you informed about your treatment | 83.1 | 0.702 | 5 |

Survey items are correlated to patient ratings of "Likelihood of your recommending this hospital to others." Represents the experiences of 1 501 672 patients treated at 1893 hospitals nationwide between January 1 and December 31, 2009.

institution's performance into context and facilitates both the setting of reasonable goals and motivating clinical and non-clinical staff for improvement. Being able to see that similar EDs have been able to achieve a higher level of patient satisfaction adds credibility to improvement efforts and offers a mechanism to reward performance in context.

Finally, having a reliable and vetted third-party administrator of patient satisfaction surveys is essential if the data are to be judged as valid for comparative purposes. While many hospitals have collected information on patient satisfaction, these surveys vary in terms of numbers of patients surveyed and the types of questions asked. A common survey instrument enables valid comparisons to be made across all hospitals. Having a governmental entity or a vendor with governmental certification and experience in statistically valid survey administration is recommended.

# The many returns of patient, physician, and employee satisfaction

## Satisfaction in the ED: a growing concern

The challenges faced by US hospitals in providing emergency care are intense. According to data from the American Hospital Association (AHA) and the US National Center for Health Statistics, from 1990 to 2008 the number of annual ED visits in the USA rose from 90 million to 123 million, amounting to about 41 visits per 100 people.[8] The number of hospitals operating EDs in the United States declined from more than 5000 in 1991 to fewer than 4000 in 2006. In March 2010, an AHA survey found that 17% of EDs at reporting hospitals were "over capacity" at some point in that month while 21% were "at capacity." Twenty-two percent of hospitals reported periods of time in which they diverted ambulances to other facilities as a result of capacity problems.

The priorities for improvement identified by patients in satisfaction survey data have remained relatively stable in recent years, led by keeping them informed about delays in care, controlling their pain, and the degree to which staff members cared about patients personally (Table 14.1). In general, the priorities identified by patients continue to suggest that how well patients are treated as human beings is more important than the quality of the facilities and equipment in the ED.

Patients indicate that they are willing to wait for care as long as they are kept informed about the wait time. Patients who reported that they received "good" or "very good" information about delays reported nearly the same overall satisfaction whether they had spent over four hours or less than one hour in the ED.[6]

## Correlations with quality

From a wide range of research, it is clear that while patients may not understand the technical details of the care they receive, their perceptions of quality from what they see, hear, and feel in the ED and elsewhere in the hospital are remarkably accurate.

A major study by Jha *et al.* looked at inpatient satisfaction and clinical data from 2429 hospitals in 2007 and found a strong positive correlation between patient overall satisfaction and clinical performance.[2] Patients admitted through the ED were included in that analysis.

Another study by Glickman *et al.* found that higher inpatient satisfaction is associated with lower inpatient mortality rates for acute myocardial infarction.[3] The research was the first on this topic to control for adherence to clinical practice guidelines. The findings were based on an analysis of clinical data and Press Ganey surveys from 6467 patients at 25 hospitals over five years.

Trucano and Kaldenberg, in a study of data from the Pennsylvania Health Care Cost Containment Council and Press Ganey Associates, found significant negative correlations between patient perceptions of the quality in the identified practices and facilities' infection rates.[4] Facilities with higher scores on cleanliness, blood-draw skills, and nurse responsiveness items tended to have lower rates of infections and infection mortality.

Not everyone, of course, believes that patient satisfaction is a valid measurement of the quality of care a patient receives, either in the ED or anywhere else. Concerns about sample sizes for smaller departments and at the individual physician level have been voiced in commentaries and other literature. Many survey organizations will provide access to data with as few as seven returned surveys despite having a stated absolute minimum sample size. This is because the data belong to the ED, and it has a right to see them. Moreover, if these data were not provided, valuable information and comments could be lost.

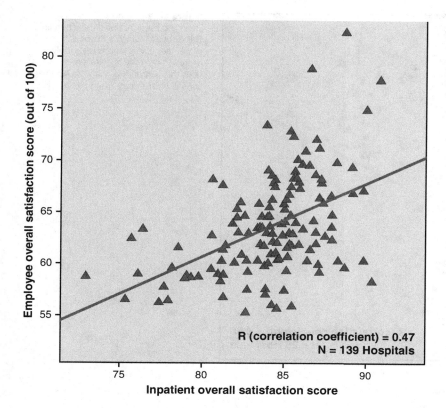

**Figure 14.1** The patient–hospital employee satisfaction link. The extent to which a hospital meets its patients' expectations for care is strongly related to how the hospital's employees feel about their workplace. Source: Press Ganey white paper, 2006.[9]

One example of the potential result of this would be not receiving a patient complaint that resulted in a lawsuit over a medical error.

Not providing data based on small sample sizes both takes ownership of the data away from the ED and potentially masks serious issues. This said, survey organizations are generally very careful to caution their clients on the interpretation of data based on small sample sizes, and recommend that these data be used to identify potentially serious issues in a qualitative/informative fashion.

## Partnerships with physicians and employees

Patients do not receive care in a vacuum. As discussed in a 2006 Press Ganey white paper, there is a complex interrelationship among patient, employee, and physician satisfaction that leads to quality care and better financial outcomes for a hospital.[9] Several studies of national databases have found:

- Strong correlations between the perspectives of physicians and patients in evaluating the hospital's quality of services.

- Strong correlations between employee and patient satisfaction, leading many clients to successfully adopt "employees first" strategies on the premise that employees will treat patients only as well as they are treated themselves.
- Strong correlations between physician and nurse satisfaction: evaluations of health service quality again converge.
- Significant relationships between measures of physician, nurse, employee, and patient loyalty, as well as actual return-to-provider, retention, and other loyalty behaviors.

Figures 14.1, 14.2, and 14.3 explore these interrelationships.

There is a variety of ways to look at these interrelationships. In the ideal situation an organization is efficient and effective in its quality and operations, and also has a strong culture of staff and physicians having good working relationships. Such a hospital is best poised to deliver great care to patients through experienced clinicians working as a team without barriers to performance. In reality,

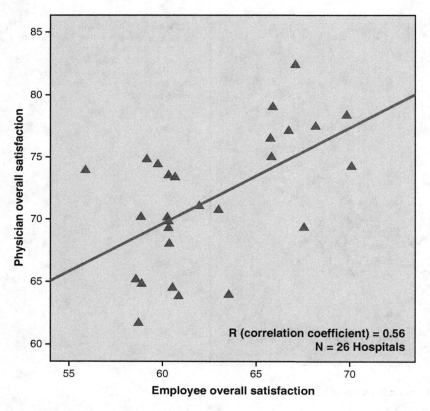

**Figure 14.2** The hospital employee–attending medical staff satisfaction link. The extent to which a hospital meets its employees' expectations is strongly related to how the hospital's medical staff rates their experience with the hospital. Source: Press Ganey white paper, 2006.[9]

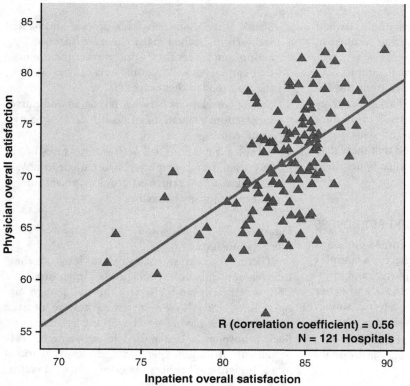

**Figure 14.3** The patient-attending medical staff satisfaction link. The extent to which a hospital meets its patients' expectations for care is strongly related to how the hospital's medical staff rates its experience with the hospital. Source: Press Ganey white paper, 2006.[9]

most organizations face some challenges in either their processes or their culture or both. Less than optimal processes create frustrations for those who work there and mean longer waits and potential gaps in care for patients.[4,6]

A struggling culture is often exemplified by a lack of teamwork and respect among caregivers, a tendency for blame, and a lack of connection with the organization as an entity. Such an environment becomes apparent to patients when they witness the attitudes and behaviors of staff interacting with one another.

On the more positive side, when an organization works to improve patient, employee, or physician satisfaction and engagement, it can realize benefits in multiple areas. When patient satisfaction issues are addressed and care is made more efficient (so patients do not have to wait) or more consistent (so patients have reduced anxiety and better communication), staff and physicians may also reap the benefits of efficiency and less stressed patients. Ideally, an organization takes into consideration these three constituent groups when working on any performance improvement initiative and, for example, works to improve care for patients by involving frontline staff and physicians, who desire more influence over their working environment.

### Case study 14.1.    Gaining ED physician buy-in to patient satisfaction at Oregon Health & Science University[6]

Oregon Health & Science University (OHSU) in Portland is Oregon's only academic medical center. OHSU operates two hospitals and numerous medical practice locations. As one of only two level 1 trauma centers in the state, OHSU provides emergency care for patients across the state and throughout the region.

The 2007 arrival of John Ma, MD, as chairman of OHSU's Department of Emergency Medicine marked a new emphasis on service excellence for both frontline staff and medical residents. All incoming residents now receive a letter from Dr. Ma discussing the role of service excellence in the ED. The letter, which has been widely adopted elsewhere, reads as follows: "At OHSU we have adopted a culture of 'always.' I promise that our department will always do what is necessary to provide you with a first-rate medical training and that you will graduate with all the necessary skills to practice as an outstanding emergency physician. One of the skills that will be strongly emphasized throughout your three years at OHSU is service excellence. The patient always comes first in the OHSU emergency department. Providing high-quality and safe patient care is always our number 1 priority. In the process, we always look to provide an outstanding experience for the patient and their family. The service excellence principles that you will learn will serve you well throughout your medical career."

The residents are trained on customer service principles their first day at the hospital. By training residents, Dr. Ma hopes to spread best practices in service excellence to other institutions.

Review of OHSU's two EDs' patient satisfaction data has led the department's service excellence group to implement a number of initiatives, including post-discharge follow-up phone calls to patients, scripting for conversations such as triage interviews, an ED expeditor program to keep patients up to date on delays, and comment cards distributed at discharge.

Most of these changes may begin by addressing patient satisfaction, but end up touching on both clinical quality and employee engagement. Post-discharge phone calls, for instance, are made by a nurse to all high-risk patients and at random to other patients.

New OHSU residents are required to follow one patient through the entirety of the patient's ED stay, from the moment he or she first arrives in the waiting room to the time of ultimate discharge. Being on the other side of the care experience helps residents understand the long wait times and uncertainty that can sometimes characterize an ED visit, and that an ability to empathize is just as important as learning medical skills, Dr. Ma believes.

## A link with financial outcomes

Reputations are built over time as word of mouth spreads through a community. A major study by the Centers for Medicare and Medicaid Services analyzed patient satisfaction in 1999 and then the subsequent changes in patient volume experienced between 2000 and 2004.[11] Hospitals were divided into quartiles based on their profitability. The least profitable hospitals had the lowest patient satisfaction scores (out of 100 points); the most profitable had the highest patient satisfaction. As patient satisfaction increased, average hospital profitability increased. Hospitals with patient satisfaction in the 90th percentile experienced nearly a one-third increase in patient volume, which was, on average, an additional

1382 patients per year. For hospitals with patient satisfaction in the bottom 10th percentile, the average volume loss was 17%.

## Solving the problems of ED patient satisfaction

Most American ED patients are satisfied with their care. In the Press Ganey ED *Pulse Report*, 6 out of 10 patients rated their ED care as "very good" and more than 8 out of 10 as "good" or "very good" on a scale of very poor to very good.[6] Given that patients are generally satisfied with their care in the ED, the challenge is converting the "good" ratings to "very good" ratings through improving the patient experience.

There can be some "quick fixes" that can lead to significant improvements in patient satisfaction with the care experience. As noted earlier, keeping patients informed of wait times and the reasons for those delays goes a long way toward enhancing the patient's experience, because it reduces uncertainty and lessens anxiety. However, addressing the underlying issues of why there are long wait times, why poor communication exists, or why patients perceive a lack of caring by the ED staff is much more difficult. These issues have been overcome by a number of EDs in the United States, leading to substantial and sustained improvements in patient satisfaction.

For example, at the Reading Hospital in Pennsylvania, placing a physician and nurse in triage, taking patients immediately from the front door to an ED patient room, standardizing treatment protocols, and communicating more effectively with patients on the progress of their treatment led to a remarkable turnaround in ED patient satisfaction scores, which increased from the low single digits as a national percentile to a sustained ranking in the 70th-plus percentile, and the 99th for EDs with comparable patient volumes.[12]

The first step is recognizing that the specific problems exist, rather than trying to explain them away through calling into question the measurement of patient satisfaction or referring to anecdotal instances where patients are clearly not appropriate in their complaints. Identifying best practices at other similar EDs, pulling together a meaningful action plan, gaining physician and nurse buy-in, creating the right incentives, and continuously monitoring improvement are important steps in the journey to a better patient experience and corresponding high patient satisfaction.

## Scripting for better communication

Many US hospital EDs use *scripting*, a term that refers to identification of target communication points that enhance patient care if delivered at a particular point in time. It should not, despite its title, mean that only a particular set of words is delivered to get the point across. Rather, it is most effectively used when these communication points are created by knowledgeable frontline staff and then delivered with individual nuances while still retaining the essence of the information. Scripts that attempt to over-emphasize words or elicit positive responses on patient satisfaction surveys diminish communication with the patient and are unlikely to help increase patient satisfaction scores in the long run. They are also demoralizing for employees to have to deliver.

On the other hand, communicating with patients in a way that is more effective, that ensures standardization of important topics or interactions, and that helps a patient understand care better will absolutely impact a patient's evaluation of care.

One example of good scripting might be when a staff member might pull a bed curtain in a semi-private room while saying "I want to give you a little bit more privacy." The nurse would have engaged in the behavior anyway, but the verbal communication provides the patient with the understanding of the concern that is being offered to them.

Another kind of scripting is exemplified by clinical staff "thinking out loud" in front of patients. A physician might describe his or her thought process while examining a patient, and might reflect back the meaning in the presence or absence of a particular symptom. Such a practice takes what could be a one-sided conversation where a physician inspects and questions the patient to come up with a conclusion and turns it into an experience where the patient feels engaged and knowledgeable about the physician's decision-making process.

## Care processes and patient satisfaction

Examining the patient experience from entry to exit in the ED can uncover multiple areas of opportunity to improve both patient flow and the patient experience. The ED is at the mercy of the inpatient capacity of the hospital, and the patient's perception of the hospital often hinges on the patient's experience in the ED. Therefore, coordination of the processes of care must be optimized both within the ED and throughout the hospital in order to realize sustainable improvement in patient experience.

At most hospitals, the patient's first contact in the ED is with a "greeter" and/or triage nurse. This initial contact is critical to the patient's perception of the hospital. In EDs in hospitals around the world, overcrowding and long waits are a common phenomenon, and now are often the norm rather than the exception. Managing this wait is key to the patient's experience. The greeter becomes an adjunct to the triage nurse and an integral part of the team. While the triage nurse's responsibility is to accurately assess and prioritize the needs of the patient, the greeter's responsibility is to warmly greet the patient and family members or visitors, help them to navigate the waiting area, and, in many cases, offer creature comforts (blankets, coffee for visitors) and information about what to expect in the waiting room. The ED manager must ensure that greeters are provided formal and ongoing education around patient satisfaction and customer service, so that this essential first impression is consistently and appropriately provided.

Most hospitals throughout the USA and Europe use a triage scale to identify the priority with which the patient will access the services within the ED. In most cases the assignment of the priority rests with a triage nurse, based on the patient's chief or presenting complaint and condition. The US Emergency Medical Treatment and Active Labor Act assures that patients are provided a medical screening examination and stabilization by a licensed independent practitioner without delays due to verification of insurance or ability to pay for the services. Proper identification of the patient is necessary, and many hospitals have adopted a "quick registration" process that allows for pertinent identification information to be obtained at the point of initial triage and then a full registration process after the patient has seen the provider. This allows the patient to be properly identified in the electronic medical record and, if that patient has accessed medical care at the facility in the past, the demographic and medical history information may be populated from past visits. The electronic medical record then improves the continuity of the patient's care beyond this visit and helps to ensure patient safety. Bachenheimer notes that additional options for capturing this information include computerized kiosk registrations whereby patients may input their own information into the kiosk, which interfaces with the electronic tracking system.[13] Another strategy that has been shown to improve patient satisfaction and wait times is the direct-to-bed triage process.[13] When treatment rooms are available the patient is taken directly to the room, bypassing triage and the waiting room. This shortens overall length of stay, and triage becomes unnecessary, as long as treatment rooms in the ED are available.

The medical screening examination and the time from patient arrival to being seen by the physician is a common metric used to determine efficiency of the ED. Patients who come to the ED are coming to see the provider. Reducing the time from arrival to provider has been shown to increase patient satisfaction.[6] Providers at triage have been shown to expedite the triage process and may be able to reduce the overall ED length of stay by allowing some patients to be discharged after the screening exam, eliminating the need to occupy a treatment room in the ED.[13]

In 2002, the NHS Modernisation Agency in the United Kingdom suggested abandoning triage and having patients seen and treated as soon as they arrive at the ED. Hospitals are increasingly using a team triage model. One such example is Gwinnett Medical Center in Georgia. This hospital implemented a rapid medical evaluation model to address patient waiting times, improve patient satisfaction and flow, and reduce the number of patients leaving without being seen. The team consists of one patient greeter, a quick registration patient access representative, a triage nurse, a medical evaluation nurse, two specialty technicians, a mid-level provider, and one physician. In this model, the triage nurse sent Emergency Severity Index (ESI) level 4 and 5 patients to one of three rapid medical evaluation rooms and discharged from there when possible. This team approach to triage resulted in a decrease in patients leaving without being seen, a decrease in time to physician, and an increase in patient satisfaction from patients who were discharged from team triage.

**Case study 14.2. An administrator takes patients from the front door to treatment**

Staten Island University Hospital is a 704-bed, tertiary care, teaching hospital in New York City with two campuses. The north campus operates as a level 1 trauma center. In June 2009, a four-year-old effort to improve patient satisfaction with the ED on the north campus had failed to deliver the desired results. The department was achieving solid clinical results, but scoring at the low end of the scale on patients' "likelihood to recommend" the facility as a good place to receive care. The staff was getting ready to move into a gleaming new 40 000-square-foot ED, but leaders feared that if they did not act quickly they would only be transferring old habits and processes to the new facility.

The solution was a revolutionary customer service program. At its heart is a new role called "administrator on duty." Each day from 10 a.m. to 3 p. m., one of a dozen ED administrators and managers takes a shift escorting patients directly to treatment areas. The process allows the administrator to provide real-time troubleshooting, noting where there are beds open or problems brewing. The program has been such a success that from 3 p.m. to 11 p.m. – peak census each day – a full-time "pavilion manager" now provides the same service.

Staff members were put through mandatory training on customer service excellence. New direct-to-bedside patient flow significantly decreased waiting times for care.

By the end of 2009, the ED had leaped to the 75th percentile nationally on "likelihood to recommend." The time from arrival to being seen by a doctor fell from 65 minutes in 2009 to 53 minutes in the first quarter of 2010. The percentage of patients who leave without being evaluated – a result of long waiting times – fell from 2.32% to 1.21%. That last statistic alone translates into nearly $400 000 in additional annual revenue to the hospital. And all of this has been achieved in the face of a 13% increase in ED utilization.

## Urgent care/fast track utilization

In many hospitals, "fast track" is really a misnomer. Patients are often not seen any faster than in the acute ED. Patients typically seen in the fast track or urgent care area are the ESI levels 4 and 5, and sometimes level 3. These patients require fewer and different resources than the more acute patient populations at levels 1–3. Separating these patients therefore often makes sense in terms of staffing and capacity in the ED. A queuing analysis, used elsewhere by restaurants and stores to avoid long lines, that differentiates the waiting times for these patients and the capacity needed to care for this population will allow the nurse manager in the ED to optimize patient care for both the more acute and less acute patient populations.

Queuing provides a level of analytics beyond what most information systems provide.[4] However, employing this analysis for the random arrivals of the ED will allow the nurse manager to determine how much staffed capacity is needed, how utilized that capacity will be, and how available the capacity (both staffing and room) will be for emergency patients. Nurse practitioners and/or physician assistants are increasingly being used as the providers for both fast track and provider at triage, with physician oversight of these roles provided by ED physicians.

## Patient flow

Understanding the role of the inpatient areas of the hospital and the impact these areas have on the ED will help nurse managers and senior leadership in the organization focus on and improve the drivers of patient flow. Boarding and overcrowding in the ED is a complex issue and one that cannot be solved by focusing solely on the ED as the solution.

> The ability to move admitted patients from the ED to hospital beds depends upon the availability of hospital beds, nursing staff, nursing ratios, ancillary service availability, local structure, and likely many other factors.[14]

Comments like the above have been cited in numerous articles across the USA with regard to ED overcrowding. However, this comment by Jayaprakash *et al.* is referencing European ED overcrowding. In countries such as the UK and Ireland, just as in the USA, elective surgical patients are vying for the same inpatient beds that the ED needs for their patients. A study by Gilligan *et al.* concluded that "the overwhelming reason for prolonged waits and overcrowding in Irish EDs is not the duplication of work inherent in the referral process but it is because of a lack of acute hospital capacity."[15]

The peaks and valleys that we see in the inpatient census can often be a direct result of the elective surgery volume and the controllable (but not well-controlled) variability in the operating room elective schedule. When the elective schedule peaks, the inpatient beds fill and thus the ED patient must board in the ED waiting for any bed available. One consequence can be inappropriate patient placement on inpatient wards when patients are moved from the ED to any bed that opens on any inpatient ward. Unfortunately, that may mean that the patient must go to a unit where the nurses are unfamiliar with his or her care, resulting in a risk of complications, errors, and extended length of stay.

This phenomenon also may mean that medical patients are "batched" so that rather than having to round all over the hospital to find their patients, physicians see all of their patients in the ED in a batch and do all diagnostic testing there rather than on the inpatient unit. This leads to increasing lengths of stay in the ED and boarding while waiting for the order or release to take the patient to the inpatient unit.

The solution is for hospital and physician leadership to take an enterprise-wide approach to patient flow and use a data-driven approach to smooth the controllable variability of the elective surgical schedule, thus allowing better management of the uncontrollable random arrivals to the ED. Queuing theory helps in the procedural areas such as the operating rooms and the cardiac catheterization lab to ensure accurate capacity in these areas for the randomly arriving urgent/emergent patients. Simulation modeling provides the ability to simulate various scheduling options for the elective volumes, focusing on utilization not only in the procedural areas but also in the destination unit to which these elective patients should go post-procedure.[16] Thus patients predictably are admitted and discharged to the downstream units, and the peaks and valleys in the inpatient census are minimized. Doing so actually increases the functional capacity of the hospital without increasing physical capacity or staff.

## Conclusion

Despite significant differences between the healthcare system in the USA and that of other nations, similarities in regards to patient experience and engagement enable many of the US ED experiences to provide potentially useful insights for other countries regarding the ED.

First, higher patient satisfaction has a number of tangible benefits for an organization. Studies have shown that organizations with higher patient satisfaction tend to have higher staff satisfaction, fewer patient lawsuits, better patient compliance with recommended care, better patient response to actual treatment, and stronger financial performance.

Second, patient satisfaction can be markedly improved through recognizing the need for improvement, putting the right processes in place to enhance satisfaction and creating a culture that rewards improvement of the patient experience.

Third, measuring patient satisfaction in the ED is not something that should be done once a year or once a quarter. Continuous satisfaction measurement provides the motivation for doctors and nurses to improve by being able to see the results of changes sooner rather than later, by having a sufficient number of surveys to draw meaningful conclusions, and by providing the means to reward improvements.

Fourth, patient satisfaction needs to be viewed as an opportunity to better fulfill the organization's mission and provide better, more compassionate care, rather than as a burden that needs to be attended to because of outside pressures from the government, other payers, or healthcare consumers themselves.

Do the unique characteristics of each country or region need to be taken into account in designing the strategies for improving patient satisfaction and measuring success in the ED? Of course, but the greater preponderance of similarities in ED care and patient perceptions of that experience across different environments should be the driving force for improvement.

## References

1. Isaac T, Zaslavsky A, Cleary D, Landon B. The relationship between patients' perception of care and measures of hospital quality and safety, *Health Services Research* 2010; **45**: 1024–40.

2. Jha AK, Orav, EJ, Zheng J, Epstein AM. Patients' perception of hospital care in the United States. *New England Journal of Medicine* 2008; **359**: 1921–31.

3. Glickman S, Boulding W, Manary M, *et al.* Patient satisfaction and its relationship with clinical quality and inpatient mortality in acute myocardial infarction. *Circulation, Cardiovascular Quality and Outcomes* 2010; **3**: 188–95.

4. Trucano M, Kaldenberg DO. The relationship between patient perceptions of hospital practices and facility infection rates: evidence from Pennsylvania hospitals. *Patient Safety & Quality Healthcare* 2007. http://www. psqh.com/enews/0807feature. shtml (accessed January 2014).

5. Valentine NB, de Silva A, Kawabata K, *et al. Health System Responsiveness: Concepts, Domains, and Operationalization.* Geneva: World Health Organization, 2003; 573–96.

6. Press Ganey. *Emergency Department Pulse Report 2010: Patient Perspectives on American*

*Health Care*. South Bend, IN: Press Ganey Associates, 2010.

7.  American College of Emergency Physicians. *The National Report Card on the State of Emergency Medicine*. http://www.emreportcard.org (accessed January 2014).

8.  American Hospital Association. *Trendwatch Chartbook 2010*. http://www.aha.org/research/reports/tw/chartbook/2010chartbook.shtml (accessed January 2014).

9.  Press Ganey. *Patients, Physicians and Employees: Satisfaction Trifecta Brings Bottom Line Results*. South Bend, IN: Press Ganey Associates, 2006.

10. Malott DL, Fulton BR. Patient satisfaction surveys are here to stay . . . so let's make sure they are valid and reliable. *Emergency Physicians Monthly* November 2010; **18**.

11. Hall M. Looking to improve financial results? Start by listening to patients. *Healthcare Financial Management*, Oct 2008.

12. Burnes B. *At the Reading Hospital, New Care Processes and a Welcoming Attitude Drive an ED Transformation*. South Bend, IN: Press Ganey Associates, 2011.

13. Bachenheimer E. Goodbye waiting room. *Emergency Physicians Monthly* January 2008; **31**.

14. Jayaprakash N, O'Sullivan R, Bey T, Ahmed SS, Lotfipour S. Crowding and delivery of healthcare in emergency departments: the European perspective. *Western Journal of Emergency Medicine* 2009; **10**: 223–39.

15. Gilligan P, Winder S, Ramphul N, O'Kelly P. The referral and complete evaluation time study. *European Journal of Emergency Medicine* 2010; **17**: 349–53.

16. Laskowski M, McLeod RD, Friesen MR, Podaima BW, Alfa AS. Models of emergency departments for reducing patient waiting times. *PLoS One*. 2009; **4** (7): e6127.

**Chapter**

# 15

# The leader's toolbox: things they didn't teach in nursing or medical school

Robert L. Freitas

## Key learning points

- Understand the importance of a systematic approach to interviewing and how to develop and use a system.
- Use quick and easy methods to have more time available and manage it better.
- Reflect on the importance of separating and balancing work and life and learn ways to better find this balance.

## Introduction

Many people in positions of leadership in the emergency department (ED) and at the hospital level who started out as clinicians tell of being unprepared for the leadership position in which they found themselves. Individuals may often be promoted to their first leadership position because of clinical prowess, or because no one more qualified was available to step into the vacant position.

Among the many management challenges with which new ED leaders sometimes struggle, three of the most common include interviewing and hiring new team members, effective time management, and balancing work and home life. This chapter will provide an overview of how leaders can step up to these new tasks.

## Interviewing

Finding the right person for a position in the ED can be difficult. As we all know, it takes a certain mindset, personality, level of training, and level of experience. Often people are hired or promoted in the ED based on a favorable recommendation by someone else or after one or more interviews that did not actually focus on the important attributes of a good ED

employee. Individuals may be promoted based on attributes important in their prior position, but less important in their new position. Finding the right person for the job is important on many levels and can even have financial consequences for the organization. One study revealed that for each year a good employee is on the job, he or she can potentially contribute monetary value of 70–140% of his/her annual salary to the organization.[1] Good employees provide better patient care, reduce patient complaints, make fewer bad decisions, cause less stress in the ED, and allow ED leaders to focus their time on important tasks. Hiring the wrong person can be a grave mistake, especially in government-funded or labor union-dominated systems, as it can be extremely difficult to fire someone once hired.[2]

Finding good employees need not be a daunting task. However, it does require planning, organization, and an understanding of what attributes you are looking for in that "ideal" employee. While some organizations may use tests, simulations, background checks, or peer and subordinate appraisals, almost all hiring and some promotions involve interviews. The goal in developing tools for interviewing should be that they are easy to implement, able to withstand legal challenges posed in union or government service environments, and consistently identify the right people to do the job at hand.

*Unstructured interviews* are very common. In this type of interview there is no set interview team, interviewers are free to ask any questions they wish, and few notes are taken, discussed, or shared among the interviewers. This approach has proven less effective than more structured interviews. A study by McDaniels *et al.* demonstrated that beneficial employees were more likely to be hired with a structured approach.[3] The structured interview uses an

*Emergency Department Leadership and Management*, ed. Stephanie Kayden, *et al.* Published by Cambridge University Press.
© Cambridge University Press 2015.

organized, step-by-step format with predetermined questions, a set interview team, and a prior review of the job description to determine which attributes are most desirable.

There are many different types of structured interviews. An interview process often starts with a *screening interview* that might be done over the phone, via email or letter, or face to face and is designed to quickly eliminate unqualified candidates who lack experience or training, who do not approve of the job hours or benefits, or whose CVs need clarification.[4] Screening interviews can be beneficial as long as they are conducted in a professional manner, by appointment, with documentation of the candidate's responses to the questions. The *situational interview*, first described in 1980, uses situational questions posed to the interviewee, such as "What would you do if the ambulance service notified you right now they were bringing in 50 patients from a chemical fire?"[5] *Stress interviews* can be a part of any of the other types of interviews, and are generally used to see how the candidate might respond to stressful environments or situations. There can be both positive and negative aspects to stress interviews. While someone interviewing for an ED job will be expected to work in stressful situations, there is no direct correlation between working under stress in the ED and sitting through a stressful experience in an interview. Be careful not to use stress interviews simply as an alternative to other interviewing techniques that require more preparation.[6,7] The last type of structured interview is the *behavioral interview*, which seeks to determine the facts behind past or present behaviors. Research indicates that the likelihood of finding the right person for the job is higher if a highly structured behavioral interview is used.[1]

Structured interviews take more time but yield better results.[8] A good interview process requires planning and preparation. Candidates may have been coached by recruiters on what to say, or they may have sat through several interviews prior to yours and thus feel comfortable with the process and simply respond with well-rehearsed answers. The first step is to determine what attributes are being sought in the new hire. Will there be technologies or protocols that are not being used now but are planned on being used in the near future that might be important? Will this person have administrative responsibilities? Establishing key components of the position up front is very important. Is creative problem solving important,

learning from mistakes, or is the ability to get things done by using influence and persuasion rather than authority key in the role?[9,10] It is advisable to do a thorough job analysis before hiring for a position, and keep in mind that jobs change over time. The job analysis should be repeated regularly if the job changes frequently.[11]

The next step is to determine who will interview the candidates. While candidates are sometimes only interviewed by the supervisor of the position, there is value in taking a team approach in which additional interviews are conducted by peers, subordinates, and others that the candidate will be expected to interact with in the ED setting. This can be accomplished either in a panel or individually, but it is best to use the same team of interviewers so that all candidates can be compared.

If a panel is used it should be small enough that the entire interview can be completed in less than one hour. A panel of more than seven or eight people becomes unwieldy. A benefit of panels is that they send the message that teamwork is important. An interview panel for an ED physician position might include a primary care physician or hospital-based specialist with whom the ED physicians routinely interact, a nurse, the direct ED supervisor, and other ED physicians. For an ED nurse position, the interview panel might consist of other staff nurses, an ED physician, a nurse from another department, and the direct supervisor.

It is advisable to meet with the team or distribute information beforehand on interviewing to ensure that everyone knows the desired selection criteria including skills, knowledge base, experience, education, and personal attributes that fit the organizational culture. If there are any relevant local human resource laws or regulations that relate to hiring, it is important that everyone on the team understands these.

Once the interviewers have been selected, a series of questions should be formulated and written down. About 10–15 good questions should allow the interviewer to elicit the information necessary to make a decision about the applicant. This is important, and should be considered one of the most important parts of the interview. The goal is to gain insight into the applicant's past behaviors in a variety of situations. Ideally these questions should be open-ended and designed to allow the candidate to talk about past experiences and how they handled them (Table 15.1).

**Table 15.1** Examples of behavioral interview questions

Tell us about a time where you thought you made an incorrect clinical decision, and what you did about it.

Describe a time when your persistence about something benefitted a patient in the ED.

How do you go about building a trusting relationship with a co-worker?

Describe the latest journal article you read about emergency medicine or emergency nursing.

Elaborate about a time when you felt overwhelmed while working in the ED.

All of us at some point in our careers have done something at work that was criticized; tell us about a time when that happened to you.

What were your most important contributions/accomplishments at your previous job?

Tell us how you approach the start of a shift in the ED knowing it is a very busy period.

What and when was the last professional educational activity you undertook?

In your previous job, what were the most difficult decisions you had to make?

What behaviors do you demonstrate in the ED to lead by example?

What was the most difficult change in work you encountered recently?

Where do you find yourself most comfortable in the ED: in a serious trauma situation, fast track or observation rooms, acute medical situation, or some other situation?

---

**Case study 15.1**

Mario was interviewing for a staff doctor position in the ED. The ED chief had assembled an interview team of both doctors and nurses as a way to improve teamwork. Silvio, one of the nurses on the interview team, forgot to ask behavioral questions and instead asked Mario how he got along with the nurses. Mario said he got along very well with everyone in his past job and he treated everyone equally. Paola, remembering to use behavioral questions, asked Mario to describe a time when he disagreed with the way a nurse was taking care of one of his patients. Mario went on to describe an incident from last month when a nurse disagreed with him about discharging a patient. The nurse, who had spent the better part of the day with the patient, suggested keeping the patient a little longer as she was not sure the patient was ready to go home. Mario wanted to clear out most of the patients before the end of his shift and was eager to discharge him. Mario recounted how at his last job there were many nurses who thought they went to medical school and often disagreed with him, but it was his responsibility to take care of the patient, and he had to be the one who made the decisions.

Effective questioning can explore both negative and positive experiences, such as, "Tell us about a time when you disagreed with your supervisor about a policy she enacted?" During the ideal interview, the candidate should do most of the talking, but the interviewers may certainly ask follow-up questions to obtain more detail on a topic. The interviewer might say, "Tell me more about this; I am very interested," or "How did this make you feel?" Ensure the responses to the questions are specific and, if the response does not answer the question, keep probing until you have an answer.

Many organizations use interview guides with rating scales that allow for more consistent evaluation among interviewers. If a guide is not used, interviewers are encouraged to take thorough notes, even though this may affect the candidates' responses. Mention at the beginning of the interview that notes will be taken and that this is a normal part of the interview process.

While it can be tempting for interviewers to talk a lot during the interview, the goal should be that most, perhaps 75%, of the talking is done by the candidate.[1] One should avoid giving advice to interviewees or telling them how they are doing. While it may be tempting to argue with a candidate if he or she says something with which you disagree, doing so usually solicits less useful information. Disagreement may actually improve the process, however, if it leads to a thorough discussion of a topic.

Immediately after the interview is over, the interviewers should document their findings and thoughts using a formal interview guide or their individual notes. It is best to convene a discussion about the candidate while the information is still fresh. Research shows that interviewers usually decide if they like a candidate within 30 seconds. While it may be tempting to rule someone in or out early in the interview, it is prudent to reserve judgment and take into consideration the other team members' findings. They may have seen or felt things you missed.[12] If there are multiple candidates, it is best to rank them so that if the most desirable candidate does not accept the position, the next most desirable candidate is clearly identified. If there are missing pieces of information after the interviews, one of the team should call the applicant for follow-up. However, be careful not to provide information to the applicant about how he or she performed in the interview, as this could be misinterpreted as a prelude to a job offer. Prior to making the job offer, an appropriate background check, including verification of references, should be carried out for all potential new hires, not just physicians and nurses.

## Time management

Hiring the right person the first time is an efficient use of time, but most leaders at some point feel overwhelmed with their responsibilities and feel that there is not enough time in the day to get all of their work done. By working smarter instead of harder, one can free up additional time to get more work done or to spend more time away from work and achieve a better work–life balance.

Leadership time can be broken down into three categories:

- boss-imposed time
- system-imposed time
- *self-imposed time*, which can be further subdivided into *discretionary time* and *subordinate-imposed time*[13]

There are few things that can be done about boss-imposed time, which involves tasks assigned by one's direct supervisor. The same is true of system-imposed time, which is, for example, the clinical shifts you are required to work or the monthly physicians' clinical shift schedule that you must prepare. It is during self-imposed time that one carries out many leadership activities: setting vision, deciding how work will be done by subordinates, and planning changes for how

care is given. Managing self-imposed time effectively is one of the keys to being an effective ED leader.

Despite widespread expectations about the working world becoming paperless, we still deal with multiple pieces of paper every day: invoices, bills, journals, and letters. Past conventional wisdom was that a piece of paper should only be dealt with once. In reality, this is impractical.[14] If papers are piling up all around you, either in the office or at home, devote some time to reorganizing these. Review each piece of paper one by one without reading it. If the paper belongs to someone else, put it in a "forward" pile. If you think you might need it, consider whether the document is available as an electronic file. If so, consider discarding it; if not, put in your "keeper" file. Your keeper file is for those things that you either need to take action on soon, or you need to keep as a record. In the latter case you should either file it immediately or scan it into an electronic file for safe-keeping. Also ask yourself, "Who sent this to me?" Chances are the original sender still has the original, allowing you to discard it.

The same systematic approach should apply to newspapers, journals, and magazines. Newspapers more than two or three days old should be discarded; if a particular article draws your interest, cut it out and save it in a file. For journals, visually scan the table of contents for interesting articles and then cut out the article, flag it for later reading, or scan it into an electronic file. In this manner, you can winnow down the pile of emergency medicine journals you keep promising to read in only minutes and get a lot of clutter off your desk. According to Mayer, up to 60–80% of all papers on and within the workspace can be discarded.[14] As you go through your piles of journals and magazines, ask yourself when you last read it and consider whether to continue the subscription. You might also see if there is an online version that you can access at your leisure.

Mayer's advice is to do away with sticky notes and use what he calls a "master list," which is just a "to-do" list.[14] He suggests that many people who use sticky notes to keep track of things either generate so many that they cannot keep track of them, or the notes are lost, crumpled, or forgotten. One approach is to use limited sticky notes for jotting down quick items such as phone numbers or names, but then sticking them on your to-do list or directly to your handheld phone or personal digital assistant so you can enter the information later to your contact list or, if it requires action, to your to-do list. Regardless of whether you keep your list electronically or on paper, remember to take things off as they are done each day and to reprioritize them as they move up or down in urgency, so you feel you are making progress. If you are using paper, or frequently forget to check your electronic list, put your list on a big piece of paper that you either keep with you or place in a prominent position on your desk so you cannot forget things that are important to do.

Learning to be realistic about deadlines is an important component of managing time. Understanding the true deadline for a project or document can save stress for both leader and subordinates. Telling a subordinate something must be done by Friday at "the close of business" if you have no intent of looking at it until the following week only adds unneeded stress to employees. If someone asks you for something "as soon as possible," try to understand more specifically when that is. Does it mean in the next two hours, anytime today, or by the end of next week? Depending on the item, do not be afraid to negotiate. If it is impossible to finish something by the imposed deadline, be honest and tell the person who imposed the deadline when you can finish, but then it is important to actually meet the deadline by the negotiated new date.

Another way to free up time is by empowering staff. While this is not widely discussed in time management books or educational programs, it can be a very effective strategy to allow staff to make decisions without seeking constant approval, but to hold them accountable for their decisions by giving them feedback. This concept was discussed by Oncken and Wass in 1974, and by Blanchard and Johnson in 1981.[13,15] All too often, subordinates come to leaders with the expectation that the leader is there to solve all their problems. Smart leaders know that by empowering subordinates to try solving problems first, and then coming to the leader only after these attempts have failed, they will in turn have more time to create vision and make strategic decisions. An investment up front in education or programs on decision making at all levels, and policies that reward initiative, is a critical step.

---

**Case study 15.2**

Inger had taken the job of ED director thinking she would have time to solve many of the longstanding problems in the ED such as overcrowding, low staff morale, and a poorly designed work schedule. She had learned in a management article the importance of keeping an open-door policy, and while her door was open her staff poured in every day to tell her about the delays in radiology and lab, problems with the old chairs in the charting room, messy ultrasound probes, and similar issues. She was finding that she could not get her own work done. After reading an article about empowering employees, she decided to enact a rule that she would still have an open-door policy, but from now on her staff could not come to her about a problem unless they had attempted to solve it themselves, they had researched possible solutions and needed her approval to try them, or the nature of the problem was such that it needed immediate action by a person at her level in the organization. At first, things did not change – until she realized she needed to be supportive of the staff's attempts at problem solving and enrolled them in a decision-making course sponsored by the Ministry of Health. In three months, she realized she had at least an extra two hours per day to solve high-level organizational problems given to her by her superiors instead of spinning her wheels trying to solve every employee's problem.

---

The use of teams to free up time for the leadership is also important. Again, this involves empowering staff to make decisions.

No discussion of time management is complete without addressing the issue of email. While originally conceived as a more efficient way to communicate than phone or the postal system, it has come to take over a large portion of our business lives and often leads to information overload. There are many studies that have looked at the negative impact of email on our lives. Microsoft researchers found in one study that on average it takes 25 minutes to return to work after an email interruption.[16] However, with just a few self-imposed rules one can adopt an improved email discipline that can save additional time for other activities. Turning off the automated notification feature in the email program on both one's desktop and personal digital assistant or smart phone will limit the constant interruptions that result from incoming new emails. If responding to email is consuming too much time, take an occasional email holiday where you do not answer any emails for a day, or limit your email time to two hours daily. It is, however, wise to inform your superiors and colleagues first that you will be doing this.

Part of the challenge with email is changing the email culture in your organization. As the leader, you might choose to declare an email-free period each week, during which no one can send internal emails. You could also decide that emails of a purely informational nature should only be posted on the company intranet, social network page, or other common platforms instead of sending as email to the whole organization. As the leader, you also can set rules or guidelines about when a telephone call is more appropriate than email: when the topic may be controversial or cause anger on the part of the recipient, or when the information is hard to convey in a brief email. Studies have shown that people interpret the tone of an email correctly only 50% of the time, and that misplaced anger or confusion about the tone of a message wastes time through distraction and lost motivation to work diligently.[17]

Old emails that are kept for reference should be organized by folders or topics in the same manner that paper files are kept, so that they will be easier to find in the future. Responding to emails as they come in will decrease the likelihood of missing an important one. Emails that have been read and acted upon or that are for information only should be deleted. Deleting emails is also important to ensure that the mailbox does not become so full that one can no longer send and receive new emails. Another strategy is to sort old email by sender and delete whole groups of email from specific senders, for example, corporate messages that are not pertinent to the ED or those that are from non-work senders such as vendors.

There are other relatively simple things to get your day jump-started. Look at your to-do list at the end of every day and decide which things are the most important to tackle tomorrow. If there are many difficult tasks to do the next day, block out the first two hours of the day, close your office door, turn off the phone, do not look at email, and schedule this time as an appointment with yourself. When you are working exclusively on administrative tasks on a given day, consider working from home all or part of the day to minimize distractions.

## Work–life balance

Effective time management also needs to factor in one's obligations and responsibilities outside of work. Much has been written about work–life balance, stress,

and burnout among emergency medicine clinicians, but little has been written about these issues among ED leaders.[18–20] Many of the participants in the International Emergency Department Leadership Institute (IEDLI) report that they are contracted to work 37–40 hours weekly, but in reality work many more hours than that.[21] In one study by the London Institute of Management of individuals in leadership positions, more than 85% of respondents were contacted by employees outside of work hours, and 75% said they worked longer than their contracted hours.[22] With smartphones, laptops, social networking websites, and other portable devices linking leaders to work 24/7, the term "weisure" has been used to describe the fact that work frequently intrudes into leisure time.[23] Another study of professionals indicated that 94% of 1000 professionals put in 50 hours weekly and, of that group, 50% worked up to 65 hours weekly, which did not include time spent checking emails on smartphones.[24] This same study showed that when people are "always on," this level of responsiveness becomes the norm, and is expected by both bosses and subordinates. However, taking predictable time off during which only significant emergencies are dealt with did not impact job performance and led to a happier, more creative workforce. As an ED leader, one must effectively manage one's own time and achieve a favorable work–life balance, but also help subordinates do the same. Subordinates should be encouraged to take accrued vacation time and days off and, when not expected to be at the ED, to take at least one day off from work every week free from work-related activities.

The demands of leadership positions, including office work, reading and understanding budgets, dealing with employees, and working an occasional off-shift can certainly lead to fatigue. Most leaders would never entertain the thought of taking a nap at work; however, one study showed that a quick nap lasting no more than 30 minutes with REM sleep improved the napper's ability to integrate unassociated information and led to enhanced problem solving.[25]

The clinical work of emergency medicine, be it at a nurse's, physician's, or any other level, is serious and often stressful work. Yet there are steps that ED leaders can take to make the work experience more enjoyable and fun, and thereby less stressful. Everyone, including ED leaders, seeks opportunity, professional development, and positive feedback.

Make your job, and those of your subordinates, less stressful by giving praise often and criticism infrequently. According to Zeff, giving those around you opportunities to improve and demonstrate their abilities improves morale, fosters creativity, reduces stress, and increases commitment.[26] In the long run, this approach makes the job of the ED leader easier, decreases the need to be "on" 24/7, and allows the leader to feel less stressed when away from work, knowing that a capable team is at the ready in the ED.

Work–life balance can also be improved by accepting that almost every day as an ED leader is going to be filled with change. On a global basis, the challenges facing ED leaders are growing and include dealing with overcrowding, reduced budgets, sicker patients who demand more care, and politicians pushing to meet these demands. Being open to this change and accepting it as part of one's daily life will also allow one to keep work in better perspective, according to Zeff, and plays an important role in enhancing our leadership abilities as well as our ability to communicate and be creative.[26]

## Summary

The three topics presented here, albeit briefly, are intended as an overview and to encourage further reading on the subjects. Finding the right people for your ED team, managing your own time effectively, and striking an effective balance between work and the rest of your life are important aspects of leadership that should be embraced by every ED leader. As important as these are for the ED leader personally, it is equally important to cultivate these skills among staff and subordinates as well.

## References

1. Turner TS. *Behavioral Interviewing Guide.* Victoria, BC: Trafford, 2004.

2. Fernandez CS, Baker EL. The behavioral event interview: avoiding interviewing pitfalls when hiring. *Journal of Public Health Management Practice* **12**: 590–3.

3. McDaniel MA, Whetzel DL, Schmidt FL, Maurer SD. The validity of employment interviews: a comprehensive review and meta-analysis. *Journal of Applied Psychology* 1994; **79**: 599–616.

4. Hoeveneyer VA. *High Impact Interview Questions.* New York, NY: Amacom Books, 2005.

5. Taylor PJ, O'Driscoll MP. *Structured Employee Interviewing.* London: Gower, 1998.

6. Matias L. *How to Say It: Job Interviews.* New York, NY: Prentice Hall, 2007.

7. Arthur D. *Recruiting, Interviewing, Selecting, and Orienting New Employees.* New York, NY: American Management Association, 2006.

8. Jenks JM, Zevnik BLP. ABCs of job interviewing. *Harvard Business Review* July 1989.

9. Ross JA. Hiring for intangibles. *Harvard Management Update* 2007. http://reporting.talent20.co.za/Harvard/HMM10/hiring/resources/U0701D.pdf (accessed January 2014).

10. Bielaszka-DuVernay C. Hiring for emotional intelligence. *Harvard Management Update* October 2008.

11. Foster C, Godkin L. Employment selection in health care: the case for structured interviewing. *Health Care Management Review* 1998; **23**: 46–51.

12. Joyce MP. Interview techniques used in selected organizations today. *Business Communication Quarterly* September 2008; 379.

13. Oncken W, Wass DL. Who's got the monkey. *Harvard Business Review* November–December 1999; 180.

14. Mayer JJ. *Time Management for Dummies*, 2nd edn. New York, NY: Hungry Minds, 1999.

15. Blanchard K, Johnson S. *One Minute Manager.* New York, NY: Berkeley Books, 1982.

16. Hemp P. Death by information overload. *Harvard Business Review* September 2009; 83.

17. Leahy S. The secret cause of flame wars, 2006. http://www.wired.com/print/science/discoveries/news/2006/02/70179 (accessed February 15, 2011).

18. Popa F, Arafat R, Purcărea VL, *et al.* Occupational burnout levels in emergency medicine: a stage 2 nationwide study and analysis. *Journal of Medicine and Life* 2010; **3**: 449–53.

19. Estryn-Behar M, Doppia MA, Guetarni K, *et al.* Emergency physicians accumulate more stress factors than other physicans: results from the French SESMAT study. *Emergency Medicine Journal* 2010; **28**: 397–410.

20. LeBlanc C, Heyworth J. Emergency physicians: "burned out" or "fired up"? *CJEM* 2001; **9**: 121–3.

21. International Emergency Department Leadership Institute (IEDLI). http://www.iedli.org (accessed January 2014).

22. Clutterbuck D. *Managing the Work–Life Balance*. London: Chartered Institute of Personnel & Development, 2003; 2.

23. Creagan ET. Don't forget the "life" in work–life balance. Mayo Clinic. http://www.mayoclinic.com/health/work-life-balance/MY01203/method=print (accessed April 3, 2011).

24. Perlow LA, Porter JL. Making time off predictable – and required. *Harvard Business Review* Oct 2009; 102–9.

25. Stickgold R. The simplest way to reboot your brain. *Harvard Business Review* Oct 2009; 36.

26. Zeff J. *Make the Right Choice: Creating a Positive, Innovative, and Productive Work Life*. Hoboken, NJ: Wiley, 2007.

## Further reading

Cydulka RK, Korte R. Career satisfaction in emergency medicine: the ABEM Longitudinal Study of Emergency Medicine. *Annals of Emergency Medicine* 2008; 51: 714–22.

Fitzwater TL. *Behavior-Based Interviewing: Selecting the Right Person for the Job*. Boston, MA: Thomson Learning, 2000.

Keeton K, Fenner DE, Johnson TR, Hayward RA. Predictors of physician career satisfaction, work–life balance, and burnout. *Obestetrics and Gynecology* 2007; 109: 949–55.

Martin F, Poyen D, Bouderlique E, *et al.* Depression and burnout in hospital health care professionals. *International Journal of Occupational and Environmental Health* 1997; 3: 203–9.

Schlenger S, Roesch R. *How to Be Organized in Spite of Yourself*. New York, NY: Penguin, 1989.

## Chapter 1

# Assessing your needs

Manuel Hernandez

## Key learning points

- Understand how to approach a comprehensive operations assessment, including what to measure and how to measure it.
- Quantify the current state of operations and the potential impact of proposed changes on clinical, operational, and financial performance.
- Effectively communicate the outcomes of the operations assessment to both clinical and non-clinical stakeholders, including those both inside and outside the emergency department.

## Introduction

Over the past four decades, emergency medicine has evolved, becoming a global component of patient access strategies. As emergency medicine has gained popularity, many advanced and developing health systems have increased the number of emergency departments (EDs), expanding the scope of their services and developing tiered and specialty levels of care such as trauma centers, chest pain units, and acute stroke centers.[1–3]

While the growth of emergency medicine and the development of EDs has favorably impacted on access to care, speed to care, and overall clinical quality and outcomes, it has also been a victim of its own success. EDs worldwide are straining to cope with surging demand and high acuity levels. Overcrowding has become commonplace. Patient volumes are growing.[4,5] Visit times are increasing, causing many non-urgent and a number of urgent and emergent patients to leave the ED without treatment and seek alternative care.[4] Ambulance diversion is a real and growing problem in some systems.[6]

While the impact of increased ED utilization on the overall healthcare system varies by delivery model,

the key themes remain the same. In market-driven systems, overcrowded and inefficient EDs can impact the financial performance of the entire hospital. In state-sponsored systems, where cost control is essential, suboptimal ED operations and crowding can siphon limited resources away from preventive and acute care services.

As emergency medicine continues its global growth and evolution, attention has turned to understanding the impact of clinical and administrative operations. A comprehensive understanding of ED operations facilitates the development of innovative practices to improve operational performance. Along with this understanding comes the need to effectively communicate the current state, potential solutions, and expected outcomes of these solutions to all stakeholders, including clinical staff, patients, and administrators.

## Performing an operations assessment

Initiating an ED operations assessment begins with developing a comprehensive understanding of the current state. This current-state assessment forms a foundation to understand which operational aspects are negatively impacting key performance metrics:

- clinical quality
- length of stay
- patient satisfaction
- revenue
- operating costs
- growth

Choosing what to assess is as important as the assessment itself. Selecting performance metrics too narrow in scope results in a limited, inaccurate understanding of ED operations, while selecting metrics too expansive creates confusion in the analysis. For the purposes

*Emergency Department Leadership and Management*, ed. Stephanie Kayden, *et al.* Published by Cambridge University Press.
© Cambridge University Press 2015.

of this chapter, the assessment will remain focused on operational principles related to patient throughput, service excellence, and fiscal stewardship. Quality metrics are addressed in detail in Chapter 7.

Comprehensive ED operations assessments should involve the following assessment tools:

- advanced data analytics
- stakeholder interviews
- direct observation and shadowing
- process mapping

## Advanced data analytics

### Timestamp analysis

Timestamp analysis is the first step in assessing ED performance data, identifying which steps in the ED throughput process have the greatest impact on length of stay and overall performance. Based on an adaptation and refinement of ED flow process models created by Asplin *et al.* and Fatovich, the ED process can be broken into three patient-care phases: (1) access, (2) evaluation and management, (3) disposition (Fig. 16.1).[6,8]

Once the key steps occurring in each phase have been identified, an appropriate timestamp analysis can be carried out, examining, but not limited to, the steps outlined in Figure 16.2.

Typically, timestamp data should be collected for a period of 12 contiguous months. Although this is time-consuming, such an analysis provides an accurate assessment of operations, and takes into account any variability that could be caused by random incidents such as:

- staffing shortages
- unanticipated inpatient capacity constraints
- seasonal volume variations due to trauma and/or infectious diseases
- ambulance diversion to/from other facilities
- mass casualty incidents

Comprehensive data capture is not always possible, particularly in EDs with limited information technology infrastructure. In such instances, directional data representing more focused time periods are appropriate for the purposes of an operational assessment. When intending to use directional data, efforts should be made to account for any volume or operational variabilities not considered characteristic during normal operations. If adequate retrospective timestamp information is available, select data from four one-week periods, with each week separated by three months (for example, January, April, July, and October).

In the absence of proper retrospective data, prospective timestamp analysis can be undertaken. In this instance, seven or thirty contiguous days of assessment, depending on available resources and patient volumes, should be undertaken. The data gathered will provide ample information for analysis and assessment.

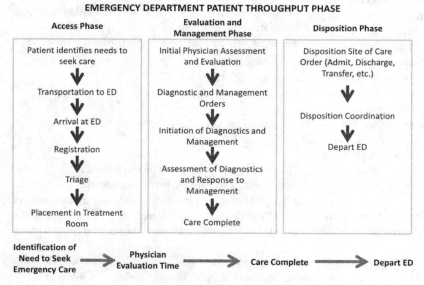

**EMERGENCY DEPARTMENT PATIENT THROUGHPUT PHASE**

**Figure 16.1** Emergency department patient throughput phase. The model illustrates "traditional" ED throughput. Steps may vary by ED.

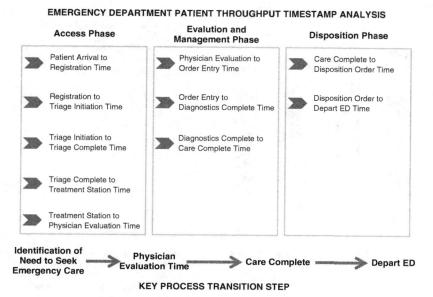

**EMERGENCY DEPARTMENT PATIENT THROUGHPUT TIMESTAMP ANALYSIS**

**Figure 16.2** Emergency department patient throughput timestamp analysis. Source: Emergency department data analysis; Confluence by CannonDesign, Chicago, IL, USA, 2011.

Once data have been collected, analysis should be completed using multiple techniques. As an operational assessment is different from a scientific research project, the goal should be to create analytic outputs that inform the current state and form a baseline for ongoing analysis and response to interventions. While traditional operational data analysis focuses on mean times, this information can be very misleading, providing department leaders with a false sense of security with respect to operations. Advanced analytic methods such as quartile regression have been effectively employed to assess throughput.[9] For the purposes of most departmental assessments, the use of median and interquartile ranges will provide ample information from which to develop a framework for understanding current operations.

## Patient satisfaction data

In many health systems across the globe, greater emphasis is being placed on ensuring that patient care meets a level of patient satisfaction considered appropriate for the ED setting. Regardless of health-system model, patient satisfaction analysis can be a useful tool to assess perceptions of quality, and also to assess responses to operational changes that are designed to expedite patient throughput, reduce costs, and enhance the patient experience.[10–12]

Multiple tools exist in the marketplace to assess patients' perceptions of their ED experience. While there is no one right approach to assessing satisfaction, a core group of metrics should be considered as essential to identifying potential operational and care delivery issues in the ED:

- time to see physician
- quality of pain management
- information concerning care status/delays
- satisfaction with perceived quality of care
- overall length of stay
- understanding of discharge instructions
- compassion/politeness of physicians and nurses
- willingness to recommend

Patient satisfaction data should be analyzed from the same time periods that are used to complete the advanced data analysis, and correlations should be made to draw parallels between operational considerations and overall patient satisfaction.[13] Additional information on measuring patient satisfaction can be found in Chapter 14.

## Staffing analysis

Building a clear understanding of ED operations mandates an assessment of existing staffing models. Often, staffing resources are not aligned to department census, resulting in overall increases in length of stay, reductions in patient satisfaction, and negative impacts on quality and outcomes.[14] While there are fixed ED staffing models, research is ongoing to develop models to identify optimal ED human resource requirements.[15]

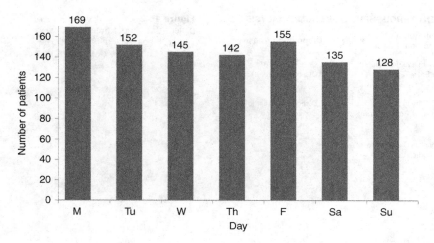

**Figure 16.3** Emergency department patient volumes by day of the week. Observations from July 1, 2010, to June 30, 2011. Source: Emergency department data analysis; Confluence by CannonDesign, Chicago, IL, USA, 2011.

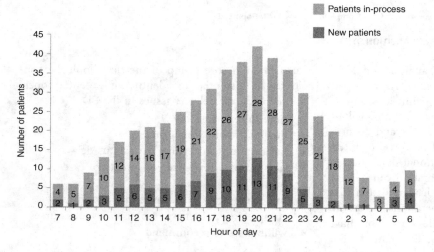

**Figure 16.4** Emergency department patient volumes by hour. Observations from July 1, 2010, to June 30, 2011. Source: Emergency department data analysis; Confluence by CannonDesign, Chicago, IL, USA, 2011.

Staffing models analysis involves a comparison of staffing against patient census at predefined intervals. As staffing and patient census are both dynamic processes, it is recommended that this analysis consider variability in patient volume and staffing levels by hour of the day and day of the week (Figs. 16.3, 16.4). In addition, staffing models should also consider all ED team members actively involved in either direct or indirect patient care.

Staff roles that should be evaluated as a part of any staffing analysis include, but are not necessarily limited to:

- physicians
- physician extenders
- nurses
- technicians
- clerical staff
- environmental services

Additional information on assessing ED staffing can be found in Chapter 20.

## Financial metrics

While the "story" of financial performance differs between a market-driven system and a state-sponsored system, the ED's financial performance is important nonetheless. As clinicians tend to focus primarily on the quality implications of operational opportunities, hospital leadership, forced to allocate limited resources across the entire clinical enterprise, is more likely to balance the quality implications with overall cost, return on investment, and competing priorities.

Data for completing the financial portion of the assessment should reflect the realities of the individual health system. In the case of systems where hospitals, and specifically EDs, receive fixed or variable revenue on a per-patient basis, both revenue and expenses should be analyzed. EDs operating on a fixed budget regardless of patient or diagnostic volumes require analysis centered on reducing the overall cost of care per patient.[16] In assessing financial performance, both fixed and variable costs should be assessed to identify opportunities to reduce the overall cost of care without compromising clinical quality and outcomes.

## Team member interviews

While using advanced data analytics to create a common understanding of the current state is an important first step, the data only tell part of the story. With the data in hand, the next component of assessing ED operations is to speak with team members on an individual basis.

While the specifics of the information to gather during interviews are beyond the scope of this chapter and will vary by department and operational model, the focus of the interview process should be to gain a diverse set of perspectives on key concepts:

- perceived current barriers to efficient patient throughput
- inconsistencies in process and workflow contributing to patient throughput challenges
- potential opportunities for throughput improvement
- previous attempts at process improvement and their outcomes

Care should be taken to ensure the interview list is comprehensive, reflecting all groups, both clinical and non-clinical, responsible for ED operations. Potential interview groups are illustrated in Table 16.1.

In addition to selecting a comprehensive group of disciplines to interview, emphasis should also be placed on ensuring that the majority of interviewees selected are frontline employees and not managers or directors. This ensures that the information collected does not have a leadership bias. Similarly, the interviewees selected should represent all shifts and include both weekday and weekend staff, to ensure that variability in operations between periods of time when leadership is and is not present is evaluated and understood.

## Shadowing and direct observation

The goal of shadowing and direct observation is to develop a comprehensive understanding of how patients move through the three phases of ED care, while developing an appreciation for how different

**Table 16.1** Potential interview list for ED operations assessment

| Functional role | Purpose |
|---|---|
| Emergency physician | Understand workflow processes<br>Assess clinical impact of operations |
| Physician extenders | Understand workflow processes<br>Determine how/where used in ED<br>Understand relationship with ED physicians |
| Nursing staff | Understand workflow processes<br>Assess clinical impact of operations<br>Review collaboration between team members |
| Technical staff | Understand workflow processes<br>Assess clinical impact of operations<br>Review collaboration between team members |
| Clerical staff | Understand workflow processes<br>Review collaboration between team members |
| Imaging staff | Understand workflow processes<br>Understand delays impacting imaging |
| Clinical lab staff | Understand workflow processes<br>Understand delays impacting lab processes |
| Admitting physicians | Understand workflow processes<br>Understand delays impacting patient admission |
| Hospital leadership | Understand hospital-wide priorities and resources |
| Ambulance services | Understand relationship with ED<br>Understand delays with EMS arrivals |

functional staff roles execute their work process in pursuit of optimal clinical care and patient throughput. In an operational assessment, shadowing and direct observation is not intended to assess *clinical* performance, but rather to understand *operational* performance.

When conducting shadowing and direct observation activities, it is best to segregate patient-centered activities from staff-centered activities while also ensuring that the ordering of such activities is logical, starting with the access phase and continuing with the evaluation and management and disposition phases.

### Patient-focused shadowing and direct observation

Patient-focused shadowing and direct observation provides a perspective on ED throughput and operations from the viewpoint of the patient. The majority of the entire ED experience occurs without the direct attendance of clinical staff at the patient's side. Given this reality, many staff members are ignorant of much of the ED care delivery process. Observation of patient throughput can be undertaken passively, to reduce patient anxiety and protect privacy. When passive observation is undertaken, observers should make certain to visualize patients at key phases of the ED care delivery process.

### Staff-focused shadowing and direct observation

A comprehensive understanding of staff workflows and their impact on patient throughput and colleague workflows is best accomplished by observing a diverse group of work roles and clinical areas. The primary goals are to understand how workflow processes interface with one another and to identify inefficient, redundant, and improperly ordered processes. In addition, comprehensive staff shadowing affords the opportunity to identify process inconsistencies that create further delays in patient throughput.

When conducting staff shadowing and direct observation, the following clinical and non-clinical functions should be targeted for inclusion:

- emergency physicians (in each clinical area of the ED)
- physician extenders
- charge/lead nurses
- clinical bedside nurses
- triage nurses
- ED technicians
- clerical staff

## Process mapping

The final component of an operations assessment should be the completion of process mapping exercises with the ED staff. The growth of "Lean" methodologies in health care has shown that process mapping exercises form a valuable aspect of understanding operations, identifying inconsistencies in processes, and developing a framework for process improvement initiatives that will flow from the operations assessment.[17,18]

The goal of process mapping exercises is to understand how the pieces of the ED experience fit together, while overlaying the information gathered from the advanced analytics, interviews, and observation activities. In its simplest form, a single, patient-centric process map can be developed showing the ED processes from the perspective of patient flow. In more comprehensive exercises, multiple process maps can be developed, detailing not only patient throughput but also key tasks impacting patient throughput such as diagnostic department workflows, nursing workflows, inpatient admission processes, etc.

Figure 16.5 illustrates a simple yet comprehensive ED process map for the patient intake process (arrival to placement in treatment station).

While there is no one right approach to process-mapping exercises, information can be gathered quickly and comprehensively through a collaborative, multidisciplinary visioning session with representatives from all work disciplines involved in a patient's ED experience. The list of potential participants includes:

- emergency physicians
- physician extenders
- charge/lead nurses

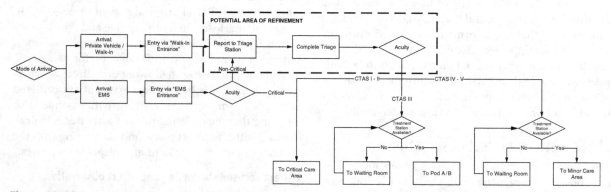

**Figure 16.5** Emergency department patient arrival process map. CTAS, Canadian Triage Acuity Score; EMS, emergency medical services. Source: Emergency department data analysis; Confluence by CannonDesign, Chicago, IL, USA, 2011.

- clinical bedside nurses
- triage nurses
- ED technicians
- clerical staff
- environmental services
- diagnostic imaging staff (x-ray and CT)
- clinical laboratory staff

It is recommended to include no fewer than two staff members from each discipline selected for inclusion. This increases the opportunity to identify inconsistencies in patient flow or workflow processes that typically form the foundation for workarounds associated with explicitly or implicitly known barriers to efficient operations. In addition, it is recommended to exclude departmental leadership from process-mapping exercises. This encourages a free exchange of information from the participating staff and avoids the desire to withhold information on workflow and processes that may be unknown to leadership.

When engaging in process mapping, a neutral third party with experience in process mapping, value stream mapping, and/or Lean methodologies should facilitate the exercise. While seemingly simple on the surface, process mapping is a nuanced exercise requiring proper facilitation skills to ensure that comprehensive and accurate information is gathered and assembled in a meaningful manner.

## Quantifying the impact

While the assessment itself forms the core of understanding how to proceed with improvement initiatives, an equally important component is quantifying the impact of the operational opportunities identified. Quantification of impact forms the backbone for justifying investment in the resources necessary to engage in performance improvement initiatives, while at the same time creating a framework for prioritizing initiatives.

Determining how to calculate and communicate impact potential begins with an understanding of the health system in which the ED operates. As was discussed earlier in this chapter, differences exist between EDs that operate in systems where funding and/or reimbursement occur on a per-patient basis, and those that operate with a fixed budget regardless of volume. In either case, most, if not all, operational opportunities can be tied to

demonstrable outcomes such that a return on investment (ROI) can be calculated for each. This ROI should be differentiated into three key areas of consideration: revenue generation, cost reduction, and increased virtual capacity.

## Revenue generation

New revenue is an ROI opportunity limited to those health systems where reimbursement occurs on a per-patient basis. Whether such reimbursement is capitated (flat fee per patient or acuity level) or based on a billing schedule, additional revenue is an important consideration for affected EDs.

**Case study 16.1. Identifying new revenue opportunities in the ED**

An example of new revenue opportunities can be illustrated in the following example showing the impact of reduced walk-out rates in the ED:

| RETURN ON INVESTMENT CALCULATION: ED WALK-OUTS | |
|---|---|
| Annual ED Volume | 55,000 |
| Walk-out Rate | 5% |
| Annual Walk-outs | 2,750 |
| | |
| Average Collections per Patient (low-acuity) | $115 USD |
| | |
| Revenue Opportunity – 25% Walk-out Reduction | $79,120 USD |
| Revenue Opportunity – 50% Walk-out Reduction | $158,240 USD |

Once ROI revenue opportunities are calculated, gathering consensus for the investments necessary to yield the projected ROI becomes easier. For example, achieving the goal of reducing walk-outs by 50% may require the addition of an eight-hour physician shift daily. To implement the physician shift, the cost of the shift must be balanced by the new revenue generated. The following calculation fails to demonstrate the feasibility of such a move:

| RETURN ON INVESTMENT CALCULATION: ADDITIONAL PHYSICIAN SHIFT | |
|---|---|
| Revenue Opportunity – 50% Walk-out Reduction | $158,240 USD |
| | |
| Annual ED Physician Salary (with benefits) | $250,000 USD |
| FTE's Required for New Shift | 1.4 FTEs |
| Annual Staffing Cost | $350,000 USD |
| | |
| Financial Impact | ($191,760) USD |

FTE = Full Time Equivalent

While the revenue opportunity fails to justify an additional physician shift, an additional ROI calculation – potential cost savings – may provide validation of the decision.

# Cost reduction

While only health systems receiving a per-patient reimbursement will benefit from revenue generation ROI calculations, all EDs, regardless of their budgeting and reimbursement model, will receive benefit from calculating the potential impact of operations improvements on their overall cost structure. When assessing cost reduction opportunities, it is possible to assess the ROI from multiple perspectives.

The largest and easiest-to-calculate cost reduction is in staffing costs. Since most EDs attempt to staff to volume, improvements resulting in reduced lengths of stay will have an immediate impact on staffing costs. Other major cost reduction calculations include, but are not limited to, supply and equipment costs, diagnostic utilization, departmental overhead, and impact of medical errors.

---

**Case study 16.2.   Establishing return on investment for process improvement initiatives**

Returning to Case study 16.1, adding an additional eight-hour physician shift to reduce walk-outs and placing the newly scheduled physician shift in the triage area may yield additional benefits beyond new revenue generation alone. Multiple studies from North America and Europe have demonstrated a quantifiable reduction in overall ED length of stay associated with placing a physician in the triage area during periods of peak census.[19,20]

Using 30 minutes as a projected reduction in overall department length of stay and its impact on staffed nursing requirements, the following ROI is calculated:

| RETURN ON INVESTMENT CALCULATION: ADDITIONAL PHYSICIAN SHIFT | | |
|---|---|---|
| Annual Volume | 55,000 | 55,000 |
| Average Length of Stay | 5.5 hours | 5.0 hours |
| Annual Care Hours | 302,500 hours | 275,000 hours |
| | | |
| Hours per Nursing FTE | 2,080 | 2,080 |
| Number of Care Hours per FTE | 6,240[1] | 6,240[1] |
| Required Staffed Nursing FTEs | 48.5 FTEs[2] | 44.1 FTEs[2] |
| | | |
| Salary per Nursing FTE | €78,000 | €78,000 |
| Annual Staffed Nursing Costs | €3,783,000 | €3,439,800 |
| Annual Cost Savings | | €343,200 |

1. Assumes 4:1 patient to nurse ratio with 75% target productivity
2. Does not include charge nurse, triage or management nurses.

When comparing the cost of adding an additional eight-hour physician shift (approximately €270 000, based on US$350 000) to the cost reductions in expected staffed nursing requirements, an ROI of over €70 000 annually can be expected, clearly justifying an additional physician resource.

## Virtual capacity

Virtual capacity is essentially the ability to care for more patients in the same space without additional treatment stations. Virtual-capacity ROI calculations are a useful consideration for all EDs, particularly those struggling with capacity constraints and those with limited financial resources to support short-term ED expansion or replacement.

**Case study 16.3.** **Establishing virtual-capacity impact of improvement initiatives**

Virtual-capacity ROI calculations should be included as a component of any ROI analysis of improvement opportunities that yield a reduction in overall length of stay. The calculations required to determine virtual-capacity impact are relatively simple to develop:

| RETURN ON INVESTMENT CALCULATION: VIRTUAL CAPACITY | | |
|---|---|---|
| Average Length of Stay | 5.5 hours | 5.0 hours |
| Treatment Station Turnaround Time | .5 hours | .5 hours |
| Total Treatment Station Time per Patient | 6.0 hours | 5.5 hours |
| Patients per Treatment Station per Day | 4 patients | 4.4 patients |
| | | |
| Annual Increased Potential Capacity per Treatment Station | - | 146 patients |
| Total Number of Treatment Stations | 25 | 25 |
| Total Annual Virtual Capacity Opportunity | | 3,650 patients |
| Virtual Beds Created | | 2.3 beds |

## Telling your story: a call to action

There are stark differences in how clinicians and non-clinical healthcare leaders interpret and respond to the data and recommendations included in an assessment.

While clinical leaders have proven their expertise at the bedside, many lack the necessary tools to successfully approach a business presentation. This section will provide a basic overview of how to present an operations assessment most favorably for all audiences, based on the author's experiences in similar settings.

## Developing your presentation

The first steps in developing a presentation focus on understanding key components forming the foundation of the presentation:

- information to be conveyed
- presentation type (written, verbal, combination)
- audience (clinical, non-clinical, combined)
- time/space allotted

In most instances, plans should be made to develop two separate deliverables: a comprehensive written report and an on-screen visual presentation detailing highlights and key points.

### Information to be conveyed

The information to be delivered in an operations assessment can be divided into six key components:

(1) presentation summary

(2) opportunities identified

(3) opportunity impact analysis

(4) recommendations

(5) summary

(6) appendix

Key to formatting a written or verbal presentation is to develop the presentation's "story" – which is essentially an expanded thesis statement for the presentation. The story should be one concept that weaves through the entire presentation, forming a cohesive and clear message. For example, the story may be as follows:

> In its current operational state, our ED has an opportunity to reduce overall length of stay by 2.5 hours. By achieving targeted reductions, the ED could expect to see operational costs decline by 15%, while reducing ambulance diversion time and walk-outs and helping to mitigate the impact of access block in the ED.

With the story established, the different presentation components can be populated with the relevant information. While the sections covering identification, quantification, and recommendations related to the opportunities should be long enough to effectively communicate the current state and proposed solutions, the presentation summary should be concise.

## Creating a call to action

The most important aspect of an operations assessment is to create a call to action that stimulates the audience to want to engage in change-management activities. The best and most comprehensive assessments are ineffective in their impact if they fail to stimulate key constituencies to act based on the findings.

In creating a call to action, the first step is developing a firm understanding of the key stakeholders in a position to allocate necessary resources, and of those who serve as potential barriers to successful implementation of change initiatives. As a component of the analysis, the value proposition each stakeholder deems important should be considered.

With the value propositions identified, the messaging behind the "story" can be tailored such that each stakeholder can clearly identify the recommendations of value to them. Ideally, the presentation would be structured to ensure that individual recommendations and their corresponding return on investment provide stakeholder benefit.

## Positioning findings for hospital administration

Administrative teams struggle daily to balance organizational mission against economic realities. In the case of systems where financial performance is based on per-patient reimbursement, this focus requires ensuring a balance between incoming revenue and outgoing expenses. In systems where finances are independent of patient volumes, focus is on ensuring expenses are kept to a minimum and resources are being utilized in the most efficient manner possible in the appropriate site of care. All of this is then balanced against governmental mandates as well as teaching and research missions and the like. Simply put, administrative leaders will seek to identify – and will be more willing to support – assessment outputs and corresponding recommendations that demonstrate a very clear business case yielding a return on investment.

At the same time that administrative leaders are looking to outcomes-based recommendations with strong return on investment, they are also seeking to receive this information in a clear and concise manner. Details of data collection methodologies, statistical power, and the different types of analysis performed are less likely to be positively received than information demonstrating impact on overall hospital performance. This author recommends the following format for visual presentations:

### Executive summary (1–2 slides)

- should detail high-level findings, with quantifiable information on impact on performance
- should include general overview of recommended solutions and their return on investment

### Operations assessment

- review of all operational metrics assessed, presented in graphic depiction
- assessment of impact of current state from all operational metrics
  - o quantifiable performance metrics such as cost, impact on staffing, impact on quality, etc.

- recommendations that tie directly back to each observation noted
  - metric to be impacted
  - cost of implementation
  - required resources
- return on investment of recommendations
  - focus on metrics of important to audience

### Summary (1–2 slides reviewing key information)

- typically similar to executive summary at beginning

**Appendix**

- largest portion of the presentation
- includes all detailed information on operations assessment
  - list of interviews
  - detailed description of data analysis including datasets and statistical methods used
  - business case for recommendations, showing calculated return on investment

# References

1. Smith J, Haile-Mariam T. Priorities in emergency medicine global development. *Emergency Medicine Clinics of North America* 2005; **23**: 11–29.

2. Anderson P, Petrino R, Halpern P, Tintinalli J. The globalization of emergency medicine and its importance for public health. *Bulletin of the World Health Orgnization* 2006; **84**: 835–9.

3. Arnold JL, Dickinson G, Tsai MC, Han D. A survey of emergency medicine in 36 countries. *CJEM* 2001; **3**: 109–18.

4. Tang N, Stein J, Hsia RY, Maselli JH, Gonzales R. Trends and characteristics of US emergency department visits, 1997–2007. *JAMA* 2010; **304**: 664–70.

5. Tsai JC, Liang YW, Pearson WS. Utilization of emergency department in patients with non-urgent medical problems: patient preference and emergency department convenience. *Journal of the Formosan Medical Association* 2010; **109**: 533–42.

6. Asplin BR, Magid DJ, Rhodes KV, et al. A conceptual model of emergency department crowding. *Annals of Emergency Medicine* 2003; **42**: 173–80.

7. Olshaker JS, Rathlev NK. Emergency department overcrowding and ambulance diversion: the impact and potential solutions of extended boarding of admitted patients in the emergency department. *Journal of Emergency Medicine* 2006; **30**: 351–6.

8. Fatovich DM. Emergency medicine. *BMJ* 2002; **324**: 958–62.

9. Ding R, McCarthy ML, Desmond JS, et al. Characterizing waiting room time, treatment time and boarding time in the emergency department using quantile regression. *Academic Emergency Medicine* 2010; **17**: 813–23.

10. Göransson KE, von Rosen A. Patient experience of the triage encounter in a Swedish emergency department. *International Emergency Nursing* 2010; **18**: 36–40.

11. Möller M, Fridlund B, Göransson K. Patients' conceptions of the triage encounter at the emergency department. *Scandinaviaon Journal of Caring Sciences* 2010; **24**: 746–54.

12. Kelly M, Egbunike JN, Kinnersley P, et al. Delays in response and triage times reduce patient satisfaction and enablement after using out-of-hours services. *Family Practice* 2010; **27**: 652–63.

13. Pines JM, Iyer S, Disbot M, et al. The effect of emergency department crowding on patient satisfaction for admitted patients. *Academic Emergency Medicine* 2008; **15**: 825–31.

14. Chan TC, Killeen JP, Wilke GM, Marshall JB, Castillo EM. Effect of mandated nurse–patient ratios on patient wait time and care time in the emergency department. *Academic Emergency Medicine* 2010; **17**: 545–52.

15. Gedmintas A, Bost N, Keijzers G, Green D, Lind J. Emergency care workload units: a novel tool to compare emergency department activity. *Emergency Medicine Australasia* 2010; **22**: 442–8.

16. Hernández M. Emergency department performance: comprehensive assessments. Presentation, European Society of Emergency Medicine 6th European Congress on Emergency Medicine, 2010.

17. Ng D, Vail G, Thomas S, Schmidt N. Applying the Lean principles of the Toyota Production System to reduce wait times in the emergency department. *CJEM* 2010; **12**: 50–7.

18. Dickson EW, Anguelov Z, Vetterick D, Eller A, Singh S. Use of lean in the emergency department: a case series of 4 hospitals. *Annals of Emergency Medicine* 2009; **54**: 504–10.

19. Holroyd BR, Bullard MJ, Latoszek K, et al. Impact of a triage liaison physician on emergency department overcrowding and throughput: a randomized controlled trial.

*Academic Emergency Medicine* 2007; **14**: 702–8.

20. Travers JP, Lee FC. Avoiding prolonged waiting time during busy periods in the emergency department: Is there a role for the senior emergency physician in triage? *European Journal of Emergency Medicine* 2006; **13**: 342–8.

## Further reading

Cohn KH. *Better Communication for Better Care: Mastering Physician-Administrator Collaboration.* Chicago, IL: Health Administration Press, 2005.

Duarte N. *Slide:ology: the Art and Science of Creating Great Presentations.* Sebastopol, CA: O'Reilly, 2008.

Duarte N. *Resonate: Present Visual Stories That Transform Audiences.* Hoboken, NJ: Wiley, 2010.

Dunn RT. *Dunn and Haimann's Healthcare Management*, 9th edn. Chicago, IL: Health Administration Press, 2010.

Smith AC, Barry R, Brubaker C. *Going Lean: Busting Barriers to Patient Flow.* Chicago, IL: Health Administration Press, 2007.

Tapping D, Kozlowski S, Archbold L, Sperl T. *Value Stream Management for Lean Healthcare.* Chelsea, MI: MCS Media, 2009.

Zidel T. *A Lean Guide to Transforming Healthcare: How to Implement Lean Principles in Hospitals, Medical Offices, Clinics, and Other Healthcare Organizations.* Milwaukee, WI: ASQ Quality Press, 2006.

# Emergency department design

Michael P. Pietrzak and James Lennon

## Key learning points

- To provide emergency department leaders with a basic understanding of the design process and planning fundamentals required to provide safe, effective, and efficient operations.
- To gain an understanding of key concepts of emergency department design in order to be able to effectively communicate with and lead a multidisciplinary emergency department design team.

## Introduction

Efficient, safe, and effective operation is highly dependent on the physical environment of the department. Emergency department (ED) managers are often called upon to be consultative experts and, indeed, to be decision makers when the physical design of the department is being determined. An understanding of the key issues surrounding current concepts in ED design and an approach to major issues will be the focus in this chapter.

## The design process

The process of architectural design is practically divided into five basic steps that, usually, are completed sequentially:[1]

(1) programming and preplanning
(2) schematic design
(3) design development
(4) construction documents
(5) bidding for construction

## Programming and preplanning

Programming is the process of developing a tabular list of spaces, which is generated through the identification of all rooms needed, the size in square feet or square meters of those rooms, and the number of each type of room needed for the entire proposed ED. Those areas are summed to equal the *net room area*:

Total sum of room areas of all the rooms in a department = Net room area

The net room area is multiplied by a "department grossing factor," which adds space for corridors, walls, and other functions that are not included in the net room area, but are needed for the ED to function. This is called the *total gross department size*:

Net room area × Department grossing factor = Total gross department size

The total gross department size is then multiplied by a *building grossing factor* (this factors in the area for elevators and connections that serve the ED and other floors, air conditioning, and corridors needed to get to the ED from other departments).

Total gross building size = Total gross department size × Building grossing factor

A key component to effective programming includes understanding the patient volume arrival patterns. That drives the number of beds needed at any given time. It also helps determine the best topology needed to array patient beds in. The arrival pattern for most EDs displays a characteristic S-shaped curve. The early morning hours (midnight to 7 a.m.) is the low ebb in arrivals, while the busiest patient arrival time is between 10 a.m. and 10 p.m. The intervals between the low and high are transitions up and down. If the

*Emergency Department Leadership and Management*, ed. Stephanie Kayden, *et al.* Published by Cambridge University Press.
© Cambridge University Press 2015.

higher volume times are consistent, the program needs to allocate a sufficient number of rooms for peak hours and not simply use an average intake over 24 hours.

The architectural program becomes the anchor and guidance for the subsequent design steps. The underlying concept of the design process is that big decisions are made first, and with each subsequent phase more detailed decisions are layered on.

A basic rule of thumb for determining the total number of ED beds in North America is that annual volume divided by total number of ED beds should be between 1200 and 1900 patients/ED bed, with 1550 patients/ED bed being normal for community hospitals in the United States. Therefore:

ED beds needed in typical ED in the USA = Annual ED visits / 1550

General method:

$$\text{Number of ED beds needed} = ((((n/365)*x\%)*\text{LOS})/12)*U$$

Where:

$n$ = Annual ED patients
$x\%$ = percentage of patients arriving during peak 12-hour period (70%)
LOS = average length of ED stay for all patients in hours
$U$ = utilization coefficient for ED rooms (1.25)

## Schematic design

After defining the site, boxes are drawn to scale within the site perimeter representing each required room in the program. They should be laid out in a pattern that achieves the desired physical relationship of each room to the other. Frequently this will involve numerous iterations to achieve the desired basic floor plan.

## Design development

This phase assumes that schematic design is complete, in that the rooms are fixed in their location and size, at which point the elements within each room are moved until they meet the specific objectives of the individual rooms. Often, additional descriptive drawings are created at a more detailed scale to allow for the precise location of important functions. Examples include the location and quantity of oxygen and vacuum outlets in patient exam rooms, or the exact type and location of ceiling lights. Only when design development is complete can the process progress to construction documents. Minor adjustments to the schematic design often occur in this phase when driven by a requirement discovered during design development.

## Construction documents

With all of the rooms fixed in position and size, equipment located, and internal functions described completely, a set of drawings is prepared that will act as an instruction kit for the builders to make the building. They are frequently called *blueprints*, but are legally referred to as *construction documents*. They comprise an integral part of the agreement between the owner and the contractor. Along with other documents, they are the basis upon which the cost of the building will be determined. Regardless of the country of origin of the design architect, it is imperative that construction documents be prepared by a local architect familiar with all local codes and building requirements.

## Bidding for construction

Once the construction documents have been fully completed, and approved by the appropriate regulatory agencies, bidding can take place. The documents are sent to several contractors. The construction documents will be the basis upon which a cost to build the project will be based. Changes to the construction documents after bidding has ended and construction has begun will alter the legal agreement between the owner and contractor, which in most cases results in cost increases.

An irony of the design process is that the most important decisions are made at the beginning of the project when the least is known about it. And when the most is known about the project (at the end of construction), the designer has the least ability to alter it.

## Emergency department planning and basic topologies

Planning refers to sizing, layout, and relations of the spaces in the ED as well as how that layout physically relates to spaces outside the ED. Planning for the ED must include all the aspects of patient arrival and intake as well as the care that occurs within the ED. While potentially there can be any number of configurations for an ED, there are a number of prototype topologies that provide basic templates from which designers can fully develop an appropriate design. Each topology has characteristics that make it more or less appealing in a particular situation. As stated in the programming section, arrival patterns can also influence design decisions. The daily expansion from low patient volume to high patient volume and back down to small volume again is the armature upon which the ED will be designed. The plan chosen should be able to demonstrate how it will expand and contract seamlessly with daily changes in patient volume. If it cannot, it is likely to suffer from inefficient staffing as well as delays in care. To put it differently, the ED must be able to "breathe" from low patient volume to high patient volume every 24 hours.

## Common topologies

The classic topology is called the "ballroom" design (Fig. 17.1a). Beds are arrayed around a central work-station, or core. The fundamental idea is that all of the beds are directly visible from the staff core in the middle of the circle of beds. This ballroom configuration has been found to be a successful topology until the number of beds exceeds 15. At that point, the circumference of beds becomes so large that the space left in the center is too large to have nurses and doctors traversing in order to accomplish their work. Often the large center space is in-filled with needed functions such as clean and soiled utilities and equipment rooms. That allows shorter walking distances to critical functions, but also fills the central core with solid walls, obscuring the views that were considered the principal advantage of the ballroom layout. The infill and view obstruction forces the establishment of multiple nurses' stations, from none of which the entire ED can be seen. Ultimately, the advantage of the ballroom is lost, and it is replaced with multiple sections of beds with separate nurses' stations called "pods" (Fig. 17.1b). Podular EDs are abundant throughout North America. However, they generally suffer from an inability to be staffing-efficient. If just one patient is in a pod, it must be staffed-up fully. The following sample topologies explore several that have the advantages of the ballroom, but expand and contract seamlessly as patient volume varies.

### The X-shape

This topology (Fig. 17.1c) is common in North America and is a variant on the ballroom. It has come into use when attempting to apply the concepts of the ballroom to a 30- or 45-bed ED. In this case, patient beds are wrapped around the perimeter of a square, rather than a circle, surrounding the central core of common services such as nurses' and doctors' work areas, soiled and clean utilities, office, medication rooms, etc. Nurses' stations are located at the vertex of each corner of the square with the idea that as patient volume increases beyond the influence of one nurses' station, the next will staff-up to meet that volume. That behavior continues around the square until all nurses' stations are in use. The difficulty with this topology is that distances between the nurses stations, in many cases greater than 100 feet (30.5 m), preclude effective communication and result in the creation of a four-pod plan. Like all podular plans, the X-shaped plan requires significant attention to staffing equity.

### The H-shape

The H-shape (Fig. 17.1d) contains a central core containing a nurses' station and emergent beds, flanked by two rows of patient rooms. Ambulances directly access the core from one side and triage from the other. As patient volume increases, staffing and patients move out to the edges of the plan. And conversely, as volume decreases, staffing contracts back to the core. Thus, the plan demonstrates that it can "breathe" over the 24-hour period.

### The T-shape

The T-shape (Fig. 17.1e) includes a central core with one arm of patient beds extending out from either side of the core. Along the arms are portable workstations (called podiums) in the corridor to reduce staff travel distances during peak times. In a teaching hospital, the central core can be subdivided into two parts, one for nurses and the other for medical staff, residents, and students. If patients enter from the middle of each arm, they will not transgress on the central core while going to and from their rooms. "Breathing" occurs in a similar manner as in the H-shape topology.

### The L-shape

A central core is located at the vertex of an L-shaped series of patient rooms (Fig. 17.1f). Emergent beds surround the core, with ambulance access from one

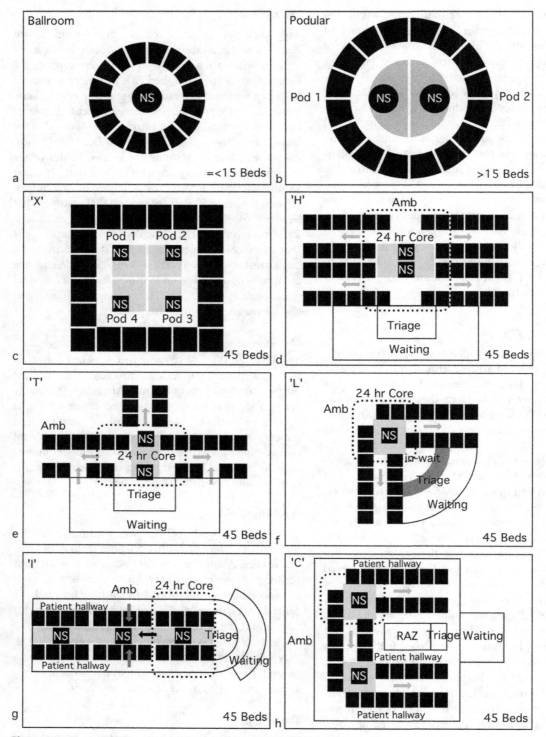

**Figure 17.1** Common ED topologies. NS, nurses' station; RAZ, rapid assessment zone.

side of the core and an inner waiting area open to the other side. Halfway up each arm of rooms is a staffing substation that is open both to the hallway of patient rooms and to the inner waiting room. In this plan type, the inner waiting area takes the form of a place that houses patients while they are waiting for test results.

### The I-shape

The I-shape (Fig. 17.1g) is significant for two elements: (1) patient beds are arranged in two parallel rows, and (2) the central core is for staff only, while patients enter from a peripheral corridor, which flanks the rows of patient's beds. Thus each patient bedroom has two doors: one for staff from the core and one for patients and family from the peripheral corridors. The rows of patient beds can be 300 feet (91 m) to 400 feet (122 m) long. The I-shape functions like a thermometer, in that one end of the rows of beds is the 24-hour hub and patients and staff progress down the length of the plan as volume increases. Then, as volume decreases, staff compress back to the 24-hour hub. This topology allows for seamless expansion without the inefficiencies associated with podular plans. Care must be given to create a truly "seamless" array of patient beds, not obstructed by utility rooms, offices, or other non-clinical functions.

### The C-shape

This is a variant of the I-shape (Fig. 17.1h), with the beds bent around a central inner waiting area. It combines the advantages of the I- and L-shapes. This plan may be used in a variety of advanced operational methods (see Case study 17.4, below).

## Physical relation of the ED to other departments and services

Effective ED operations are reliant on the support provided by other departments. These ancillary services include but are not limited to imaging, laboratory, other diagnostics, and pharmacy. In some cases, where a key clinical service is a prevalent component of the services provided to the ED patient population, the co-location or full integration of that specialty service may be desirable. The most common elements are laboratory and imaging services, but other services can be involved. For example, if there is a high incidence of ophthalmology referrals due to an occupational hazard of a nearby industry then proximity to the ophthalmology department may be desirable. However, more typical examples are operating rooms and catheterization suites.

The location, physical relationship, and accessibility of these services and departments can profoundly impact coordination, interoperability, and manning requirements of the ED. And each needs to be considered as a business case analysis as well. The results impact cost and staff satisfaction, and total time needed to provide the needed care is a critical element in the design process of an ED. From the standpoint of labor, the saving of one full-time equivalent (even a low-cost employee) has an impact of millions of dollars over the life of the facility. Thus, efforts to optimize the physical proximity of these departmental or service lines are well worth intensive efforts. In terms of potential savings, this ranks just behind the general layout or topology of the ED itself.

## Emergency department staff needs

The workload intensity in the ED imposes significant demands on staff, both physically and emotionally. In many cases, during a shift physicians and other caregivers can find it very difficult to leave the proximity of the clinical area. Thus the department needs to provide appropriate support spaces for the human needs of staff. This is not an unimportant endeavor, as human factors are the leading cause of medical errors in the ED and hospitals in general.[2] Thus the environment provided for the staff is an important factor and plays a key role in human performance. Some have applied the use of certain research tools, such as Q methodology, which allows for subjective staff input to evaluate the needs.[3]

There is no set formula to determine what is needed for staff, as staffing models and local cultural habits can dramatically change the potential needs. For example, some EDs that have a very low volume at night and are staffed with 12-hour shifts may require sleeping quarters, while other EDs with short shifts and high volumes 24 hours per day may find the sleeping area not useful. In any case, starting to determine the staff needs is to consider the known human needs – rest, food, physiologic functions, communication, socializing, space for personal items, privacy, and security in the context of the ED volumes, the staffing models, and the surrounding environment including the proximity of services available in the hospital.

In an existing ED, the first approach might be simply to survey the existing staff with questions regarding the deficiencies of their current ED environment. However, one might find that what was needed for the staff in an old ED might not be needed in a new ED because the security of the new location might be different, etc. In an entirely new project, a reasonable approach is to list each type of staff member working in the department – physician, nurse, technician, clerical, etc. – and evaluate their potential needs: rest, food, physiologic functions, communication, socializing, space for personal items, privacy, and security, based on shift length, workload, equipment or records they may need to bring with them, cultural needs, etc. That lends itself to a simple matrix. Once those needs are established, one can evaluate what is provided in proximity to the ED that is readily available and accessible by the staff. For example, if the hospital has a break area immediately adjacent to the ED with snack machines, refrigerator, and microwave, it might not be necessary to replicate this in the ED break area (assuming accessibility, availability, and security are appropriate). While the hospital may have public bathrooms immediately adjacent to the ED, it is often important to provide private facilities for ED staff, not only for their convenience but also for security and infection control purposes. Often overlooked in ED planning is the area for sufficient and secure storage for individuals' personal items such as laptop computers, personal digital devices, documents, etc. Many ED staff do not have personal offices, so that space is very critical. One could even consider a power source for recharging personal devices inside the locker, so that this can be done in a secure fashion without the need for such personal devices to add to the clutter of the ED.

## Surge capacity

EDs are programmed and designed to meet projected needs and requirements. These are targeted capabilities and capacities based on historical and projected volumes as well as patient mix. Such projections also allow for peak hours and seasonal variations, as well as some reasonable growth factors based on population projections. Typically, ED managers and decision makers would hope their ED could efficiently accommodate these variations of volume the vast majority of times. However, during disasters or contingency events large numbers of casualties may present, exceeding the capacity of the design. Robust surge capacity is needed.

Surge capacity is the additional volume that can be accommodated for a limited period of time (typically, 24 hours to one week). Surge capacity is achieved both through operational methods (staffing and process) and enabling design features. These design features should be reasonable in scope and cost. Generally, it is not practical to create contingency space to accommodate patient volumes that could be created by every potential scenario or event that might occur. Designed surge capacity should be a thoughtful consideration of the more likely contingency scenarios, considering the expected role of the ED in the community disaster plan. Based on those potential scenarios, some level of desired surge capacity can be determined. The insertion of these considerations prior to initiating schematic design will enable the designer to find opportunities within the layout, structure, and landscape to provide some cost-effective surge solutions. The goal is to have a minimal incremental increase of square footage to provide a robust capacity.

---

**Case study 17.1.   Project ER One: optimizing surge capacity**

Project ER One provides a prototype case study for surge capacity. Shortly after the 9/11 attacks, the Department of Health and Human Services became highly interested in surge capacity in multiples of normal ED capacity.[4] Project ER One studied this extensively and was able to develop a fivefold static capacity with approximately a 15% increase in required space.[5]

The ER One design study uses a number of strategies to integrate surge capacity into a functional ED. Each treatment/examination room can be moderately increased in size to allow double occupancy in contingency. The 176 square-foot (16 m$^2$) room footprint allows this to occur without congestion. In the single-bed configuration, an additional contingency bed is positioned on the posterior wall and lowered to function as a seating area for family members or attendants of the individual patients (Fig. 17.2a). The medical gases are preconfigured for the second bed. Therefore when patient volumes or contingency demands exceed normal capacity, double capacity is instantly available (Fig. 17.2b).

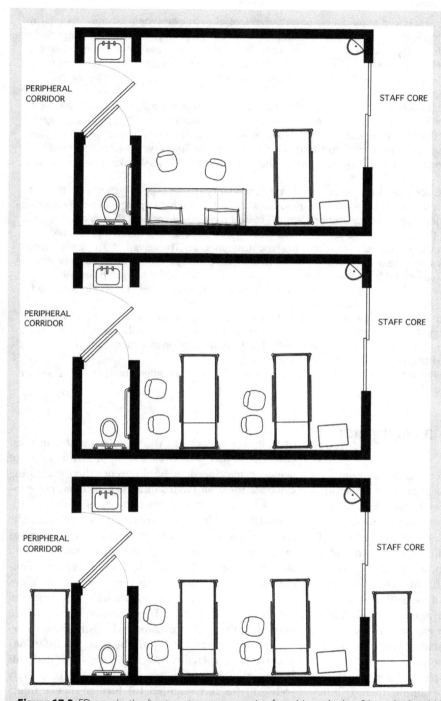

**Figure 17.2** ED examination/treatment room: conversion from (a) one-bed to (b) two-bed and (c) four-bed capacity.

A third bed can be placed and serviced immediately outside the door of each exam room, as three feet (c.1 m) extra circulation space was allotted in the design of the core space. This reconfiguration can also be accomplished in rapid fashion, allowing a three-fold scalability of the ED in minutes. The department was further designed with a peripheral circulating hallway behind the treatment rooms. Thus a fourth bed can be added very quickly to achieve a four- to fivefold static surge capacity (Fig. 17.2c). Additional "dynamic" surge capacity can be achieved via augmented manning and process.

However, scaleable throughput requires the ability to disposition patients more rapidly. Typically the hospital will not be able to admit as rapidly as the ED can process patients in these situations. Thus, the project design included strategies for rapid intake and transfer of patients. Rapid intake and transfer were facilitated by multi-lane unidirectional access right of ways similar to an airport terminal. Contingency helipads were nicely disguised in green areas using under-surface pavers for underlying support. That allowed for increased intake and dispersion of patients.

The concept of dual use of spaces was adopted because large contingency spaces kept as warehouses that may never be used most likely are not the most cost-effective way to prepare for disaster. If the space had a daily use that was not likely to be needed during a disaster (e.g., sitting lobby) it could be effectively used in the contingency (if it were located properly and had the appropriate electrical and plumbing infrastructure). Lobbies, atriums, wide hallways, and conference rooms were designed "pre-wired" to allow such functions. Those were strategically located in a way to be usable by the ED and accessible to ancillary services. This was actually incorporated into a number of EDs around the world, including a university hospital in northern Italy. In this case the university hospital strategically selected waiting areas and hallways and inserted the applicable medical gases and wiring to allow for surge clinical care in these spaces.

Even the ambulance garage offers a contingency use. During a disaster one would assume the ambulances would not stay in the garage – and thus that rather large space would be available. Typically, the garage would have excellent ventilation, plus water and drains, making it also useful for decontamination in a protected area. That concept was also extended to covered parking areas.

Since the completion of the Project ER One design study numerous facilities have implemented one or several of these features to increase surge capacity.

# Evidence-based design in emergency medicine

Similar to medicine, the design world is adopting the application of various fields of science, engineering, and statistical analysis to help determine which design concepts or features can improve the performance of the built environment.[6–8] The desired outcomes of this effort include (but are not limited to) quantifiable clinical improvements, financial benefits, safety enhancements, and patient/staff satisfaction. Most in the design sector now refer to this field as *evidence-based design*, but the term *performance-based building design* has also gained favor. In either case, the intent is to apply the best available science, data, or information to inform design decisions.

Just as in medicine, there are challenges with an evidence-based approach. For example, there is little "body of evidence" established or available for any particular design decision that one might face. Even more challenging than in the medical realm, randomized controlled trials of the built environment will usually be financially prohibitive and "blinding" to

one's built environment will be unachievable in most cases. Thus the standards one applies for levels of evidence may need to be different when evaluating evidence for built environments. Moreover, environments are very complex interactions of multiple variables (the building, the environmental systems, the effect of the exterior environment, and the various people in it) and it is very difficult to control for all these variables. This usually limits the predictive conclusions one can make regarding clinical outcomes from any particular study of the built environment. For example, it is very difficult to develop a study to determine the impact of a new self-disinfecting door-handle surface material on the rate of infections occurring in a facility. At the same time that this intervention is put in place the facility is actively trying to (in fact required to) further reduce infections as much as possible, confounding any attempt to measure the contribution made by the new surface. Often one will need to rely on intermediate or surrogate indicators, such as surface contamination (colony counts) on the door handle. On the other hand, engineering data and statistics can often be very reliable and reproducible. One can reliably calculate return on investment for windows that have been designed and engineered to reduce heat transfer, translating into significant energy savings. On the other hand, it is much more difficult to quantify the effect of this glass on patient comfort.

The ED is unique, for the simple reason that individual patients are only in this environment for a limited period of time. Thus the physical environment is unlikely to have a significant opportunity to promote "healing" of a disease state. On the other hand, the physical environment of the ED might indeed have an impact on the general comfort of a patient, which, in turn, might have an effect on the amount of pain medication needed. Perhaps more than other departments, the physical environment of the ED has a major impact on operational efficiency, worker satisfaction, and safety. These elements lend themselves to measurement and validation and thus are an appropriate area of focus for evidenced-based efforts in ED design.

As this field of study and application is growing, a number of institutions have dedicated themselves to building the body of evidence and improving the application of the principles of evidence to design efforts. These organizations and others have developed a variety of tools, including "post-occupancy evaluations," which can be valuable in developing evidence for design. Others have promoted intensive analyses of quality-improvement costs to assist with evidence-based medicine (EBM) decision making. Similar tools can be applied to develop return on investment (ROI) analyses for building design decisions. This can be fairly straightforward when evaluating the cost of a material against energy savings, but it is a little more involved when one is trying to determine the value of a cost of the material to achieve a patient outcome.

In the end, all must realize that evidence-based design is still in the developmental stage. The body of evidence is incomplete, the tools are not fully mature, and the methods of application have not been fully agreed upon. Yet, in the future, it will be important for ED managers to contribute to the body of evidence and to develop tools to improve application. In working with your design team, challenge them to provide evidence of best practices, and at the same time offer to participate in the evaluation and validation of your chosen design solutions. The ultimate goal is for future ED leaders to be able to predict the outcome of their design decisions.

## Conclusion

Successful ED design requires effective integration of ED leaders into the design team. An understanding of the fundamentals of ED design and the design process will improve the ability of those ED leaders to function in that role.

---

**Case study 17.2.  Door-to-Doc: getting more capacity from an existing ED**

In the early years of the twenty-first century, Phoenix, Arizona, was the fastest-growing metropolitan area in the United States. That resulted in a significant burden on the EDs throughout the city. Patients waited for hours, only to be placed in a hallway bed once they finally entered the clinical area. One multi-hospital system was very interested in relieving the problem, but understood that construction of new EDs would take years. The hospital system wanted to get relief from the crowding during the five years it would take to construct new EDs.

A consulting/research team studied potential solutions to improve waiting times, a project called "Door-to-Doc." Their recommendations included dividing the incoming stream of patients into two types: *horizontal*, which was considered to be any patient who absolutely needed to be in an emergency bed (usually Emergency Severity Index [ESI] 1 and 2), and *vertical*, meaning any patient who could tolerate being in a chair for the entire stay (ESI 3, 4, 5). Their work had three primary goals: (1) make minimum architectural changes to their existing EDs, (2) reduce the time it took for a patient to see a physician, and (3) reduce the need for ED beds within the existing hospital. This was accomplished by restructuring the triage process to decide only if the patient was horizontal or vertical. That required them to convert the space that was used for multiple triage rooms into intake spaces for physicians to see patients with no waiting after triage. Secondarily, they used a section of their existing waiting room as a "results lounge." Hence, their solution involved minimal remodeling of the ED coupled with operational changes necessary to implement the Door-to-Doc strategy.

Further refinements divided the incoming flow of vertical patients into those who required only one resource and those who required more than one. Those who required only one resource were sent to a separate zone called

"Qtrack" (quick track) and the remainder were shunted to the results waiting area, which was actually just a large room with comfortable chairs and positive distractions such as TV. That allowed one nurse to watch all of the patients in that room. The Qtrack concept, on the other hand, identified those patients that could be seen and treated by a physician's assistant, or other trained professional other than a physician and discharged directly after treatment without utilizing the results lounge. Q-track zones can be carved out of existing fast track, or minor patient spaces.

It should be noted that the Door-to-Doc process was not aimed at reducing length of stay, but rather at redistributing the incoming flow of patients to effectively utilize main ED beds. The Door-to-Doc and Qtrack processes have demonstrated the ability to significantly reduce the time between a patient arriving at the ED and being seen by a physician, while at the same time reducing the number of ED beds needed. The major variables contributing to success are: (1) having a large number of patients that do not need to be in an ED bed, and (2) appropriate medical and nursing staff processes. It is important to note that the best physical design can be frustrated by inefficient processes.

Figure 17.3 diagrammatically illustrates the flow concept in relationship to the basic spaces needed for implementation.

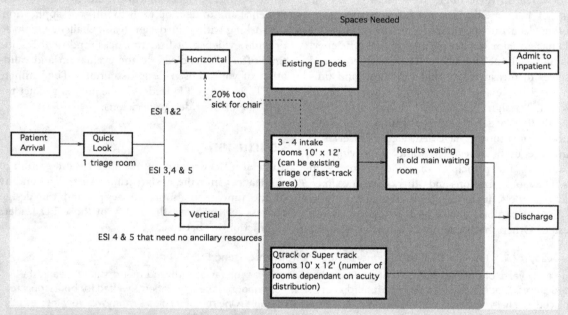

**Figure 17.3** The Door-to-Doc process: patient flow through the ED.

## Case study 17.3.   Designing for flexibility: volume and patient acuity

In the ED setting, flexibility refers to two dimensions: (1) the ability to easily flex to changing volume demands on a daily basis (largely a function of layout and staffing) and (2) the adaptability to accommodate different patient types and acuities (largely a function of the room design).

There are three important drivers of change that influence ED planning: (1) staff can work in a more distributed fashion, closer to patients, rather than from centralized points, (2) the proliferation and ever-changing nature of medical equipment calls for spaces of accommodation closer to patients than traditional nurses stations, and (3) demographic shifts with attendant increasing acuity of patients require a more flexible patient room design than ever before. The linear concept combined with flexible (universal) room configuration (Fig. 17.1g) brings many of those considerations together. It allows for ease of volume flexibility as well as adaptability to patient type and acuity. Pioneered at a hospital in the Midwestern United States,[9] the concept was realized via a double row of patient rooms surrounding a large, linear central space for staff and equipment. Critical to the success of the design scheme was having undifferentiated (universal) patient rooms, which were, by necessity, of sufficient size to address the needs of most patient types.

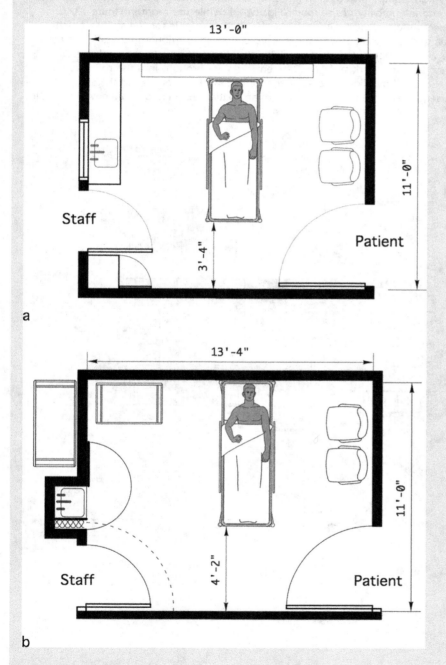

**Figure 17.4** ED examination/treatment room.

185

Figure 17.4a shows the original patient room. designed in 2000. The room was 143 square feet (13.3 m$^2$) (larger than United States minimum standard of 120 square feet [11 m$^2$]). The additional 23 square feet (2 m$^2$) allowed the room to accommodate most patient types and care requirements comfortably, and since all rooms (except resuscitation rooms) were the same, any room could accommodate any patient. The floor-plan configuration that the rooms were arrayed in increased the space for staff to work by more than double a traditional "ballroom" ED (Fig. 17.1a). It also allowed for increased direct contact between staff and patients and anticipated the effects of future computerized informatics on staff deployment. Later work was done to further increase the efficiency and adaptability of the room (Fig. 17.4b). While the room in Figure 17.4b is virtually the same size and aspect ratio as that in Figure 17.4a, the space available for the staff to function within the room is 20% greater, and that additional space is more effectively distributed for staff. The room presents as a simple rectangle with no elements (counters, sinks, etc.) penetrating into the work area. Carts exclusively serve as the storage and work surfaces. Different carts are brought into the room as needed for individual patient needs. All mobile elements of the room can be removed, and the sink, TV, cubicle curtain, etc. can be sequestered behind a door, to turn any patient room into a safe environment for psychiatric patients.

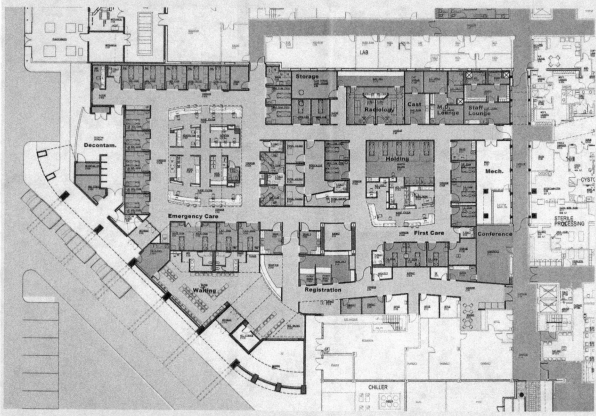

**Figure 17.5** (a, b) ED floor plans.

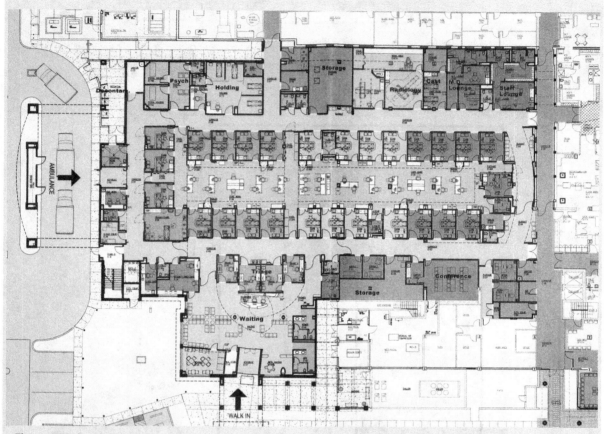

**Figure 17.5** (*cont.*)

Figure 17.5 displays two floor plans in which the same construction area is designed in a pod-like topology (Fig. 17.5a) and a linear topology (Fig. 17.5b). These plans are significant for several reasons:

(1) In Figure 17.5a, the plan presents as a diffused collection of rooms without a defined pattern. Figure 17.5b, on the other hand, appears to be a clear, unified, logical arrangement
of rooms.

(2) The staff work area in Figure 17.5b is significantly larger than in Figure 17.5a.

(3) The individual patient rooms are larger in Figure 17.5b than in Figure 17.5a.

(4) Patient spaces in Figure 17.5a are inconsistent, with some being five-bed rooms separated by curtains, whereas in Figure 17.5b the topology of the rooms is consistent and easy to
understand.

As a note, the plan shown in Figure 17.5b was constructed and is in service in the southern part of the United States,[10] and has reported lower length of stay, 20% less travel distances, and more efficient staffing.

---

**Case study 17.4. Replacement ED design: optimizing efficiency through effective planning choices**

There is no such thing as a perfect ED floor plan. However, individual floor plans represent a balance between operational objectives and the real-world constraints of site and budget. To that end, Figure 17.6 represents one way to address many of the operational features mentioned in this chapter.

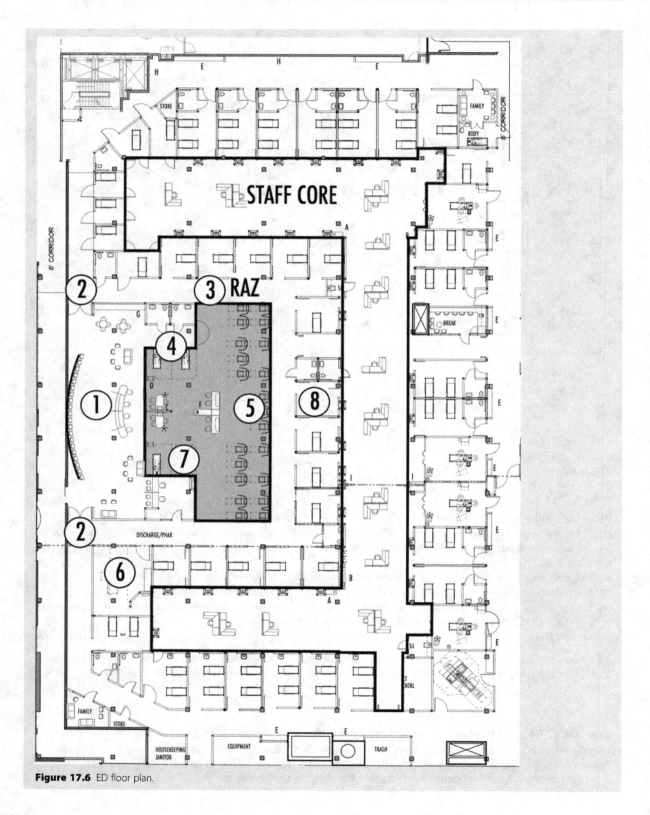

**Figure 17.6** ED floor plan.

A hospital system in Erie, Pennsylvania, saw a need to implement a quick-track, non-ambulatory (horizontal)/ ambulatory (vertical) split, streamlined triage, universal rooms, peripheral circulation, contingency planning, and a linear operating model in one plan.[11] Patients flow directly to a counter which houses two quick-look triage positions (Fig. 17.6, 1). From there patients are divided into non-ambulatory and ambulatory streams. The horizontal patients are accompanied to the main ED beds via the peripheral circulation system (Fig. 17.6, 2). Ambulatory patients enter the *rapid assessment zone* (RAZ), where several options for care are present. ESI 4 or 5 patients with need for only one resource are sent to a four-bed quick-track zone (Fig. 17.6, 3) directly behind triage and close to the results lounge. All other vertical patients are given a comfortable recliner, with personal distraction devices such as TV, computer access, educational materials, and their visit status information all displayed on an LCD screen similar in design to aircraft entertainment systems (Fig. 17.7). The recliners act as the home base for those patients during their entire stay, but they are routed to conveniently located ancillary support (Fig. 17.6, 4 x-ray, 5 phlebotomy) and procedure spaces (Fig. 17.6, 6, 7) ringing the RAZ area. Intake functions can take place in any bank of three contiguous rooms anyplace around the RAZ core. On some days there may be a need for more than three intake rooms, while on other days fewer may be needed, and the plan allows for complete flexibility between busy and slow days of the week, as well as between peak and minimum times of the day. A significant number of patient rooms (Fig. 17.6, 8) are capable of housing two patient beds, thus allowing the ED to flex from the design goal of 46 main ED beds to 65 beds without having to use hallways or peripheral circulation space. Integral to the design of the triage counter is sufficient space for automated triage kiosks that could work in conjunction with the quick-look triage functions. The entire clinical program was designed within a 34 000-square-foot (3159 m$^2$) shell; additional space was required for teaching and administrative functions.

**Figure 17.7** Patient recliner chair.

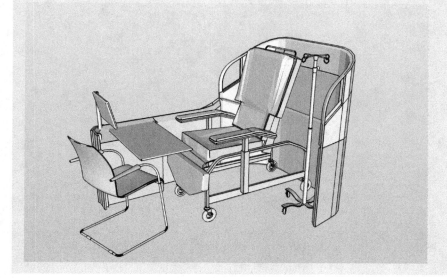

# References

1. Huddy J. *Emergency Department Design: a Practical Guide to Planning for the Future.* Dallas, TX: American College of Emergency Physicians (ACEP), 2002.

2. Landrigan CP. Temporal trends in rates of patient harm resulting from medical care. *New England Journal of Medicine* 2010; **363**: 2124–34.

3. Chinnis AS, Paulson DJ, Davis SM. Using Q methodology to assess the needs of emergency medicine support of staff employees. *American Journal of Emergency Medicine*, 2001; **20**: 197–203.

4. Pietrzak MP. Notes from meeting with Secretary of Health and Human Services, the Honorable Thomas H. Thompson, January 2002.

5. Pietrzak MP, Smith MS, Feied C, et al. *ER One Technical Report.* Published by Mitretek and submitted to Department of

Health and Human Services, June 2002.

6. Ulrich RS. Effects of healthcare environmental design on medical outcomes, in design and health: the therapeutic benefits of design. Proceedings of the 2nd Annual International Congress on Design and Health, Karolinska Institute, Stockholm, June 2000.

7. Zimring CM, Augenbroe GL, Malone EB, Sadler BL. Implementing healthcare excellence: the vital role of the CEO in evidence based design.

White Paper Series 3/5, Evidence-Based Design Resources for Healthcare Executives, the Center for Health Design, September 2008.

8. Ulrich RS, Zimring CM, Zhu X, *et al.* A review of the research literature on evidence based healthcare design. White Paper Series 5/5, Evidence-Based Design Resources for Healthcare Executives, the Center for Health Design, September 2008.

9. Lennon JA, design architect under project direction of Raana

Ponstingle, MD, Medical Director, Department of Emergency Medicine, St. Anthony's Medical Center, St. Louis MI; 2000.

10. Haynes Architects, PA. Tampa, Florida: design architect.

11. Lennon JA, design architect under project direction of Wayne Jones, DO, Medical Director, Department of Emergency Medicine, St. Vincent Health System, Erie, PA; Rectenwald Architects Erie, PA, Architect of Record; 2010.

Chapter

# 18

# Informatics in the emergency department

Steven Horng, John D. Halamka, and Larry A. Nathanson

## Key learning points

- Information technology provides critical tools to help enhance the flow of emergency department patients and improve medical decision making and the quality of care.
- Decision support such as computerized provider order entry (CPOE) systems are proven to decrease errors, but can have unintended negative consequences.
- Partnerships between clinical and information systems staff are one of the best ways to overcome the many challenges to effective emergency department information systems implementation.

## Introduction

The practice of modern emergency medicine can be extremely challenging. Emergency physicians see the full spectrum of human maladies, treating patients with a wide range of ages, social situations, and acuity. Available resources are often constrained, including physical space and personnel, and "overcrowding" has become commonplace. An efficient emergency department (ED) operation is not just a business matter; even short delays in treatment can result in precious minutes being lost, to the detriment of the patient. Optimal medical care hinges on rapidly gathering, sorting, prioritizing, and synthesizing large amounts of data. The ED is a collaborative environment often requiring coordination and communication among multiple other services within the hospital. Computers can help manage all this information and improve the quality, safety, and efficiency of emergency care.[1] In this chapter we will discuss how information technology (IT) helps enhance the

flow of patients through the ED, assists in documentation and communication of the encounter, helps clinical staff make better decisions, and assists in the monitoring and improvement of quality of care. We will also discuss a number of challenges in deploying these systems.

## Management of patient flow

### Dashboards

Dashboards (otherwise known as "tracking boards" or "electronic whiteboards") improve the efficiency of patient flow by enhancing the situational awareness of ED staff. They replace the dry-erase marker systems that formerly served as the primary method for tracking patients. The old way, staff members were responsible for manually updating the whiteboard as patients arrived, departed, and changed status. These manual boards were only visible from one location and could not be viewed outside the ED. As the department became busier, staff assigned to update the board became overwhelmed with other tasks and the data on the board became stale. This system would systematically break down at the time it was needed most, causing a vicious cycle of inefficiency. Computerized dashboards eliminate many of the problems associated with these boards. Effective systems are interfaced and draw critical operational and clinical parameters from the underlying hospital information systems, such as laboratory, radiology, and admissions. Patient flow is enhanced as the triage nurse is able to immediately see what rooms are open, and physicians can tell at a glance whether the lab results are back and x-rays complete. Hospital communication systems such as paging, as well as on-call schedules and resource management, can be integrated directly into the dashboard.

*Emergency Department Leadership and Management*, ed. Stephanie Kayden, *et al.* Published by Cambridge University Press.
© Cambridge University Press 2015.

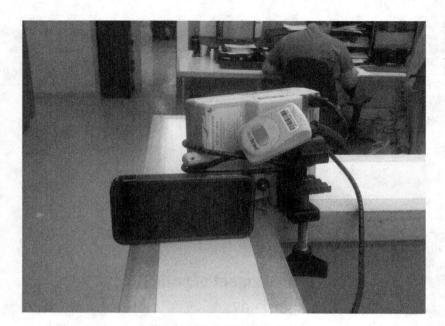

**Figure 18.1** An example of an active RFID tag attached to an automated intravenous pump. It is positioned next to the latest-generation smartphone so the reader can gauge its relative proportions.

There are a number of different ways that these types of systems provide an overview of the department. The most common is tabular, with each row representing a patient and the columns representing various attributes such as location, status of diagnostic tests, inpatient bed status, and names of current providers. The other major style of dashboard is geographical, where patients are depicted as icons on a visual map of the department. The status of the various attributes is shown pictorially: e.g., an icon of a bone indicating that an x-ray is complete or a flashing test tube to indicate a lab result. While each approach has its strong proponents, there are currently no studies available to indicate if one is better than the other.[2]

## Tracking systems

Process improvement in health care requires high-fidelity data to drive improvement efforts, as well as to monitor the effects of interventions. Data sources must be resilient, precise, and automated. Both barcodes and radiofrequency identification (RFID) tracking systems have been successfully used to supply these data.

Barcodes have long been used in industry for inventory management. In health care, they have been successfully deployed for inventory control,[3] as well as for the prevention of potential adverse medication administration errors.[4–6] Barcodes are inexpensive to print and therefore have a low marginal cost. Unfortunately, this technology is limited by user compliance and requires line-of-sight between the scanner and the object. Furthermore, it is often difficult to find a universal scanner that can support the multiple barcode formats already being used in a hospital. This incompatibility has forced some hospitals to discard expensive first implementations because they were unable to read the majority of barcodes in the hospital.[3] Pilot testing can mitigate the risk of incompatible scanners.

RFID tracking systems are quickly replacing barcodes as their startup and maintenance costs continue to fall. They enable complete automation of real-time location services without the need for user compliance. RFID tracking systems can use either passive or active tags. Passive RFID tags, like the ones found in identification access cards, require 1–2 centimeter proximity, as they are powered by induction from a nearby RFID sensor. Passive tags are best suited for access control and inventory management applications. Although active RFID tags have a much larger range, they are orders of magnitude more expensive to purchase and to maintain, as their battery source will eventually require replacement.

Active RFID tags (Fig. 18.1) are often used in patient, personnel, and asset tracking applications. They provide automated, high-fidelity data about location and time, which can be used to perform time-flow studies and provide ED performance metrics not otherwise possible, such as time to stretcher, time to clinician, or total time spent per patient. They can also be used to track high-cost ED assets that are often temporarily misplaced in the hospital, such as cardiac monitoring equipment and defibrillators. Active RFID tags can also automate patient location information on electronic ED whiteboards, freeing up ED personnel for other tasks, as well as providing location information for process improvement efforts. The improvements attained using this information must be weighed against the high recurring costs from the need to maintain tags, as well as their high loss rate. Furthermore, active RFID tags are often unable to discriminate between stretcher bays and patient rooms, information critical to using data for analysis and clinical care. Hybrid active RFID/infrared systems overcome these limitations, but as a proprietary technology they have much higher startup and maintenance costs.

---

**Case study 18.1.   Active RFID in the emergency department**

The ED at an academic teaching hospital in Boston, Massachusetts, USA, utilizes an active RFID tracking system. Their experience has been that it has approximately a 10-foot (3 m) range and can have trouble with the physical layout of the ED, such as determining which side of a wall a tag is on. This is not adequate for detailed time–motion studies of staff and patients, but it has proven valuable to keep track of high-value assets such as ventilators, portable monitors, and rapid volume infusers. The ability to track critical resources allows patients to move seamlessly from the ED to the operating room to the intensive care unit (ICU). Patient care is no longer delayed while equipment is exchanged or tracked. Instead, ED staff use this technology to locate critical pieces of equipment that inevitably become scattered in emergent cases. For example, the aforementioned hospital had frequent issues keeping track of its rapid infuser (used for critically ill trauma patients). It was not uncommon for the day staff to arrive after a chaotic, trauma-filled night and have to start calling around the hospital to locate this important piece of equipment. After it was tagged, it was easy either to locate its present location, or if for some reason that was not possible to identify the time and trajectory that it left the department. The 10-foot (3 m) resolution proved quite adequate to enable quick retrieval.

## Bedside registration

Information technology can support streamlined patient flow through the use of wireless mobile computing devices, such as tablet computers and computers on wheels (COW) (Fig. 18.2). In most EDs, patients are first seen by a triage nurse. If stable, they wait to be registered by a clerk who collects demographic, financial, and other administrative data, prior to being brought to a bed for the initiation of medical treatment. With a bedside registration model, the patient is moved from triage directly to an available bed, where care can proceed without delay. The full registration process then occurs in parallel with medical care, eliminating a bottleneck. Moving patients directly to a bed using a bedside registration model can improve patient satisfaction and decrease wait times, ED length of stay, and walk-out rates.[7–12]

Although it is advantageous, there are some pitfalls to this approach. While most of the information captured by the registration clerk is not necessary to initiate patient care, there are a few critical administrative tasks that must occur very early in the visit. These include uniquely identifying the patient in the system and creating an associated medical record number/visit number, as well as physical creation of a chart. If the registration clerk does not complete these tasks, then someone else must fulfill that function. That will most likely be the triage nurse, who is usually overloaded and maximally extended. If the patient is misidentified at initial presentation, there is a chance that the information from two patients could become mixed in the same record, putting both at risk.

For the most critically ill patients, many hospitals have pre-generated charts that are already entered into the system. Pre-generated charts allow for instantaneous care of critically ill patients, immediately upon arrival. Unfortunately, use of such records is a barrier to the integrated use of previously collected safety information such as allergies or medication history. While expeditious, this approach may bypass many built-in safety functions in the most complex, sickest patients. At a later time, these pre-generated charts must eventually be merged with existing records, providing an additional source of potential confusion and error.

The bedside registration model makes it possible for the clinical components of care to be

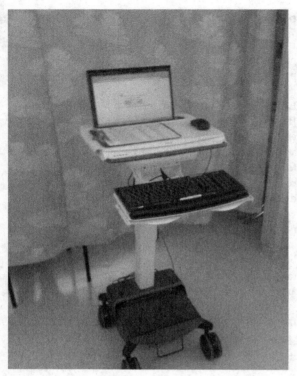

**Figure 18.2** An example of a computer on wheels (COW). These contain long-life batteries and can be wheeled to any needed location.

completed prior to the capture of complete registration information. This is more likely during times of surge when the clerks may be delayed and the physicians will feel particularly pressured to discharge patients as quickly as possible. If this occurs, there is a risk patients could leave the ED without the hospital having critical information on file. This can put patients at risk if they cannot be reached to report a delayed test result such as a change on a radiology reading or critical lab finding. There is also the financial risk of patients leaving without capture of their billing information. If not carefully managed, friction could develop between the clinical staff and the clerical staff trying to capture the registration information. This can further delay registration and increase the odds of the patient leaving prior to full registration. This can be mitigated by showing a symbol or flag on the tracking system, and also by building clear warnings into the discharge planning to prevent unregistered patients from leaving prior to complete registration.

# Electronic health records (EHR)
## Clinical documentation

Clinical documentation of the ED visit serves a number of very important purposes.[13] Emergency care is usually the initial care and stabilization of an acute condition. The record serves as a communication tool to subsequent providers, documenting the circumstances of the visit, the physical findings, and rationale for the care rendered. Secondly, it provides some measure of the complexity of the medical encounter, as justification for a certain level of payment. Thirdly, it records the thinking process and rationale of the providers in order to support or refute allegations of negligence in the event of an untoward outcome. Lastly, it provides an important public health service, facilitating important public endeavors such as syndromic surveillance, communicable disease reporting, and all manner of medical research. While the medical record has become a critical component of modern medicine, there are significant difficulties in collecting, storing, and sharing the information therein.

Well-received computerized systems for nursing and physician documentation have been described in the literature.[14,15] Storing the data within computer systems makes it easy to quickly retrieve and share information with other providers without the need to waste time hunting around for a paper record. The computer can analyze the electronic chart and make suggestions about missing critical information, and can potentially detect errors automatically.[16] It can lead to lower costs, as staff no longer need to collect, collate, and photocopy the various portions of a paper record.

However, the switch to electronic documentation is not without downsides. Most sites report a sharp decrease in efficiency when switching to an electronic system. After an adjustment period, users regain some speed, but do not return to baseline. Some EDs attempt to mitigate this by the use of scribes. Scribes are relatively inexpensive clerical workers, often premedical students, who follow the physician around and handle data-entry tasks. This is controversial, with proponents favoring the increase in efficiency and detractors noting that it circumvents the clinical decision-support benefits of having the provider interact with the computer.

Another strategy for improving the efficiency of clinical documentation is the use of voice recognition software, where the user dictates into a microphone attached to the computer. The computer analyzes the audio and enters the user's words as if they had been typed. The user then reads the generated narrative in real time and corrects it, which allows the computer to hone its algorithm and decrease future errors. After decades of development, this technology finally has an accuracy rate that is suitable for clinical use. The downsides to this approach include relatively high cost and the risk that poorly proofread dictations will be confusing or indecipherable.

## Clinical data exchange

Many countries, including the UK, Canada, and the USA, have committed billions of dollars to the implementation of electronic health records and data sharing for coordination of care. Several hospitals in Massachusetts (USA), have implemented this kind of healthcare information exchange.

Here's how it works:

When a patient registers for care, he or she is asked to identify the primary care giver and referring clinicians. As a patient is evaluated in the ED, the patient's problems, medication history, and allergies are documented, diagnostic studies such as labs and imaging are ordered, and medications are administered. Upon discharge, a summary document is created with a narrative of the care, diagnosis, treatment, prescriptions, and recommended follow-up. A printed copy of this summary is provided to the patient and an electronic copy is transmitted to the primary care giver and referring clinicians.

In Massachusetts, the New England Healthcare Exchange Network (www.nehen.org) has provided a secure means to send information among payers and providers since 1997. Although, ideally, these summaries would be routed to the EHR of the primary care provider (the patient's "electronic medical home"), some providers do not have an EHR. In that case, they are routed via the provider's preference, which could be fax or secure email.

This mechanism of sending data from the ED to community providers is called "pushing" data, and it is the most common form of healthcare information exchange currently in use.

Another type of healthcare information exchange is possible, the "pulling" of data, with patient consent, from multiple community data sources. Today, in the USA, EDs can easily retrieve comprehensive medication lists using a network that connects various pharmacies to produce an electronic history of all dispensed and reimbursed medications. Laws can be quite variable regarding privacy protections. For example, in Massachusetts, it is not permitted for some pharmacies to transmit summaries of mental health/substance abuse/HIV-related medications.

In the future, it is likely that patients will opt in on a facility/institution basis to share their data, so that an ED will be able to pull data from hospitals, labs, and clinician offices to assemble a "just in time" record that will inform emergency care. Pulling data to ensure safe care and pushing data to ensure continuity of care with primary care providers will one day be the standard of care for all emergency providers.

## E-prescribing

When an ED professional prescribes a medication, e-prescribing ensures that the medication is safe, affordable, and conveniently available for the patient.

Here's how it works:

Using an ED information system, a clinician begins to prescribe the medication.

First, the patient's insurance status is checked to identify medications at various levels of reimbursement. As the clinician continues, the list of preferred medications is displayed. For example, if the clinician wants to prescribe an $H_2$-blocker, the generic omeprazole will be shown as a fully reimbursed medication while the expensive brand-name Nexium will be shown as a non-preferred and not-reimbursed medication. The clinician can choose any medication, but the patient will likely prefer one with a low co-pay and high reimbursement.

Second, the patient's history of dispensed and reimbursed medications is extracted from the e-prescribing network. The medication being prescribed is compared to the history, and all drug–drug interactions and therapeutic duplications are shown.

Third, the medication, once safely prescribed, is routed to the retail pharmacy or mail-order pharmacy of the patient's choice.

Thus, the prescription has gone from the ED clinician's brain to the "patient's vein" without paper, handwriting, or an intermediary. It is checked for reimbursement and interactions along the way and then is made available to the patient via a convenient retail or mail-order pharmacy.

This works very well for non-controlled substances, but what about narcotics?

A substantial portion of the medications prescribed in the ED are controlled substances. Ideally, one workflow will be used to electronically prescribe controlled and non-controlled medications. However, many countries impose special protections upon the controlled-substance prescribing process, such as the use of "two-factor authentication," something you know (a password) and something you have (a known cell phone, a thumbprint, or a smart card).

It will become increasingly important for ED information systems to support fully automated electronic prescribing workflows of controlled and non-controlled substances over the next few years.

## Decision support

### Computerized physician order entry

Computerized physician order entry (CPOE) presents a unique challenge to the ED. The advantages of CPOE systems are well established in health care for improving the accuracy of medication orders, increasing patient safety, improving compliance to dosing guidelines, and improving documentation.[17]

The ED has arguably the largest information needs and information turnover in a hospital. CPOE systems deployed in the ED must be specifically tailored to work in this environment. For example, the ED places only a small subset of possible medication, radiology, nursing, and other orders. These orders are often ordered urgent or stat for the ED, with often only one or two dosages.

The inpatient and ED settings have a very different range of common therapeutic and diagnostic modalities. It is extremely important to bear this in mind when planning the deployment of an ED CPOE system, particularly when considering a system primarily used in the inpatient setting. Most emergency providers will use a relatively small subset of the choices available to those who work on the wards. Good design will increase the efficiency of the common choices (such as aspirin, cardiac biomarkers, chest x-ray, ECG) at the expense of less common choices. Treating a wide variety of choices as equals means most of the options are superfluous and will cause confusion, delays, and errors. Ideal systems are optimized around the safe, rapid entry of the tests and interventions most commonly used.

As with any technological intervention, there is always the potential for unintended consequences, both positive and negative. In a survey of 176 hospitals across the United States that had implemented inpatient CPOE, respondents overwhelmingly reported changes in workflow (88%), communication (84%), dependence on technology (83%), system demands (82%), emotions (80%), and more or new work (72%).[18]

**Case study 18.2. CPOE implementation in the emergency department**

The ED at an academic teaching hospital in San Diego, California, USA, implemented CPOE in 2003. For more than a decade, crowding has been identified as a significant issue in EDs in the USA. In addition to improving the accuracy of medication orders, this ED was interested in reducing lab turnaround times to improve ED efficiency. Laboratory tests are one of the most commonly ordered tests in the ED and often the rate-limiting factor in the workup of a patient. Improving ED operational efficiency improves patient flow and consequently can reduce crowding. This ED used a sequential process improvement approach, changing both how specimens were handled and how laboratory tests were ordered. They were able to achieve a reduction in median lab turnaround times after the implementation of the electronic system for sodium (9.5 minutes), CBC (5.9 minutes), and troponin-I (11.2 minutes) tests. The authors attributed this decrease in turnaround times to changes in specimen handling and workflow made possible by CPOE, which enabled tasks to be performed in parallel.[19]

### Clinical decision support systems

Modern patient care is continuously becoming more complex as researchers discover better ways to provide high-quality care. Despite these advances in scientific knowledge, translation into clinical practice can be slow and inconsistent. Clinical decision support systems (CDSS) are an elegant way to produce sustainable knowledge translation.[20]

Clinical decision support systems have been shown effective in changing clinician behaviors for diabetes care, cardiovascular disease, depression, cancer screening, vaccinations, and ventilator management, among others. These systems have been used for disease diagnosis, preventive care, disease management, and drug prescribing across this broad spectrum of disease processes.[21–23]

In the ED, they can be used as a way to improve compliance to departmental clinical and operational guidelines. For example, CDSS can be used as a way to decrease unnecessary testing, enforce admission and discharge protocols, and improve compliance with treatment protocols. As a side effect, a formally defined pathway can establish a local standard of care and consequently reduce overall practice risk.[24]

## Outbreak detection alerts and population surveillance

EDs have always been on the front line of disasters. Newer threats to public safety have arisen in the form of bioterrorism and emerging disease epidemics such as novel influenza types. In traditional mass casualty incidents such as bomb explosions, the nature and location of the incident is obvious and victims present to a small number of facilities over a relatively brief period of time. With newer threats, such as intentional release of anthrax spores, there can be a wide variation in the time and location of initial presentation, which can be so great as to significantly delay the realization that there is an outbreak going on. Syndromic surveillance is a name given to a group of techniques being used to aggregate and analyze visit data from a cohort of EDs.[25] By linking together the data from multiple EDs it is possible to detect emerging illness much sooner than was previously possible, speeding the response and possibly saving lives. It is also possible to provide reassurance that a small number of unusual cases do not represent a wider outbreak.

In addition, the data generated by syndromic surveillance systems can be particularly useful to EDs. Novel sources of information such as internet search-engine results have been found to provide a reliable early warning that an outbreak is under way.[26,27] Related data sources such as convenience-store purchases of cold medication, tissues, and orange juice have all shown promise as a means of predicting disease outbreaks.[27]

ED leaders can use syndromic surveillance data to predict the short-term demand for emergency services. These new systems will enhance global situational awareness to proactively increase staffing, accurately assess current and surge capabilities, and coordinate within a region to provide a comprehensive public health response.

## Quality improvement

### Throughput reporting: provider efficiency, matching staffing to volume

Quality improvement often requires combining multiple disparate data sources. These data can originate from ED information systems, pharmacy information systems, radiology information systems, hospital admit–discharge–transfer (ADT) systems, cardiology systems, physician and nursing scheduling systems, real-time location systems, and many others. Business analytic dashboards can be used to present key performance indicators (KPI) in a way that is insightful, actionable, and compelling. These business analytic dashboards can monitor KPIs such as provider efficiency, facility utilization, and performance metrics.

Queuing theory can use actual throughput data to model different processes (see Chapter 23 for details). Leadership can then use this model to simulate the effect of different process interventions. Process simulation allows administrators to test different process interventions without the expense, chaos, and frustrations of real-world trials.

At an academic teaching hospital in New York City, investigators used a queuing model to guide provider scheduling. The reallocation of providers based on a queuing model resulted in a 21.7% decrease in patients left without being seen despite a 5.5% increase in patient volume. This study demonstrates the importance of collecting and analyzing arrival patterns, in order to adjust daily staffing levels to match changes in demand across the week.[28]

### Clinical quality metrics

A key advantage to the integrated ED information system is the ability to combine different data sources to automate the rapid report of clinical quality metrics. At a basic level, a computer system can automatically scan prior visits, alerting the clinicians as well as the quality assurance (QA) team that a patient was seen in the same ED within the prior 72 hours. A more complex example would involve combining the data from CPOE orders and automated medication dispensing, cross-referenced with chief complaint and final diagnosis codes. Such a system could provide real-time and retrospective QA data on the timeliness of antibiotic administration in pneumonia.

For institutions that have protocols and special response teams for acute myocardial infarction and stroke, computer systems have been developed that can automate the process of notifying the response team, as well as recording the time of the notification, the time of the response, and critical milestones such as obtaining a head CT or administering thrombolytics.

Compiling and reviewing clinical quality metrics in many institutions is a manual process often requiring extensive manual review and weeks of effort. With an automated process, comprehensive information is easily available for QA review, and even more importantly, deviations can be recognized during the actual visit, thus immediately rectifying the situation.

## Training and simulation

EDs often have a high turnover of rotating residents, medical students, and other staff members. This creates a need for repeated, consistent orientation and training sessions. Asynchronous learning methods are student-centered techniques that allow learners to participate at personally convenient times, without needing to synchronize to a teacher's schedule. Web-based didactic programs are well suited to deliver this type of standardized training to a revolving group of staff. Furthermore, web-based synchronized learning, such as webinars, can be leveraged to deliver just-in-time (JIT) training for rare events such as chemical or bioterrorism disasters. JIT training can be used to quickly disseminate to staff critical operational and clinical information during crisis. For example, JIT modules can be created on how to use personal protective equipment, identification of early symptoms of a suspected biological weapon, or treating a victim of a nerve-agent attack. JIT training compliance can be tracked and deployed in real time without removing trainees from their clinical responsibilities.

Simulators have long been used in aviation training to allow pilots to safely experience unusual and difficult situations. Simulation can similarly be used in emergency medicine to practice complex, rarely performed, and/or time-critical procedures such as managing cardiac arrest or performing an emergent thoracotomy or lateral canthotomy. Computer simulation can increase exposure to rare diseases such as neonatal cyanotic heart disease and other rarely seen life-threatening conditions. Simulation provides an ideal environment for participants to analyze the medical decision process, team dynamics, and communication. These cases can be observed by experts, and can provide valuable feedback to improve care. They can also be used as an additional method for subjective and objective evaluation of clinical knowledge, skills, and attitudes.

## Discharge instructions

For most patients who are discharged home, their ED visit represents the initiation of care of an acute condition. By their very nature, most of these encounters are unplanned and patients may be preoccupied, distracted, and possibly even sedated by the end of their stay. It is unlikely that they will be able to remember and follow a comprehensive treatment plan unless it is provided in written form.

One of the most common uses for software in the ED setting is for the generation of printed discharge instructions. These software packages can be standalone or fully integrated into an ED information system. They usually have a large number of standardized instructions for the most common conditions seen. Some have variations that will print in multiple languages, and often they print pictures or diagrams to help explain the condition. Most instructions should include the patient's diagnosis, the recommended treatment, the warning signs that should result in seeking immediate care, and what follow-up should occur, including when and with whom. Advanced integrated systems can incorporate features such as e-prescribing, clinical data exchange, and clinical decision support, as described previously in this chapter.

## Challenges

### Integration of ED information systems into hospital information systems

The ED information system must not be an island of data or an informatics silo within the hospital. The ED serves many purposes: it is a referral center for primary providers in the community, it is an entry point for patients on the way to the wards and the ICU, and it is an important outpatient care center. In order to fulfill those disparate functions, it must include full integration into its hospital information system. ED systems must be able to receive data from hospital information systems, including patient demographics, insurance information, problem lists, medication lists, allergy information, notes/reports, and diagnostic studies such as labs, images, and pathology reports. In many ways, the ED system is the integration hub for the hospital, pulling data as needed from multiple departmental applications and databases.

Many hospitals have deployed CPOE, and ideally ED clinicians would adopt CPOE as part of their workflow, since it enhances safety. However, hospital order entry systems may not be ideally suited to the workflow of the ED clinicians, who need a quick way to order from a battery of a few dozen labs, imaging studies, and medications. Full adoption and integration will require compromises and accommodations on both sides.

Once a patient is evaluated, the ED clinician creates clinical documentation for the encounter. That documentation should be stored as part of the patient's permanent lifetime record and should be available to all subsequent clinicians, particularly hospitalists who will be caring for admitted patients. Thus, ED integration with hospital information systems must be bidirectional – pulling from all inpatient and outpatient data sources and pushing the finished documentation back to hospital information systems for all to read. CPOE integration is ideal, as it supports medication reconciliation, ensuring all orders from the ED are appropriately continued once patients are admitted.

Many enterprise software vendors provide ED modules that are fully integrated into inpatient and outpatient systems. Other vendors provide ED-specific ("best of breed") packages that include inbound and outbound interfaces to hospital information systems. Running a standalone database that supports ED workflow but does not communicate with hospital registration, clinical, and CPOE segregates the data among different departments and does not support safe, high-quality, and efficient care.

## Financial

Hospital IT departments' budgets are always constrained. No matter how large the budget, demand will exceed supply. Departmental software purchases such as ED information systems may need to compete for scarce finances in hospital capital allocation committees against ventilators for neonates and the latest MRI for brain imaging. Since an ED information system may be seen as an expense and not a source of revenue,

ED leaders need a strategy to obtain funding for the automation they need. Here are a few suggestions:

- Create a governance committee. Hospital IT departments are likely to have committees of stakeholders who help set project priorities for the year. Although the IT department may not be able to unilaterally convince senior management of the importance of an ED information system, a guiding coalition of clinicians and hospital stakeholders is likely to have substantial influence.
- Join the hospital's capital allocation committee. Hospitals allocate capital based on strategic importance, quality/safety impact, regulatory/compliance requirements, return on investment, and employee/patient/clinician impact. By framing an ED information system as essential for continuity of care, supporting efficient throughput of patients, and necessary for compliance with national documentation requirements, the odds of receiving funding will be substantially increased.

In addition to arguing for financial support, it is also important to partner with IT departments to get their support for the project. There are three ways to enhance your relationship with the hospital IT department:

- Make the ED implementation low-impact, by choosing an internet-based remotely hosted system. Suggesting that an ED information system implementation will not require resources from an already overburdened IT department will enhance your chance of success.
- Choose a module that is already part of your enterprise hospital information system. It may be lower-cost and easier for the IT department to implement an ED module that is part of the hospital system they already support.
- If you choose to implement a new system that interfaces to, rather than integrates with, the existing hospital information system, you may want to choose a phased approach. Start with an ED dashboard, which requires modest integration, and progress to an order entry and documentation system, which requires a more significant integration effort. IT department projects are a function of scope, timing, and resources. Since IT resources are often fixed, reducing scope and extending timing for the ED information system may lead to enhanced support from IT leadership.

## Usability

Careful attention to the user interface and how the computer system fits in with the workflow of the clinician is of paramount importance. Yet this critical issue often receives too little attention.

Some systems are designed with mandatory data elements that must be completed in order to proceed. However, there are times in the ED when the answer may not be known. Mandatory fields do a good job of collecting data, but experience has shown that users will often make up answers in order to circumvent the block and continue with their work.

Human–computer interface design and usability are critical to user satisfaction and implementation success. Unfortunately, these two elements are difficult to quantify and evaluate, specifically in a contract or work scope document. Good usability and interfaces are unfortunately often neglected in favor of providing additional features and functionality that are easier to quantify. This often leads to a phenomenon known as "feature creep," where extraneous features continue to be added, further making interfaces more complex and less intuitive.

The nature of the software industry dictates that ED information system products are designed to be generic in order to increase the number of potential clients. Having a large client base can reduce product costs and aggregate user experience. However, this one-size-fits-all approach forces clinicians to alter workflow to accommodate a product rather than the other way around. These changes in workflow can fundamentally disrupt ED operations and lead to implementation failure.

## Types of systems

Hospitals often invest in enterprise systems to support the clinical and administrative functions of a hospital. Many of these products offer modules for the ED as well. These modules provide integration with the rest of the hospital enterprise systems without significant overhead. Although these systems do provide the potential for improved communication across transitions of care, ED modules are often poorly adapted to the unique workflow of the ED, and are often modifications of existing modules for outpatient settings. The mismatch between product workflow and clinical workflow can lead to loss of efficiency, a decrease in provider satisfaction, and possibly a risk to patient safety.

Best-of-breed models are those ED information systems specifically designed for use in the ED and its unique workflow. These products can better model an individual site's unique workflow and ease the transition to electronic systems. Unfortunately, most of these systems cannot natively communicate with other hospital information systems. Instead, these systems require extensive and expensive interface engineering that can require months of work. Changes to software on either side of the interface could require additional planning and expense.

## System reliability and downtime

One of the greatest dangers of advanced technology is that the clinical and clerical staff becomes so dependent on computerized systems that they are unable to effectively take care of patients without them. Computer outages, or downtime, can occur for a variety of reasons: software programming errors, failures of computer or network hardware, human error, and disruption of infrastructure, either natural or intentional, can all cause systems to be unavailable. Computer data centers are highly dependent on stable infrastructure, and if the power, coolant, or network connectivity is compromised, it will likely impact the users.

Redundancy and efficiency are of critical importance to prevent downtime. Critical servers can be "multi-homed," with multiple physical computers all sharing the load, and if one crashes the users barely realize it. Modern data centers have multiple independent power feeds and backup generators protected by bridging systems made up of batteries and/or newer kinetic-energy flywheels. One of the biggest challenges in a data center is heat management. Techniques such as cold aisle containment, floor tile ventilation, and hot air recapture can make the cooling systems more efficient and allow for more modular deployment. Network outages can be as devastating to the users as computer failure – connectivity is a mission-critical component and requires both multiple robust physical network paths without a common point of failure and a backup method such as point-to-point microwave.

Even when all precautions are taken, downtime is sometimes unavoidable, either due to maintenance that cannot be done on a running system or due to catastrophic failure. It is imperative that well-defined procedures ensure that care continues, for emergencies will continue despite a computer outage, and in fact a large-scale event, such as an earthquake or bomb explosion, could cause both a computer disruption and a large influx of patients.

So called "downtime kits," replete with copies of the necessary forms, information guides, key contact information, and other critical supplies, can go a long way to mitigating the effects of an unexpected outage.

# References

1. Feied CF, Handler JA, Smith MS, *et al*. Clinical information systems: instant ubiquitous clinical data for error reduction and improved clinical outcomes. *Academic Emergency Medicine* 2004; **11**: 1162–9.

2. Aronsky D, Jones I, Lanaghan K, Slovis CM. Supporting patient care in the emergency department with a computerized whiteboard system. *Journal of the American Medical Informatics Association* 2008; **15**: 184–94.

3. Hanson LB, Weinswig MH, De Muth JE. Accuracy and time requirements of a bar-code inventory system for medical supplies. *American Journal of Hospital Pharmacy* 1988; **45**: 341–4.

4. Poon EG, Keohane CA, Yoon CS, *et al*. Effect of bar-code technology on the safety of medication administration. *New England Journal of Medicine* 2010; **362**: 1698–707.

5. Poon EG, Cina JL, Churchill W, *et al*. Medication dispensing errors and potential adverse drug events before and after implementing bar code technology in the pharmacy. *Annals of Internal Medicine* 2006; **145**: 426–34.

6. Wright AA, Katz IT. Bar coding for patient safety. *New England Journal of Medicine* 2005; **353**: 329–31.

7. Spaite DW, Bartholomeaux F, Guisto J, *et al*. Rapid process redesign in a university-based emergency department: decreasing waiting time intervals and improving patient satisfaction. *Annals of Emergency Medicine* 2002; **39**: 168–77.

8. Morgan R. Turning around the turn-arounds: improving ED throughput processes. *Journal of Emergency Nursing* 2007; **33**: 530–6.

9. Chan TC, Killeen JP, Kelly D, Guss DA. Impact of rapid entry and accelerated care at triage on reducing emergency department patient wait times, lengths of stay, and rate of left without being seen. *Annals of Emergency Medicine* 2005; **46**: 491–7.

10. Bertoty DA, Kuszajewsk ML, Marsh EE. Direct-to-room: one department's approach to improving ED throughput. *Journal of Emergency Nursing* 2007; **33**: 26–30.

11. Takakuwa KM, Shofer FS, Abbuhl SB. Strategies for dealing with emergency department overcrowding: a one-year study on how bedside registration affects patient throughput times. *Journal of Emergency Medicine* 2007; **32**: 337–42.

12. Gorelick MH, Yen K, Yun HJ. The effect of in-room registration on emergency department length of stay. *Annals of Emergency Medicine* 2005; **45**: 128–33.

13. Davidson SJ, Zwemer FL, Nathanson LA, Sable KN, Khan AN. Where's the beef? The promise and the reality of clinical documentation. *Academic Emergency Medicine* 2004; **11**: 1127–34.

14. Bourie PQ, Ferrenberg VA, McKay M, Halamka JD, Safran C. Implementation of an on-line emergency unit nursing system. *Proceedings, AMIA Symposium* 1998: 330–3.

15. Likourezos A, Chalfin DB, Murphy DG, *et al*. Physician and nurse satisfaction with an electronic medical record system. *Journal of Emergency Medicine* 2004; **27**: 419–24.

16. Schenkel S. Promoting patient safety and preventing medical error in emergency departments. *Academic Emergency Medicine* 2000; **7**: 1204–22.

17. Bates DW, Leape LL, Cullen DJ, *et al*. Effect of computerized physician order entry and a team intervention on prevention of serious medication errors. *JAMA* 1998. **280**: 1311–16.

18. Ash JS, Sittig DF, Poon EG, *et al*. The extent and importance of unintended consequences related to computerized provider order entry. *Journal of the American Medical Informatics Association* 2007; **14**: 415–23.

19. Guss DA, Chan TC, Killeen JP. The impact of a pneumatic tube and computerized physician order management on laboratory turnaround time. *Annals of Emergency Medicine* 2008; **51**: 181–5.

20. Holroyd BR, Bullard MJ, Graham TA, Rowe BH. Decision support technology in knowledge translation. *Academic Emergency Medicine* 2007; **14**: 942–8.

21. Garg AX. Effects of computerized clinical decision support systems on practitioner performance and patient outcomes: a systematic review. *JAMA* 2005; **293**: 1223–8.

22. Chaudhry B, Wang J, Wu S, *et al*. Systematic review: impact of health information technology on quality, efficiency, and costs of medical care. *Annals of Internal Medicine* 2006; **144**: 742–52.

23. Shea S, DuMouchel W, Bahamonde L. A meta-analysis of 16 randomized controlled trials to evaluate computer-based clinical reminder systems for preventive care in the ambulatory setting. *Journal of the American Medical Informatics Association* 1996; **3**: 399–409.

24. Lewis MH, Gohagan JK, Merenstein DJ. The locality rule and the physician's dilemma: local medical practices vs the national standard of care. *JAMA* 2007; **297**: 2633–7.

25. Mandl KD, Overhage JM, Wagner MM, *et al.* Implementing syndromic surveillance: a practical guide informed by the early experience. *Journal of the American Medical Informatics Association* 2004; **11**: 141–50.

26. Wilson K, Brownstein JS. Early detection of disease outbreaks using the Internet. *CMAJ* 2009; **180**: 829–31.

27. Ginsberg J, Mohebbi MH, Patel RS, *et al.* Detecting influenza epidemics using search engine query data. *Nature* 2009; **457**: 1012–14.

28. Green LV, Soares J, Giglio JF, Green RA. Using queueing theory to increase the effectiveness of emergency department provider staffing. *Academic Emergency Medicine* 2006; **13**: 61–8.

# 19

# Triage systems

Shelley Calder and Elke Platz

## Key learning points

- Identify the core components of a triage model.
- Understand various triage models, including novel approaches.
- Understand how to evaluate your triage process and measure your success.

## Introduction

Emergency departments (ED) around the globe are faced with issues of crowding, acuity, staffing, and financial challenges. The Centers for Disease Control and Prevention (CDC) reported nearly 117 million ED visits in the USA in 2007, a 23% increase over the last decade.[1] Time to provider, as reported by the National Center for Health Statistics, increased from 38 minutes in 1997 to 56 minutes in 2006.[2] In response to this growing crisis the Institute of Medicine (IOM) recommends improvements in hospital efficiency and patient flow in addition to more coordinated emergency care systems with increased resources.[3]

Current and future ED leaders will be challenged to develop innovative systems that will withstand the pressures of healthcare restructuring without deviation from patient care and safety. Evaluation of current triage practices is a potential area of opportunity for process improvement. Triage is most often the point of entry to the healthcare system and can largely impact crowding, flow, and resource management.

Triage, meaning separation, sorting, or selecting, was first defined in the early nineteenth century on the battlefield.[4] Soldiers and medical personnel used triage to prioritize care and resources for wounded soldiers. The Emergency Nurses Association (ENA) describes the primary goal of triage systems as a systematic approach to rapidly identifying patients with urgent or life-threatening conditions.[5] An efficient triage system ensures that patients get to the right place at the right time with the right care provider. In the twenty-first century triage has evolved from a rapid sorting mechanism to a dynamic process incorporating patient acuity, resource utilization, patient flow, quality, and patient satisfaction.

In today's hectic EDs the role of the triage provider and the function of the triage system have become critical. Multiple triage systems are identified throughout the literature, and there appears to be a lack of consistency or standardization in triage around the globe. The ENA and American College of Emergency Physicians (ACEP) recognize the profound influence of triage and believe that quality of patient care can be largely impacted by utilization of a standardized ED triage scale and acuity categorization process.[6] As leaders in emergency medicine we must begin to understand the role of a standardized triage system as part of a solution to improve patient flow, safety, and quality of care in our EDs.

## Traditional triage models

Currently 96% of EDs use some form of triage system as a basic framework to sort patients.[7] Three common triage systems are described throughout the literature:

- **Greeter** or **traffic director** is the simplest form of triage system described in the literature. On arrival the patient is greeted and a chief complaint is collected. This role is often performed by a non-medical person. This model is most frequently used in lower-volume EDs with open bed access.
- **Rapid triage** or **spot check** is completed by collection of a limited dataset allowing for rapid assignment of a triage acuity level. Data collected

*Emergency Department Leadership and Management*, ed. Stephanie Kayden, *et al.* Published by Cambridge University Press.
© Cambridge University Press 2015.

during rapid triage or spot check will include, but is not limited to, chief complaint, pertinent past medical history, and vital signs. Rapid triage ensures that the highest-acuity patients are quickly identified and treated. This type of triage is best suited for facilities with lower volume and immediate provider and bed access.

- **Comprehensive triage** allows for a more in-depth data collection process including assessment of physical, developmental, and psychosocial needs. If the patient appears critically ill, the assessment is stopped and the patient is immediately triaged to a care area. The ENA recommends comprehensive triage as a preferred model for triage.[5] Comprehensive triage is most successful in facilities with high volume and frequent delays in the time it takes for a patient to be seen by a provider. This assessment system provides additional information that can be used to determine appropriate clinical diagnostics and pathways to be initiated at triage.

## Three- and five-level triage acuity systems

Triage acuity, also referred to as severity or urgency in the literature, is a communication tool used by healthcare providers to identify which patients can safely wait and those who need immediate care.[8] If triage acuity systems are utilized appropriately they can also assist leaders in trending data for patient acuity, morbidity and mortality, length of stay (LOS), and staffing. Hospitals using similar triage acuity systems may also share data to benchmark. Numerous triage acuity rating scales are identified in the literature,

and they exist throughout the United States, Canada, Australia, and Europe.

## Three-level triage systems

In the late 1980s and early 1990s, EDs primarily used triage systems with three or four acuity categories (Table 19.1). Colors or numbers were used to identify emergent, urgent, and non-urgent patients.

There is currently little support in the literature for the adoption of three-level systems, because of lack of reliability.[9] When inter-rater agreement was measured in a three-level triage system by Wuerz et al., the findings showed a poor agreement between nurses in acuity assignment.[10]

## Five-level triage systems

Currently there is a progressive movement toward adopting five-level triage acuity systems, based on evidence of increased reliability, sensitivity, and specificity in comparison to three-level systems.[11] In 2010 the ENA and ACEP issued a joint statement advocating for the implementation of a standardized five-level triage system and acuity scale.[12] The following are the most common five-level triage systems currently used throuinghout the USA, Canada, Australia, and Europe:

- The **Australian Triage Scale (ATS)**, developed in Australia in 1993 by emergency medical staff, was the first nationally recognized five-level triage systems (Table 19.2). ATS is now a mandatory requirement for all Australian hospital and triage reports.[13] Each category of the five-level system lists clinical descriptors or conditions that correspond to a specific acuity level. Time to treatment is defined and the performance threshold for meeting treatment times is outlined.
- The **Canadian Triage Acuity System (CTAS)**, developed in the 1990s by a group of Canadian

**Table 19.1** Three-level triage systems

| Triage level | | |
|---|---|---|
| Emergent | Red or Level I | Requires immediate care Threat to life, limb, or organ |
| Urgent | Yellow or Level II | Care is required as soon as possible Patient condition is acute but not immediately life-threatening |
| Non Urgent | Green or Level III | Minor condition or routine care |

**Table 19.2** Australian Triage Scale (ATS)

| Triage level | Time to treatment | Performance indicator threshold |
|---|---|---|
| ATS 1 | Immediate | 100% |
| ATS 2 | 10 minutes | 80% |
| ATS 3 | 30 minutes | 75% |
| ATS 4 | 60 minutes | 70% |
| ATS 5 | 120 minutes | 70% |

physicians, is the nationally recognized tool used for triage in Canada (Table 19.3).[14] Use of CTAS has also been reported in a few US and European hospitals. Each triage level is associated with a list of presenting complaints. Acuity is assigned using the acuity scale level, with 1 being the highest and 5 the lowest acuity. Similar to ATS, the time it takes for a patient to be seen by a physician is outlined in addition to the fractile response. The fractile response represents the frequency at which the nurse and physician are required to meet response times. CTAS developers have recently reported the launch of an effective electronic training program.[15]

**Table 19.3** Canadian Triage Acuity System (CTAS)

| Triage level | Time to physician | Fractile response |
| --- | --- | --- |
| CTAS Level 1 | Immediate | 98% of the time |
| CTAS Level 2 | Within 15 minutes | 95% of the time |
| CTAS Level 3 | Within 30 minutes | 90% of the time |
| CTAS Level 4 | Within 60 minutes | 85% of the time |
| CTAS Level 5 | Within 120 minutes | 80% of the time |

- The **Manchester Triage System (MTS)**, developed in 1997 in the United Kingdom, consists of 52 flowcharts each representing a chief complaint (Fig. 19.1). Each of the 52 charts contains discriminators that allow the triage nurse to choose the patient's urgency based on a color-driven acuity scale. The colored acuity represents the maximum amount of time for a patient to be seen by the physician. Patients triaged red are seen by a physician immediately, orange wait times may be up to 10 minutes, yellow 60 minutes, green 120 minutes and blue 240 minutes.[16] An interesting feature of the MTS is the inclusion of a specific discriminator for pain using visual, behavioral, and verbal descriptors to assess and assign the patient's urgency category. The MTS includes a handbook for training and reference.

- The **Emergency Severity Index (ESI)** was developed by a group of physicians and nurses in the USA in the late 1990s. The ESI uses a five-level scale similar to CTAS. The ESI is unique in its approach, integrating acuity and resource utilization. In contrast to most of the other described triage systems ESI uses *one* flowchart and does not define maximum wait times. Patients requiring immediate life-saving

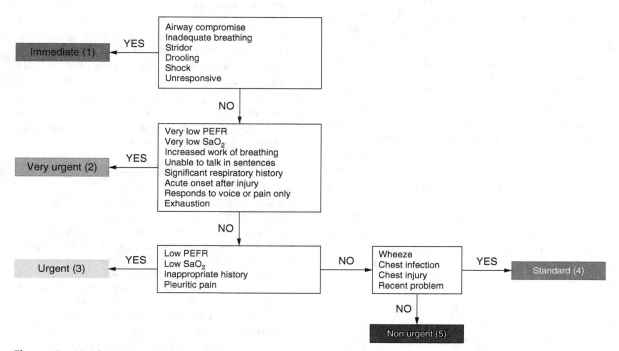

**Figure 19.1** Manchester Triage System (MTS) flowchart example: asthma. PEFR, peak expiratory flow rate.

intervention will be triaged as ESI 1. Patients at high risk for deterioration, severe pain, distress, or changes in level of consciousness will be triaged as ESI 2. Less severely injured or ill patients are triaged into the remaining three categories. Vital signs in the danger zone in addition to required resources are calculated to determine ESI 3, 4, or 5 assignment. Resources are defined as: laboratory test, radiology, medications, and specialty consultation.[8] A major strength of the ESI is the training and implementation material provided in the ESI handbook, as well as a single-chart triage algorithm.

## New triage models

Novel processes have been developed and implemented in countries across the globe in recent years in an attempt to improve patient flow through the ED, and in some instances not only to expedite care but also to decrease care variability among practitioners.[17]

## Practitioner in triage

Adding a practitioner, that is, a physician or mid-level provider (MLP) (e.g., physician assistant or nurse practitioner, in countries where these professions exist), to the triage team during peak patient arrival times can reduce ED length of stay (LOS) and left without being seen (LWBS) rates.[18–20] In one study mean ED LOS was decreased by 23 minutes for discharged patients and by 31 minutes for admitted patients, while the LWBS rate dropped by 1.7%.[18] The role of these providers is to initiate diagnostic testing and treatment during times of high ED patient volumes or for lower-acuity patients from triage prior to the patient's placement in an ED treatment room. In some instances patients can be discharged directly from the waiting room without ever being placed in the main ED. Frequently, practitioners in triage are paired with a nurse or medical assistant to take care of patients.

**Advantages** of this approach include the ability to initiate the diagnostic and treatment process from the triage area at times when the ED is crowded. This system can decrease the need for ED beds if patients are discharged directly from triage.

**Disadvantages** include the additional cost of staffing triage with a physician or MLP and "tying" this scarce and high-cost resource to the triage area, which is often physically separated from the main ED. Moreover, if patients who were initially managed

in the triage area then require admission, without an ED bed available, this may create a high-risk or at least challenging situation for the providers. In lower-volume EDs where only one or two physicians are scheduled per shift, placing one of them in triage may not represent a feasible option.

## Advanced triage-based care protocols and pathways

In EDs with long arrival-to-provider times, triage-based care protocols can facilitate earlier initiation of diagnostic testing (e.g., urine pregnancy test in female patients with abdominal pain) and treatment (e.g., pain management protocols). These orders can be initiated by a triage nurse with appropriate training.

In settings where clinicians from various medical specialties are practicing in the ED, a protocol-driven triage model may be useful not only to initiate diagnostic testing and treatment from triage but also to decrease management variation amongst clinicians. One such example is the Adaptive Process Triage (ADAPT) system that has been implemented in Scandinavian countries.[21]

**Advantages** that have been reported with the implementation of advanced triage protocols include, for instance, decreased length of stay,[22] decreased time to pain treatment,[23,24] decreased time to antibiotics in patients with pneumonia,[25] and decreased time to ECG in patients with chest pain (Case study 19.1).[26]

**Disadvantages** can include triage nurse over- or under-ordering of tests despite implementation of advanced care protocols.[27] Both carry the risk of unintended consequences, including administration of unnecessary medications or performance of imaging studies that may not be indicated.

> **Case study 19.1. Implementation of a triage chest pain protocol**
>
> An academic ED had recently participated in the successful establishment of a citywide transfer and treatment protocol for patients with ST-elevation myocardial infarction (STEMI). Door-to-balloon times for patients arriving to this ED by ambulance were consistently falling within the 90 minutes recommended by national guidelines. However, a protocol for identifying walk-in patients with STEMI was lacking, and door-to-balloon times in this population were less consistent. STEMI guidelines were recommending that the ECG be performed

within 10 minutes of arrival to the ED,[28] but this goal was rarely achieved with walk-in patients, particularly at times when the ED was busy.

The ED leadership team developed a simple protocol whereby a 12-lead ECG would be performed immediately upon arrival for any walk-in patient over the age of 40 presenting with a complaint between the umbilicus and nares, including chest discomfort with or without radiation to the arms(s), back, neck, jaw, or epigastrium; shortness of breath; weakness; diaphoresis; nausea; abdominal pain; lightheadedness; or palpitations. This ECG was to be hand-delivered to an ED attending physician on duty. If a STEMI was identified, the attending physician would be able to activate the cardiac catheterization team directly with a single page. If there was no STEMI identified, the patient would continue through the standard triage process.

Following implementation of this protocol, the overall percentage of qualifying walk-in patients for whom a door-to-balloon time of 90 minutes or less was achieved rose from 70% to over 90%.

# Immediate bedding and bedside registration

Immediate bedding is based on the concept of placing patients immediately in a treatment room, as soon as one becomes available. As trivial as this may sound, implementing this approach in an ED in which all patients have been undergoing a comprehensive triage process prior to placement in a room requires re-thinking of the basic idea of triage and establishment of a new process for registration staff, nurses, technicians, and physicians. It is important for everybody in the team to understand that ED triage is a *process* rather than a *place*, and that it only needs to occur when the number of new patients exceeds that of treatment rooms or providers. How does this process work? When a new patient arrives in the ED a "medical greeter" (usually an experienced triage nurse) asks for the patient's name, a unique identifier (such as date of birth), and the chief complaint. This information is usually sufficient to generate a chart or enter the patient into the electronic medical records. If a room is available, the patient is immediately placed into an empty ED bed. The patient's initial assessment then takes place by the nurse and physician who will be caring for the patient while he or she is in the ED. Full registration of the patient (for insurance information, etc.) is then undertaken by a clerk at the bedside. If all rooms are full, new patients

undergo a traditional triage process, for example with a five-level triage system. Moving from successive to parallel processes can have beneficial effects on patient flow.

**Advantages** of immediate bedding and bedside registration include decreased wait times,[29,30] LOS,[29–31] LWBS rates,[29,30] and improved patient satisfaction.[29]

**Disadvantages** include the need for a "backup" triage process when no empty ED beds are available and the need for ongoing reinforcement of this triage model in order for it to be sustained. These process changes do require staff buy-in to be successful (Case study 19.2).

---

**Case study 19.2. Implementation of immediate bedding and bedside registration**

An academic ED with an annual census of 58 000 patients was struggling with long waiting and LOS times and high LWBS rates, as well as low patient satisfaction scores.

After visiting several "best-practice" EDs across the country where novel approaches to front-end operations had been successfully implemented, the leadership team decided to move from a traditional model of full registration and five-level triage to immediate bedding and bedside registration. In the new process, if a bed was available in the ED, only the patient's name, date of birth, and chief complaint would be collected, enough for an electronic record to be generated. The patient would then be directed to a bed, where an initial nursing assessment would take place, often simultaneously with a physician or physician assistant. Full registration was relegated to the back-end, and would be performed at the bedside whenever possible.

In order to facilitate this change, the leadership team created work groups, consisting of attending physicians, residents, nurses, medical assistants, and registration staff, that developed a stepwise implementation plan for the new process. Prior to "going live," they performed simulations that allowed participants to experiment with the new process, identify potential problems, and propose solutions. These tabletop exercises also helped create buy-in among providers who were initially skeptical about the new initiative.

With just these simple process improvements, the ED was able to reduce average waiting-room time by 18 minutes, and saw the LWBS rate drop by nearly 50% over a six-month period. Not surprisingly, patient satisfaction scores improved at the same time.

---

## Kiosk self check-in

Airlines and hotels have long discovered the utility and efficiency of kiosks for check-in processes, and have implemented them over the past years. Not surprisingly, this technology has been adapted for health care, and triage solutions are now commercially available. Their functions range from basic collection of registration information to collection of past and present medical history and even the measurement of vital signs. While literature on the safety and efficiency of self check-in kiosks and wireless registration devices is sparse, the availability of these emerging technologies will likely generate more evidence in the near future.

## Choosing a triage model

Choosing a triage model that is appropriate for your patient population and meets your departmental needs is critical. Prior to choosing a triage system, leadership must carefully evaluate the systems available. The literature strongly suggests the superiority of five-level triage over three- or four-level systems.[11] Other factors to consider in the selection process should include ease of implementation, reliability, and validity, in addition to the required training and resource required for implementation.

## Triage providers and training

### Providers

Identifying the appropriate individuals to perform triage, and providing them with adequate training, is as important as choosing a triage model. Proper triage assessment and acuity assignment is critical and can largely impact patient safety, flow, and resource utilization. A mis-triage, an inappropriate acuity categorization, can take the form of over- or under- triage.[32] Over-triage, an overestimation of a patient's acuity, may lead to a critical patient waiting or not receiving the necessary treatments as quickly as needed, in addition to poor resource utilization. On the other hand, under-triage may leave a patient waiting who is at high risk of clinical deterioration.

### Qualifications

The qualifications and type of provider utilized to perform triage vary in the literature. The ENA and ACEP recommend the use of a clinical nurse with a minimum of six months of emergency experience.[33] Alternatively, paramedics, physicians, and physician extenders have been identified as potential options. Provider combinations such as a nurse and physician are gaining popularity in current practice models.

## Characteristics

Regardless of your choice of qualifications for the providers who perform triage, these individuals will require a unique skill set that may differ from that of clinicians providing direct patient care. Characteristics of a skilled triage provider include advanced assessment, decision making, critical thinking, and customer service skills.[34] These individuals should also demonstrate excellent clinical judgment and communication skills.

## Training approach

A combined didactic and clinical orientation to triage will provide a practice framework for the skilled practitioner.[35] Fortunately, many of the five-level systems developed in recent years provide training tools and guidelines for implementation. Institution-specific policies, clinical pathways, and a briefing on disaster management should also be included in the curriculum.

## Triage competency assessment

Upon completion of triage training, competency may be evaluated using one or more of the following methods: written exam, chart review, and/or clinical observation. The literature recommends periodic competency evaluation of new triage nurses and an annual assessment for all nurses (Table 19.4).[35]

Triage is a challenging position that requires specific education and skills. Leaders can significantly decrease the risk of frequent mis-triage in their departments by choosing appropriately skilled individuals to triage and by providing adequate training and ongoing supervision.

## Measuring success

Measurement of process improvements at triage will vary depending on the departmental goals identified in the reorganization or implementation of a new

**Table 19.4** Triage competency standards, as specified by the Emergency Nurses Association[33]

The emergency registered nurse triages each healthcare consumer, utilizing age-appropriate, developmentally appropriate, and culturally sensitive practices to prioritize and optimize healthcare consumer flow, expediting those healthcare consumers who require immediate care.

**The emergency registered nurse:**
- Obtains pertinent subjective and objective data while providing physical, emotional and psychosocial support to the health care consumer, family, and others as appropriate.
- Interprets data obtained incorporating age appropriate physical, developmental and psychosocial needs of the health care consumer.
- Utilizes a valid and reliable triage system to designate triage acuity.*
- Implements appropriate interventions according to established organizational policies/protocols, as warranted by the health care consumer's status.
- Documents relevant data and triage acuity for every health care consumer in a retrievable form.
- Communicates significant findings to team members,

**In a disaster the emergency triage registered nurse:**
- Collaborates with appropriate disaster personnel and Incident Command for situational awareness, safety, and security measures.
- Identifies the nature of the disaster and resources required.
- Utilizes a rapid triage system to determine priority of emergency treatment, categories, and mode of transport.
- Documents according to established organizational policies/protocols
- Modifies the triage decision depending on the circumstances, as either by routine operations or disaster management.

triage system. Wuerz *et al.* identify the following frequent drivers in triage reorganization:[36]
- reduction of variation of assigned triage categories
- decreased risk of negative outcomes due to mis-triage

- data collection
- transition form a three-category to a five-category triage system to better "sort" the increasing number of ED patients
- improvement in patient flow and care

Whatever the rationale for the journey of triage process improvement, you will want to collect data both pre- and post-implementation to support the process change. Quality markers frequently evaluated at triage include:[8]
- length of stay
- time to provider
- triage acuity accuracy
- rates of over- or under-triage
- performance thresholds or fractile response times if using a five-level triage system with indicators

Regular measurement of quality markers allows us to celebrate our successes, identify opportunities for improvement, and benchmark with other facilities.

## Conclusion

With increases in patient volume, acuity, and demands on resources, emergency leaders will benefit from close examination of current triage practices and/or implementation of a standardized triage model. There are several triage frameworks available for consideration, with many new and innovative solutions and technologies to improve patient care. A standardized triage system will ideally provide a common mechanism for providers to identify and communicate patient acuity, improve patient care, and allow for data collection.

## Acknowledgments

The authors thank Dr. Joshua Kosowsky (Brigham and Women's Hospital, Boston) for editing the case studies.

## References

1. Niska R, Bhuiya F, Xu J. *National Hospital Ambulatory Medical Care Survey: Emergency Department Summary*. Hyattsville, MD: National Center for Health Statistics; 2007. http://www.cdc.gov/nchs/data/nhsr/nhsr026.pdf (accessed January 29, 2011).

2. Burt C, McCaig C, Rechtsteiner E. *Ambulatory Medical Care Utilization Estimates for 2005.* Hyattsville, MD: National Center for Health Statistics, 2007.

3. Institute of Medicine. Hospital-based emergency care: at the breaking point. IOM, 2006. http://www.iom.edu/~/media/

Files/Report%20Files/2006/ Hospital-Based-Emergency-Care-At-the-Breaking-Point/ EmergencyCare.ashx (accessed January 29, 2011).

4. Robertson-Steel I. Evolution of triage systems. *Emergency Medicine Journal* 2006; **23**: 154–5.

5. Emergency Nurses Association. *Triage: Meeting the Challenge*, 2nd edn. Park Ridge, IL: ENA, 1998.

6. Fernandes CM, Tanabe P, Gilboy N, *et al*. Five-level triage: a report from the ACEP/ENA Five-level Triage Task Force. *Journal of Emergency Nursing* 2005; **31**: 39–50.

7. Emergency Nurses Association. *Nursing Companion Guide to Data Elements for Emergency Department Systems*. Park Ridge, IL: ENA, 1997.

8. Gilboy N, Tanabe P, Travers D, Rosenau A, Eitel DR. *Emergency Severity Index, Version 4: Implementation Handbook*. AHRQ Publication No. 05-0046-2. Rockville, MD: Agency for Healthcare Research and Quality, 2005. http://www.ahrq.gov/ research/esi (accessed January 29, 2011).

9. Gill JM, Reese CL, Diamond JJ. Disagreement among health care professionals about the urgent care needs of emergency department patients. *Annals of Emergency Medicine* 1996; **28**: 474–9.

10. Wuerz R, Fernandes CM, Alarcon J. Inconsistency of emergency department triage. Emergency Department Operations Research Working Group. *Annals of Emergency Medicine* 1998; **32**: 431–5.

11. Travers DA, Waller AE, Bowling JM, Flowers D, Tintinalli J. Five-level triage system more effective than three-level in tertiary emergency department. *Journal*

of Emergency Nursing 2002; **28**: 395–400.

12. Emergency Nurses Association. Standardized ED triage scale and acuity categorization: Joint ENA/ ACEP statement. Joint position statements, 2010. http://www.ena. org/about/position/ jointstatements/Pages/Default. aspx (accessed January 29, 2011).

13. Australasian College for Emergency Medicine. The Australasian Triage Scale. *Emergency Medicine (Fremantle)* 2002; **14**: 335–6.

14. Canadian Association of Emergency Physicians. The Canadian Triage and Acuity Scale (CTAS) for emergency departments. CAEP, 2002. http:// www.caep.ca/template.asp? id=B795164082374289 BBD9C1C2BF4B8D32 (accessed January 29, 2011).

15. Atack L, Rankin JA, Then KL. Effectiveness of a 6-week online course in the Canadian Triage and Acuity Scale for emergency nurses. *Journal of Emergency Nursing* 2005; **31**: 436–41.

16. *Emergency Triage: Manchester Triage Group*. 2nd edn. Plymouth: BMJ Publishing Group, 2001.

17. Wiler JL, Gentle C, Halfpenny JM, *et al*. Optimizing emergency department front-end operations. *Annals of Emergency Medicine* 2010; **55**: 142–60.e1.

18. White BA, Brown DF, Sinclair J, *et al*. Supplemented Triage and Rapid Treatment (START) improves performance measures in the emergency department. *Journal of Emergency Medicine* 2012; **42**: 322–8.

19. Han JH, France DJ, Levin SR, *et al*. The effect of physician triage on emergency department length of stay. *Journal of Emergency Medicine* 2010; **39**: 227–33.

20. Russ S, Jones I, Aronsky D, Dittus RS, Slovis CM. Placing physician orders at triage: the effect on

length of stay. *Annals of Emergency Medicine* 2010; **56**: 27–33.

21. Goransson KE, von Rosen A. Interrater agreement: a comparison between two emergency department triage scales. *European Journal of Emergency Medicine* 2011; **18**: 68–72.

22. Lee KM, Wong TW, Chan R, *et al*. Accuracy and efficiency of x-ray requests initiated by triage nurses in an accident and emergency department. *Accident and Emergency Nursing* 1996; **4**: 179–81.

23. Campbell P, Dennie M, Dougherty K, Iwaskiw O, Rollo K. Implementation of an ED protocol for pain management at triage at a busy Level I trauma center. *Journal of Emergency Nursing* 2004; **30**: 431–8.

24. Seguin D. A nurse-initiated pain management advanced triage protocol for ED patients with an extremity injury at a level I trauma center. *Journal of Emergency Nursing* 2004; **30**: 330–5.

25. Cooper JJ, Datner EM, Pines JM. Effect of an automated chest radiograph at triage protocol on time to antibiotics in patients admitted with pneumonia. *American Journal of Emergency Medicine* 2008; **26**: 264–9.

26. Graff L, Palmer AC, Lamonica P, Wolf S. Triage of patients for a rapid (5-minute) electrocardiogram: A rule based on presenting chief complaints. *Annals of Emergency Medicine* 2000; **36**: 554–60.

27. Seaberg DC, MacLeod BA. Correlation between triage nurse and physician ordering of ED tests. *American Journal of Emergency Medicine* 1998; **16**: 8–11.

28. Antman EM, Anbe DT, Armstrong PW, *et al*. ACC/AHA guidelines for the management

of patients with ST-elevation myocardial infarction: a report of the American College of Cardiology/American Heart Association Task Force on Practice Guidelines (Committee to Revise the 1999 Guidelines for the Management of Patients with Acute Myocardial Infarction). *Circulation* 2004; **110**: e82–292.

29. Spaite DW, Bartholomeaux F, Guisto J, *et al.* Rapid process redesign in a university-based emergency department: decreasing waiting time intervals and improving patient satisfaction. *Annals of Emergency Medicine* 2002; **39**: 168–77.

30. Chan TC, Killeen JP, Kelly D, Guss DA. Impact of rapid entry and accelerated care at triage on reducing emergency department patient wait times, lengths of stay, and rate of left without being seen. *Annals of Emergency Medicine* 2005; **46**: 491–7.

31. Gorelick MH, Yen K, Yun HJ. The effect of in-room registration on emergency department length of stay. *Annals of Emergency Medicine* 2005; **45**: 128–33.

32. Howard PK, Steinmann RA, eds. *Sheehy's Emergency Nursing: Principles and Practice*, 6th edn. St. Louis, MO: Mosby Elsevier, 2009.

33. Killian M. *Standards of Emergency Nursing Practice*, 4th edn. Park Ridge, IL: Emergency Nurses Association, 1999.

34. Funderburke P. Exploring best practice for triage. *Journal of Emergency Nursing* 2008; **34**: 180–2.

35. Gilboy N, Travers D, Wuerz R. Re-evaluating triage in the new millennium: a comprehensive look at the need for standardization and quality. *Journal of Emergency Nursing* 1999; **25**: 468–73.

36. Wuerz RC, Milne LW, Eitel DR, Travers D, Gilboy N. Reliability and validity of a new five-level triage instrument. *Academic Emergency Medicine* 2000; **7**: 236–42.

# Staffing models

Kirk B. Jensen, Daniel G. Kirkpatrick, and Thom Mayer

## Key learning points

- Define the key variables in staffing an emergency department.
- Identify the key concepts that define strategies for meeting staffing needs.
- Consider how to build staffing models based on different priorities.
- Describe the subtleties of staffing academic emergency departments.
- Examine case studies illustrating fundamental building blocks of a staffing model and how to optimize flow and resources.

## Introduction

Focusing on staffing in your emergency department (ED) is necessary, and even crucial, in order to optimize what amounts to 75% or more of professional staff expenditures in delivering ED services. In this chapter, we will analyze how best to determine staffing needs, examine how to optimize and leverage your current staff, and, finally, review alternative staffing models.

## What are your staffing needs?

Let us look briefly at the key factors that drive your staffing needs, keeping in mind that they are often interrelated. We will also define key terms that will be used throughout this chapter.

## Patient volume

Certain efficiencies are achieved once the ED delivers more than 20 000 visits annually (as well as 30 000, 40 000, 50 000, etc.) As these volume marks are achieved, EDs find they can better utilize physicians and physician extenders (physician assistants, medical assistants, and nurse practitioners, generally speaking, are healthcare professionals licensed to practice medicine under the supervision of a licensed physician) and can become even more efficient through segmenting different patient flow streams (through acuity or through various triage and intake criteria based on volume at different presentation times). We will assume patient volume data come from registration logs.

## Patient acuity

Higher-acuity patients require additional staffing resources for evaluation, management, treatment, and disposition.[1]

## Patient length of stay (LOS)

Longer LOS requires more staffing time and attention, although not necessarily more clinical staff; longer LOS also reduces the available beds. This will reduce capacity to treat higher volumes. It is crucial that we fully understand our LOS and available bed capacity in order to understand whether we have a capacity problem in treating incoming patients. We calculate LOS by measuring the time from registration until ED departure (treat and release LOS) or departure from ED to an inpatient unit (treat and admit LOS).

## Boarded patients

If we are responsible for "boarding patients" (those awaiting admission to an inpatient unit but who are still located in the ED), our staffing resources will be reallocated in order to monitor these patients. Also, each boarded patient reduces our ability to better utilize bed capacity. We calculate boarding time as the number of minutes beyond 120 after a physician has documented a decision to admit.

---

*Emergency Department Leadership and Management*, ed. Stephanie Kayden, *et al.* Published by Cambridge University Press.
© Cambridge University Press 2015.

## Capabilities of clinicians (physicians and physician extenders)

More experienced physicians will be in a better position to treat patients in a more efficient manner. Also, physicians more experienced in dealing with the local medical staff, understanding transfer issues, and more familiar with the current hospital, will be able to more consistently achieve efficiencies in treating patients. When using rotating physicians, or residents, establishing standard operating procedures (SOP) can help reduce variability and improve practice reliability.

## Role of non-physician staff

How the physician group utilizes physician extenders both for less acute patients and as supplements for more acute patients will have a significant impact on staffing needs.[2] Physician extenders are not an option in many countries. Development of SOPs and collaboration with nursing staff in developing and adopting advanced treatment protocols (e.g., clinical pathways for diagnostics ordering) are two excellent approaches for improving physician effectiveness.

## Hospital's expectations

The hospital's expectations for physician involvement with all patients, door-to-doctor time, and the physician's involvement with all aspects of decision making and communications with attending staff, transfer orders, transfer organizations, etc. can markedly change the staffing requirements.

## Nursing expectations and nursing skills

The nursing culture and engagement with the clinical staff will have a major impact on staffing needs. The scope of nursing care will impact clinical staffing. Many nurses and physicians come from a variety of backgrounds and training experiences, and thus the use of routine evaluation protocols, SOPs, and advanced treatment protocols can create greater consistency for the ED team. The greater the consistency amongst the nurses and physicians, the greater the effectiveness of medical assistants.[3]

## Into practice: creating your schedule

As you better understand your tactical drivers, the next step is to determine how, in practice, staffing decisions actually get made. Most hospitals establish staffing goals through an annual budgeting process. Many times the budgeting process is based on historic patterns and/or algorithms taking into account historic and benchmarked service hours per patient visit. For the professional staff, changes in staffing patterns should result from careful analysis of patient demand.

## Patient arrivals

You must thoroughly understand your ED's patient arrivals. From a macro perspective, review annual arrivals over the past five years in order to understand trended historic growth and anticipate future growth. Review average daily visit volume for each of the most recent 24 months to determine seasonal fluctuations. Review patient arrivals by hour of the day (HOD) and by day of the week (DOW). While we know that Sundays, Mondays, and the day following a holiday are generally heavier-volume days, you will want to compare average volumes and variation from the average for each day. We recommend identifying "heavy" (greater than average) and "light" (less than average) days. Creating different staff schedules for these days is prudent resource use. By reviewing your patient arrival curve by HOD and DOW, you can schedule staff to stay ahead of the patient arrival curve.

## Benchmarking

Establish goals for how many patients per hour your physicians will treat by benchmarking externally and internally. The following groups are recommended for external benchmarking: Medical Group Management Association (www.mgma.com); Emergency Nurses Association (www.ena.org); The International Conference on Emergency Medicine (www.icem2010.org). You should also do your own benchmarking. This may be done by discussing staffing patterns and visiting local colleagues who direct EDs. This can also be expanded outside of your immediate market area to colleagues within the region. As you compare your ED staffing needs, be sure to understand similarities and dissimilarities with hospitals with which you are benchmarking, e.g. admission percentage, LOS, etc.

## Performance metrics and determinants of staffing needs

As we are assessing our staffing needs, some reasonable performance metrics, which will allow us both to establish goals and to determine whether we are effectively meeting them, include the following:

- bed placement to clinician exam
- test results available to clinician review
- total ED length of stay
- percentage of admitted ED patients
- treat-and-release ED length of stay
- left without being seen (LWBS) rate
- overall customer satisfaction with the ED

Each of these metrics helps fully illuminate successful patient flow. Understanding the hospital's goals surrounding patient flow will be crucial in order to create goals for the professional group staffing.

In summary, as we look at what is determining our staffing needs, we need to capture historic data and goals or expectations on the following:

- Patient complexity (we recommend a comparative metric of average RVUs per E/M code for the USA; we recommend admission rate for other EDs).[4] Note: RVU (relative value unit) refers to a methodology of normalizing work done by medical providers; in the United States it has been widely adopted in reimbursement policy. E/M codes (evaluation and management) refer to the current procedural terminology codes that describe physician–patient encounters.
- Customer service (understand your patient satisfaction survey tool and metric relating specifically to clinician performance).
- Skilled workforce shortages (fully understand your supply of experienced nurses, new nurses, nursing technicians, paramedics, unit secretaries, medical assistants, transportation technicians, etc.).
- ED crowding or boarders awaiting admission and occupying scarce beds.
- Current practices that may contribute to high-risk situations.
- The group's preference on using physician extenders independently or only under direct physician supervision.[5]
- The viability of using scribes.
- The current medical record and hospital information management system.

## Determining your staffing strategy

Ultimately, each ED should allocate staff by anticipating patient demand, and ensuring that a reasonable asset velocity (patients evaluated per hour) is employed

for the clinician treating the arriving patients. Patient arrivals should be broken down by HOD and preferably by Emergency Severity Index (ESI) or some indexing algorithm to understand acuity. Additionally, as you look at allocating staff, you need to take into consideration 24-hour/7-days-a-week coverage and whether you have clinicians who want to work only nights versus those that will rotate nights, evenings, days, weekends, etc. Ease of recruiting and your group's historic staff retention are crucial drivers to understanding your flexibility in creating staffing allocations.

Certain EDs are easier to staff than others. Staffing in the heart of a major city with several emergency medicine training programs and plenty of physicians and nurses is vastly different than staffing and scheduling an ED in a rural area with no training programs and fewer amenities.

In planning and managing your ED team, you will be more successful if you develop an overall strategy and if you leverage tactics driving your staffing and scheduling goals prior to establishing the best staffing numbers for you and your department. Questions you need to ask include:

- Do you want to staff safely despite a shortage of physicians?
- Do you need to minimize the number of physicians in your department?
- Do you want to maximize patient satisfaction?
- Do you want to have a waiting room full of patients ready for the clinician?
- Do you want to have a LWBS rate approaching zero?

Agree upon an asset velocity (how many patients per hour treated) and then start to back in to duration of shifts and how many hours annually you expect your clinicians to work. Once you have assembled key strategies for these questions, you can begin both generating a schedule and clearly identifying needs for your department.

## Adding coverage

There are several different ways of looking at both assembling core coverage and identifying trigger points for adding extra coverage. The most fundamental way is looking at patients seen per hour. If your asset velocity (number of patients treated per hour) is two patients per hour and you begin routinely exceeding two patients an hour, you should look towards adding an additional provider. Normally, single coverage (24 physician hours per day) will be able to handle an ED volume of 18 000 visits annually. You should also budget or forecast monthly volume against monthly clinician hours so that, as volume is growing, you can identify thresholds indicating trigger points for adding staff. Other key drivers that are indicative of the need to consider additional staff include:

(1) Turnaround times are becoming progressively higher.
(2) LWBS rate is unacceptably high.
(3) Your clinicians are concerned that the shifts are too long.
(4) Patient satisfaction survey results are unacceptably low.
(5) There are frequent concerns or complaints about clinician behavior in a stressful environment.
(6) Heavier-volume days (usually Sunday, Monday, Tuesday) become days that both clinicians and nursing staff do not want to work, and key performance metrics are unacceptable on these heavier volume days.

It is important to differentiate routine variation in patient volume from trended or progressive increases in volume. While both of these result in additional demand and complexity for the ED clinician, the solutions will be different. In the case of routine variation, it is essential that patient arrivals be analyzed by both HOD and DOW in order to forecast and adequately project additional staffing in anticipation of patient surges. The entire ED clinician team should be in agreement on a surge capacity plan (on call, ability to open additional beds, ability to re-deploy both clinicians and nursing staff to handle a newly created patient stream).

Different staffing models offer different solutions for different EDs, and for the same ED at different times in its staff's development and evolution, as well as when transitioning to different models. Patient flow is clearly predictable. With 80–85% accuracy, you can forecast when patients are coming, what the diagnoses are, and what sort of lab and x-ray needs they are going to have. Again, this is the reason we collect and analyze arrival data, plotting patient arrivals by HOD, DOW, acuity, diagnoses, and tests required.

## Staffing with other clinicians

You should always seek to employ the least expensive resource to accomplish the mission. In the case of an ED, 25–35% of the cases can be adequately and successfully seen independently by physician extenders. In countries where physician extenders are not a viable alternative, SOPs and advanced treatment protocols developed and implemented with nursing participation should be explored. Family practitioners or internists can see 75% or more of the cases that emergency physicians see in the ED. Normally, the use of residents in the ED is only a net gain when you are using senior-level residents (final year). In general, new residents only add complexity and slowness to the EM clinician's day. See below for more discussion on academic training considerations.

## Single coverage with 12-hour shifts

This approach can accommodate anywhere from 18 000 to 20 000 visits per year. This will require the ED to treat 2–2.5 patients per hour. Groups often try to push their asset velocity up to three patients per hour, allowing single coverage to accommodate up to 26 000 patients per year. Unfortunately, while many physicians think they can see three patients an hour, rarely can they sustain seeing three patients an hour for an entire 12-hour shift, let alone 12-hour shifts for an entire year. One of the significant challenges in an ED is to deal with the patient arrival curve and the necessary asset velocity during different times of the day. In fact, 64% of the daily ED volume arrives between 10 a.m. and 10 p.m. Consequently, in the typical ED, with 18 000 annual visits, patients are being processed at 2.63 patients per hour during this peak presentation period. During the remainder of the day (10 p.m. to 10 a.m.), patients are seen at less than two per hour. Most EDs cannot function at 2.63 patients per hour. And the resulting dysfunction includes increased wait time, poor patient satisfaction, and dissatisfaction amongst the team. Workable strategies to accommodate this increased demand during the 10 a.m. to 10 p.m. shift include productivity-based compensation, template-based charting, ED efficiency initiatives, scribes or personal productivity assistants, rapid medical evaluation, on-call clinician backup, and transition to eight-hour flex length shifts (shifts that can be two or more hours shorter or longer depending on patient demand).

Scheduling methodologies center on an understanding of five key questions:

(1) What is the volume coming in?
(2) What is the workload?
(3) What is the acuity?

(4) What are your performance measures?

(5) What are your priorities for meeting performance measures?

Once you have an understanding of these questions, and have developed strategies depending on their answers, you can begin establishing approaches to scheduling. The approaches to scheduling include a review of historical staffing patterns and an understanding of advantages and disadvantages. This allows establishment of the best fit by trial and error. Rule-based computer programming allows efficient generation of draft schedules that follow prescribed rules and allow better "fairness" as it relates to weekends, nights, holidays, etc.

Clearly, clinicians operate more effectively and efficiently when performance and compensation are more closely aligned. The caveat to remember here is that the lowest-cost staffing resource should always be maximized first.

Team-based processes should be employed and are characterized by front-loading your care, having a physician or medical assistant in the front seeing patients, ordering diagnostic and treatment protocols, and then handing them off to the fast-track or fast-track-like environment. This approach leverages the sensitivity and specificity of the diagnostic skills of the physician, while also leveraging the expertise of the physician extender in procedural-type services.[2]

---

**Case study 20.1.   Demand capacity: determining patient arrivals and aligning physician staffing**

This study walks the reader through the process of gathering sufficient data to plot a patient arrival curve (demand) and align physician staffing (capacity).

- **Step 1**. Gather patient arrival data by hour of the day (HOD) and by day of week (DOW). You should be able to collect these data from the patient registration system; if the data are not available from a registration system, use a spreadsheet to tally one month's patient arrivals by documenting date and time of arrival for each visit to the ED. Calculate averages for each hour of the day and each day of the week. These data points lead you to the next step.

- **Step 2**. Plot HOD and DOW patient arrival curves (Figs. 20.1, 20.2).

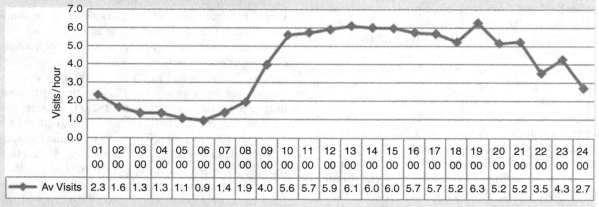

| | 01 00 | 02 00 | 03 00 | 04 00 | 05 00 | 06 00 | 07 00 | 08 00 | 09 00 | 10 00 | 11 00 | 12 00 | 13 00 | 14 00 | 15 00 | 16 00 | 17 00 | 18 00 | 19 00 | 20 00 | 21 00 | 22 00 | 23 00 | 24 00 |
|---|---|---|---|---|---|---|---|---|---|---|---|---|---|---|---|---|---|---|---|---|---|---|---|---|
| Av Visits | 2.3 | 1.6 | 1.3 | 1.3 | 1.1 | 0.9 | 1.4 | 1.9 | 4.0 | 5.6 | 5.7 | 5.9 | 6.1 | 6.0 | 6.0 | 5.7 | 5.7 | 5.2 | 6.3 | 5.2 | 5.2 | 3.5 | 4.3 | 2.7 |

**Figure 20.1** Average visits by hour of the day (HOD).

- **Step 3**. Initial analysis. The HOD curve reveals the consistent patient arrival pattern replicated by EDs throughout the world. The DOW graph reveals heavy days (visits > average) as Saturday, Sunday, and Monday and lighter days (visits < average) as Tuesday, Wednesday, Thursday, and Friday. This pattern, too, is consistent with most EDs. We should note that our patient arrival "ramp up" begins at 8 a.m. and arrivals quickly increase to six per hour, which is sustained until 9 p.m. until receding to a level of one visit per hour from 2 a.m. to 7 a.m. In this example, 75% of patient arrivals occur from 10 a.m. to 10 p.m.; this fact alone has huge ramifications for staffing.

- **Step 4**. Decide on staffing model. We will assume that our physicians can treat two patients per hour. We will also assume, for the purposes of this example, that we have adequate beds and nursing staff. So, 90 patients/day divided by 2 patients/hour = 45 hours of daily clinical coverage.

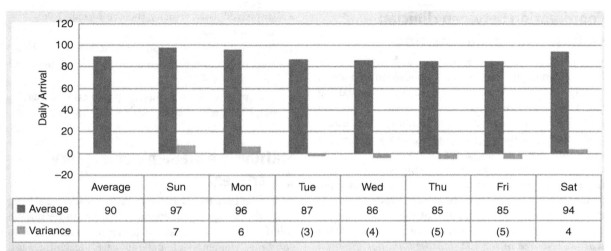

**Figure 20.2** Average visits by day of week (DOW).

| | Average | Sun | Mon | Tue | Wed | Thu | Fri | Sat |
|---|---|---|---|---|---|---|---|---|
| ■ Average | 90 | 97 | 96 | 87 | 86 | 85 | 85 | 94 |
| ▨ Variance | | 7 | 6 | (3) | (4) | (5) | (5) | 4 |

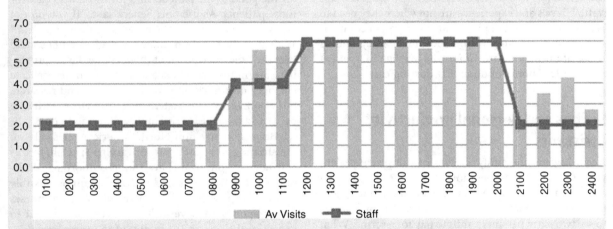

**Figure 20.3** Staffing model.

The model shown in Figure 20.3 was developed by using two 10-hour, two 9-hour, and one 7-hour shifts. Our challenge is the < 2 patient/hour arrivals during the early morning hours, which does not allow our night clinician to achieve our goal. Consequently, we are not able to accommodate the "ramp up" (10 and 11 a.m.), nor are we able to better staff the evening hours (9 p.m. through 12 a.m). A better variation of this model could be achieved by scheduling five 8-hour shifts and one 5-hour shift. You and your physician group will need to decide on staffing issues which will include: length of shifts, how many patients/hour physicians are expected to treat, whether physicians will have to rotate shifts or whether you have "night" coverage that allows others to not have to work nights, and what type of on-call backup system to implement.

# Backup systems

The best physician backup systems are formalized and focused on expediting bed placement to physician exam. A backup system should be resisted unless the hospital provides its members of the backup team to support the ED when the ED is overwhelmed. In other words, having a physician on-call when there will not be additional nursing staff to support the additional physician is both inefficient and unsuccessful at accomplishing the goal of heightened treatment services. Backup systems are most effective when they have predefined thresholds, triggers, and next-actions that have been trialed and agreed upon before the crisis ever happens.

## Coordination between clinician staffing and nursing staffing

While the clinicians cannot control nurse staffing, there is a fundamental management paradox incorporated herein: you need to know what your physician staffing levels are and you need to know what the nursing staffing levels are. You also need to know what benchmark staffing data are being used, and you need to know how many nursing shifts are going unfilled. Even though the clinicians do not have control over it, nursing staffing severely impacts what clinicians can do. Emergency physicians may be the scarcest resource in the ED, but they are certainly not the most valuable. That bears repeating: *Emergency physicians may be the scarcest resource in the ED, but they are not the most valuable.* In many EDs, nurses often run the department, and it is nurses who keep things flowing. If nurse staffing levels and experience are not where they need to be, then no amount of physician coverage can compensate for it. According to the 2001 Emergency Nurses Association *Benchmark Guide*, the average ED patient requires 1.57 hours of direct ED nursing care.[3]

## Scribes and personal productivity assistants

According to one study, scribes can improve patient velocity or patients per hour from 2.2 to 2.5.[6] On average, a good scribe program will add half a patient per hour. From a different perspective, one only needs to see two extra patients a shift to pay for a scribe. What will the scribe do for you? The scribe will complete the chart, order x-rays and labs, and keep you on task. They allow more complete charting, they prompt you for elements that will result in optimizing your coding, and they assist you in promptly getting test results, particularly when they relate to multiple patients. Additionally, the scribe can assist in real-time problem solving by being an extender for the physician, can improve coding, and can improve overall asset velocity. The scribe can act as an assistant to perform patient rounding for comfort and follow-up with patients and assist nursing and medical-assistant team members in improving overall patient flow. The following data from a hospital in Virginia certainly defends the case for using scribes.

- 18–20% increased charge capture (reduction in downcodes; downcodes occur when record documentation fails to substantiate care rendered).
- Improved asset velocity (before scribes 1.9; after scribes 2.3).
- Improved RVU per hour production of 15–20%.
- Improved lab documentation (before scribes 55%; after scribes 89%).
- Improved ratio of compliments to complaints per 1000 visits (before scribes 5 : 1; after scribes 9 : 1).

## Staffing the academic emergency department

Providing care to ED patients in the academic setting produces unique challenges, which require unique solutions. Like all areas of academic medicine, EDs combine elements of patient care, teaching, and research, all of which must be effectively combined for the good of the patients and for those who care for those patients. As the poet Seneca said, "If you do not know where you are going, no wind is the right wind." With that wisdom in mind, each academic ED should take the time to ensure that those charged with providing care not only understand the sometimes delicate balance between clinical care, education, and research, but also have a clear statement of the vision (why we exist) and the mission (what we are trying to do).

Because many non-North American EDs rely on physicians and residents from varying specialties, this constancy of purpose is even more important. Without it, the physicians and residents cannot possibly know what is expected of them, nor can the nurses and support staff have a clear conception of what to expect of the physicians in any of the three areas.

The leadership of the academic ED must also have data on the types and numbers of patients who will be cared for, what their acuity is, when they will arrive, and what they will need in order to receive appropriate care. The type, number, and time of arrival of patients seen should not be a surprise to the ED staff. Once those data are known, ED managers should assess the resources that will be required, from both a clinical and a support-staff standpoint, to meet these needs (Fig. 20.3). The educational mission is a related but distinct part of that analysis, since providing education to residents, medical students, and nursing students requires additional time and resources, over and above those needed for effective patient care.

Evidence-based medicine (EBM) approaches to emergency patients are increasingly a core part of the provision of effective ED care, but they are even more essential in EDs with educational missions, for several reasons. First, many of the earliest and most widely adopted EBM approaches arose from critically ill or injured patients, including those with major trauma (advanced trauma life support), myocardial infarctions (advanced cardiac life support and "time to open artery" protocols), stroke (thrombolytic and interventional therapies), and pediatrics (advanced pediatric life support and pediatric advanced life support protocols). Each of these is an example whereby a collegially developed EBM protocol was married to a widely accepted educational program, which ensures that patients receive consistent care with consistent results, but also ensures that those who provide that care have the confidence, derived from effective training, to provide the care. Second, rotating residents and students should be provided with training in these EBM approaches, which effectively ensures that both consistent clinical care and education are met proactively. Third, an EBM approach ensures that the nurses and support staff know what to expect when faced with certain clinical situations, which makes both clinical care and education more effective. Fourth, in those settings in which attending physicians are not available in the department during night hours, EBM approaches

are even more important, since those providing the care better understand both what is expected of them and how to provide care efficiently and effectively.

The downstream effect that such an EBM approach can have on the education of residents, medical students, and nursing students is extremely important. Regardless of the specialty or the setting in which physicians and nurses eventually practice, they will have received an invaluable education in how to evaluate, approach, and treat patients with the most acute illnesses and injuries.

Finally, the academic setting is an excellent place in which non-clinical aspects of the art of medicine can and should be taught. Whether they are called service or communication skills, students and residents should be mentored in building the skills and techniques required to address patients' psychological and spiritual needs, as well as their clinical ones. As the great physician, musician, and theologian Albert Schweitzer said, "One can save one's life as a human being, as well as one's professional existence, if one seizes every opportunity, however unassuming, to act humanly towards another human being. The future of the world depends on it." Perhaps there is no better place to teach these skills than in the ED.

---

**Case study 20.2. Patient flow: flow symptoms and staffing analysis**

Hospital A is a community-based private organization in northern Virginia, USA. The ED treats 60 000 patients annually with an admission rate of 12%. Boarding admitted patients in the ED, a left without being seen (LWBS) rate of > 8%, patient satisfaction survey results < 50th percentile, and fast-track treat and release LOS > 170 minutes (Table 20.1) were characteristics precipitating a thorough patient flow analysis and construction of a demand–capacity staffing model.

**Table 20.1** Baseline ED metrics

| Metrics | Trend: before | Goal | Your ED |
|---|---|---|---|
| LWBS | 8.5% | < 3% | |
| Fast-track LOS | 171 min | < 100 min | |
| Admitted LOS | 394 min | < 252 min | |
| Overall physician satisfaction percentile | 11th percentile | > 75th percentile | |
| Monthly boarding hours | > 500 hours | < 100 hours | |

## Patient arrival analysis

Data were captured in order to fully analyze patient arrivals by hour of day (HOD) and day of week (DOW) (Fig. 20.4). Additionally, patient arrivals were segmented by severity, or acuity.

We identified sufficient daily variation to categorize "heavy" and "light" days to drive our staffing allocation. Next we built our staffing model by plotting our patient demand (arrivals-based) against the current clinical staffing. This ED staffs three areas: the main room (24 hours/day × 7 days/week), the fast track (19 hours/day × 7 days/week), and a pediatric ED (10 hours/day × 7 days/week) (Fig. 20.5).

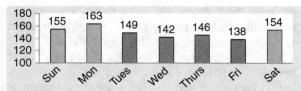

**Figure 20.4** Patients seen per day.

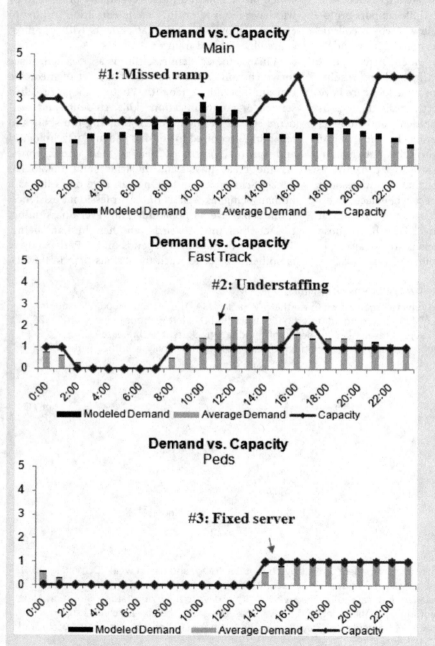

**Figure 20.5** Demand versus capacity in various units.

## Findings

The patient arrival and staffing (demand vs. capacity) graphs above highlight the following mismatches:

- **Main** – missing the patient arrival ramp-up (begins at 10 a.m.) and overstaffing twice later in the day (2 p.m. and 10 p.m.).
- **Fast track** – understaffing from 10 a.m. to 4 p.m.
- **Pediatrics** – seems to be a fixed server that can treat approximately 2 patients per hour; as such, it is inelastic to surges and cannot readily adjust to assist either the main or the fast track.

## The intervention

Currently, fast track and pediatrics demonstrate little capacity to flex to accommodate volume surge. Pediatrics treats roughly 20 patients per day and fast track treats roughly 35 patients per day. We reorganized these two services into one (Table 20.2). Lower-acuity patients have testing started in the post-triage area ("results waiting" area) and are staged awaiting test results. Patients are not being kept in a bed for purposes other than being evaluated or while having a procedure performed, e.g., suturing. Fast-track beds are the first to be used, and when additional beds are needed, pediatric beds are used. Pediatric patients requiring procedures can be treated in pediatric or fast-track rooms, as appropriate.

**Table 20.2** Revised staffing model

| Main ED | | | |
|---|---|---|---|
| | **Current** | **Heavy** | **Light** |
| Physician | 7 a.m. – 5 p.m. | 6 a.m. – 4 p.m. | 6 a.m. – 3 p.m. |
| Physician | 2 p.m. – 12 a.m. | 9 a.m. – 8 p.m. | 9 a.m. – 8 p.m. |
| Physician | 4 p.m. – 2 a.m. | 3 p.m. – 1 a.m. | 3 p.m. – 12 a.m. |
| Physician | 9 p.m. – 7 a.m. | 8 p.m. – 6 a.m. | 8 p.m. – 6 a.m. |
| Physician extender | 7 a.m. – 5 p.m. | 6 a.m. – 3 p.m. | 6 a.m. – 3 p.m. |
| Physician extender | 9 p.m. – 7 a.m. | 9 p.m. – 6 a.m. | 10 p.m. – 6 a.m. |

| Fast-track/pediatric | | |
|---|---|---|
| | **Current** | **Revised** |
| Physician | 2 p.m. – 12 a.m. | 8 a.m. – 6 p.m. |
| Physician extender | 8 a.m. – 6 p.m. | 11 a.m. – 10 p.m. |
| Physician extender | 4 p.m. – 2 a.m. | 6 p.m. – 2 a.m. |

## Outcomes

These recommendations were implemented, allowing us to better align staffing (capacity) with demand (patient arrivals and clinician treatment requirements), which resulted in initial reductions of LWBS to < 5%. Treat-and-release LOS in the fast track is < 120 minutes and door-to-doctor time decreased by 25% (Table 20.3).

**Table 20.3** ED metrics two months after staffing changes were implemented

| Metrics | Trend after | Goal |
| --- | --- | --- |
| LWBS | 4.6% | < 3% |
| Fast-track LOS | 111 min | < 100 min |
| Admitted LOS | 286 min | < 252 min |
| Overall physician satisfaction percentile | 51st percentile | > 75th percentile |
| Monthly boarding hours | < 90 hours | < 100 hours |

# References

1. Jenkins PF, Barton LL, McNeill GB. Contrasts in acute medicine: a comparison of the British and Australian systems for managing emergency medical patients. *Medical Journal of Australia* 2010; **193**: 227–8.

2. Patrick VC, Lazarus J. A study of the workforce in emergency medicine: 2007 research summary. *Journal of Emergency Nursing* 2010; **36** (6): e1–2.

3. Twigg D, Duffield C, Bremner A, Rapley P, Finn J. The impact of the nursing hours per patient day (NHPPD) staffing method on patient outcomes: a retrospective analysis of patient and staffing data. *International Journal of Nursing Studies* 2010; **48**: 540–8.

4. Albrecht R, Jacoby J, Heller M, Stolzfus J, Melanson S. Do emergency physicians admit more or fewer patients on busy days? *Journal of Emergency Medicine* 2011; **41**: 709–12.

5. Unterman S, Kessler C, Pitzele HZ. Staffing of the ED by non-emergency medicine-trained personnel: the VA experience. *American Journal of Emergency Medicine* 2010; **28**: 622–5.

6. Arya R, Salovich DM, Ohman-Strickland P, Merlin MA. Impact of scribes on performance indicators in the emergency department. *Academic Emergency Medicine* 2010; **17**: 490–4.

**Chapter**

# 21

# Emergency department practice guidelines and clinical pathways

*Jonathan A. Edlow*

## Key learning points

- What practice guidelines are, and what they are not.
- Why creating them can help leaders lead.
- Practical tips for writing practice guidelines.

## Introduction

Practice guidelines are primarily documents that help clinicians to employ the best medical evidence available to guide patient care in a given situation. These documents are also called clinical policies or pathways, practice parameters, care maps, and clinical decision rules, among other terms. Some have suggested a hierarchy of flexibility between different types of documents (policies being less flexible and guidelines being more flexible), and other differences.[1] Because there are no clear, agreed-upon distinctions, we will simply use the term *practice guidelines* in this chapter, unless a distinction is required in a specific instance.

In the ideal world, practice guidelines aim to improve clinical care, but in the real world they are sometimes used for other objectives. The wise leader will understand that in addition to a purely clinical purpose, guidelines can also have administrative and political implications and ramifications.

Therefore, in order to profit from both of these elements, the leader must understand precisely what practice guidelines are and how to use them. This knowledge will not only help to better manage physicians and nurses within the unit, but will also help to better protect the department from political assaults from outside, and to collect information to better understand quality within the emergency department (ED).

Finally, the time spent researching and creating a perfect guideline is rendered meaningless without proper implementation. Furthermore, proper implementation also does not achieve the ultimate goal if the guideline does not lead to improvements in practice. In turn, these practice improvements should result in measurable improvements in actual patient-centered outcomes. Much of the current leading-edge research on practice guidelines is on how they actually impact patient outcomes.

This chapter will discuss exactly what practice guidelines are, what they are not, how to design and implement them, and how they can help the chief to better manage his or her unit. A number of case studies are included.

## What practice guidelines are

Practice guidelines are documents that provide individual clinicians, both nurses and doctors, with a rational, systematic, and standardized way to respond to a given clinical situation. Institution-specific guidelines can be developed by staff within the ED, but often guidelines are developed externally and then adopted by (or imposed upon) the ED. Guidelines can be based upon expert opinion, consensus, other societies' guidelines, or analysis of the medical literature.

Some practice guidelines, or parts thereof, may merge with "policies and procedures." For example, an ED policy to "obtain an electrocardiogram (ECG) on all patients over the age of 35 years presenting with chest pain" is a policy that usually impacts the triage nurse and possibly an ED technician. However, this policy (ECG in < 5 minutes) would be but one very small step of an ED practice guideline (on the approach to patients presenting with chest pain). Obtaining vital signs on all ED patients would be another example. It is important to draw distinctions

*Emergency Department Leadership and Management*, ed. Stephanie Kayden, *et al.* Published by Cambridge University Press.
© Cambridge University Press 2015.

between policies and procedures on the one hand, and practice guidelines on the other, since the former are generally steps that "must" occur, which is not always the case for the latter (see Chapter 8).

Different organizations may use different methods in grading evidence in order to determine the strength of a recommendation. For example, the American College of Emergency Physicians (ACEP) uses a single three-point scale for measuring quality of data to determine the "class" of evidence (Table 21.1). The American Heart Association (AHA) uses two schemes for grading evidence (level and class)

(Table 21.2). The "level" of evidence is based upon the "certainty of treatment effect" whereas the "class" of evidence is based upon size of treatment effect. In the ACEP classification scheme, a recommendation based solely upon expert opinion or case reports would rarely be above a class 3 recommendation, whereas in the AHA scheme, it could be a class 1 recommendation.

Another good example of different organizations assigning different weight to the same data would be the use of tPA in acute ischemic stroke with the 3–4.5-hour window. The AHA gives this recommendation

**Table 21.1** ACEP scheme for classification and grading of the literature (adapted from ACEP clinical policies)

| Class | Therapeutic study [a] | Diagnostic study [b] | Prognostic study [c] |
|---|---|---|---|
| | | Study type | |
| 1 | Randomized controlled trial (RCT) or meta-analysis of randomized trials | Prospective cohort using a criterion standard | Population prospective cohort |
| 2 | Non-randomized trial | Retrospective observational | Retrospective cohort case control |
| 3 | Case series and reports, consensus reviews, other | Case series and reports, consensus reviews, other | Case series and reports, consensus reviews, other |

[a] Studies measuring therapeutic efficacy comparing multiple interventions
[b] Studies that determine sensitivity and specificity of diagnostic tests
[c] Studies that predict outcomes

**Table 21.2** AHA scheme for classification and grading of the literature (adapted from AHA policies)

| | Class 1 | Class 2a | Class 2b | Class 3 |
|---|---|---|---|---|
| | Benefit >>> risk Action "should be taken," is effective | Benefit >> risk Action "reasonable to take" | Benefit ≥ risk Action "may be considered," not well-established | Risk ≥ benefit Action "should not be taken," may be harmful |
| Level A [a] Multiple (3–5) population strata studied | Sufficient evidence from multiple RCTs or meta-analyses | Some conflicting evidence from multiple RCTs or meta-analyses | Greater conflicting evidence from multiple RCTs or meta-analyses | Sufficient evidence (of harm) from multiple RCTs or meta-analyses |
| Level B Limited (2–3) populations studied | Limited evidence from 1 RCT or non-randomized studies | Some conflicting evidence from 1 RCT or non-randomized studies | Some conflicting evidence from 1 RCT or non-randomized studies | Limited evidence (of harm) from 1 RCT or non-randomized studies |
| Level C Very limited (1–2) populations studied | Expert opinion, case studies or "standard of care" | "Divergent" expert opinion, case studies or "standard of care" | "Divergent" expert opinion, case studies or "standard of care" | Expert opinion, case studies or "standard of care" |

RCT, randomized clinical trial
[a] Level of evidence is an estimation of the certainty of treatment effect.

a class 1 level B recommendation, whereas the European Stroke Organization (ESO) gives the same recommendation a class 1 level A recommendation. Both organizations used the exact same studies,[2–4] but the ESO gave more weight to the one meta-analysis of stroke patients treated within six hours than did the AHA.[2]

Some guidelines may describe processes that are fully within the purview of the emergency physician. An example of such a guideline would be one on the approach to the febrile infant. The emergency physician controls all the elements subsumed by this guideline (taking the history, doing the physical examination, and performing and interpreting diagnostic testing). Some examples of guidelines that cross departments within a given institution include a massive blood transfusion guideline, one for the diagnosis of acute back pain, the approach to patients with acute coronary syndromes. Finally, there are policies that are created by national professional societies or government organizations that cross specialties and geography.

ED leaders must understand that some practice guidelines that are written by non-emergency medicine organizations impact, or try to impact, emergency medicine practice. Consider the administration of clopidogrel to patients with non-ST-segment-elevation myocardial infarction (NSTEMI). The 2002 AHA guidelines included a major change in this practice, calling for giving clopidogrel "on admission."[5] Some physicians interpreted this as "in the ED," but one needs to first decide if the patient is being treated surgically or medically, which generally does not occur in the ED.

In many institutions, the cardiology mandate became "give clopidogrel in the ED," which is not what the AHA guideline said. This highlights the importance of knowing the details of the data. If one is going to debate the cardiologist, then it is important to know not only what the guideline said, but also what it was based upon. In this case, that portion of the AHA document was based on the CURE study, which was not a study of ED-administered clopidogrel at all.[6] As a general principle, a leader's best weapon is information. In this specific example, the best solution is an institution-specific guideline, or an accord, in which emergency medicine, cardiology, and cardiac surgery (if present) all have input. Clopidogrel is important; the issue is when is the best and safest time to give it to an individual patient.

We will discuss this in more detail below, but, in general, practice guidelines should be directed at important clinical problems – high frequency, high risk, and/or high cost.[1] Remember too that just because there is no national or professional societal guideline on a given subject, that does not mean that an individual ED cannot create one. There may be various local reasons why this would make perfect sense.

## What practice guidelines are not

As stated above, the first thing that guidelines are not is a substitute for ED policies and procedures. The latter should impact intradepartmental workflow. These are steps that the ED leadership believes should always occur, unless there is a very good reason to bypass them (see Chapter 8).

They are also not methods by which the leadership forces the staff to perform certain tasks. This is likely a recurring theme in this book, but staff should be motivated by other means than being forced to follow a guideline that is not logical or adds unnecessary steps in workflow.

Finally, and crucially important for ED leaders, practice guidelines should not be used as means by which outside departments (administrative or clinical) try to get their needs met. If they are not patient-focused and data-driven, the ED staff will quite rightly rebel against them, and the leader loses both credibility and political power.

## Why use practice guidelines, and what is their purpose?

There are many reasons to create or use practice guidelines, but the most important by far is better patient care. Although physicians, especially physician leaders, are motivated by all sorts of factors, we all have an inherent desire to provide the best-quality care possible for our patients. To the extent that guidelines have been well researched and well designed, implementing them will probably improve quality, and there is some evidence that this is true.[7,8]

The second and third major purposes of practice guidelines, especially important to a leader, are inextricably linked. They are standardization of process and reduction of cost. Physicians sometimes liken themselves to artists, who treat each patient individually, and while there is some truth to this, there is also truth to the fact that the amount of variance should be relatively low. Within a given department, medical center, region, and across different countries, there can be enormous variation in the approach to a given clinical problem.[9–11]

An Australian study documented considerable variation in the treatment of acute agitation.[11] This same study found that the emergency physicians would welcome a guideline from the Australasian College of Emergency Medicine (ACEM) dealing with acute agitation. Interestingly, another Australian group found that a standardized protocol for treating acute agitation led to more rapid control of the patient.[12] In a study of different pediatric EDs, case-adjusted hospital admission rates by physician varied by eightfold at one ED.[9] There was significant practice variation for lab testing and computed tomography (CT) scan testing, both of which led to increased length of ED stays.

Importantly in that study, there was no difference in 72-hour return visits.[9] This could be the "hook" for leaders to convince physicians to change their practice. Seeing that their "artistic" approach to practice may not have any clinical advantage (and may have disadvantages such as increased testing or increased hospitalization rates) over more guideline-based practice may be enough to convince a doctor to practice closer to the mean.

Another example is the approach to ED patients presenting with abrupt onset of severe headache. The differential diagnosis for this common problem includes several high-risk problems, such as subarachnoid hemorrhage (SAH), and other diagnoses whose evaluation may be resource-heavy. Should these patients undergo brain CT, lumbar puncture (LP), and CT angiography (CTA)? The ACEP 2008 clinical policy on headache addressed these questions.[13] One indication that such a policy would be useful is the fact that in such cases only 50% of patients have an LP performed after a negative CT scan.[14]

The ACEP 2008 document states as a level B recommendation, "in patients presenting to the ED with sudden onset, severe headache, and a negative non-contrast head CT scan result, LP should be performed to rule out SAH." This would be expected to improve the rate of SAH diagnosis, but only in patients in whom one considered doing a CT in the first place and only in patients whose CT scans are normal. Therefore that part of the guideline might help improve quality, but probably not by very much.

Another question addressed in that same guideline was the importance of CTA in patients with normal CT and LP results. For this question, the level B recommendation was that patients with normal CT and LP "do not need emergency angiography and can be discharged from the ED with follow-up recommended." Based on a meta-analysis of over 800 patients,[15] this portion of the guideline clearly has the propensity to improve quality and reduce length of stay, radiation, and contrast dye exposure, while at the same time reducing financial costs. As well, the policy may curb the "technology creep" that might lead to increased use.[16,17]

Adherence to guidelines also might help emergency physicians to avoid legal actions, which is another reason to use practice guidelines. Of course, this may be more or less important country by country, depending on the local prevalence of legal actions. There is some indication in the obstetric literature that adherence to clinical guidelines does reduce malpractice exposure.[18]

Of course legal protection from guidelines can be a double-edged sword, because if you have them, but do not follow them, they can be used against a doctor in a legal action.[19] Therefore, it is important to create and use guidelines that are not overly prescriptive. After writing a guideline, think about it from the perspective of a lawyer and try to use language that does not box a physician in to a specific action unnecessarily – "unnecessarily" being the key word.

There are times when a guideline is intended to be specific ("use tPA for acute ischemic stroke patients who can be treated in under three hours from symptom onset") and others when one should be purposefully a bit vague ("consider a radiation therapy consult for patients with acute back pain and cord compression"). Most guidelines will contain some standard "boilerplate" language stating that the document is designed to be used in a general sense and not to replace physician judgment in the individual case.

Finally, in addition to improving quality, reducing variability in practice, reducing costs, and possibly offering protection from legal actions, another potential purpose of using practice guidelines is to help with compliance with various regulatory bodies. For example, incorporating aspirin use into a guideline for acute coronary syndromes is better patient care, but if (or when) governmental and other regulatory agencies begin to measure this as a quality metric (or reimbursement metric), your department will be a step ahead in terms of compliance. Case study 21.1 illustrates how this can work.

## Case study 21.1.   Acute ischemic stroke

In the USA, governmental regulators have begun collecting data about patients with acute ischemic stroke (AIS) and transient ischemic attack (TIA). In Massachusetts, the Department of Public Health (DPH) measures (amongst other metrics) time from arrival to the ED to activating a "code stroke" (15 minutes is the target), to ordering a brain CT scan (25 minutes), to thrombolytic use (60 minutes). At one large hospital, the ED senior physician can activate a "code stroke" which electronically notifies the neurologist, radiologist, lab technician, and others.

A team from neurology, radiology, emergency medicine, and emergency nursing met monthly when the system was implemented. That monitoring group found several issues. The first was that there was a delay in ordering the CT, even when the activation of the "code stroke" was rapid. When the audit team spoke to individual practitioners, it was clear that the neurologist thought the emergency physician was going to order the CT, and vice-versa. This was easily fixed by simply defining that the emergency clinician would order the CT at the same time as activating the "code stroke" – a simple action, since both are accomplished at the same location.

The monitoring group also found instances in which the "code stroke" was activated very late in the patient's ED course. When these were analyzed as a group, there were two types of patients. The first were patients with isolated or predominant visual or speech symptoms. Correction of this was more difficult but involved an educational component for the triage nurses and the physicians. Some of these patients, for example those who presented with a visual-field deficit or dysarthria, were simply not being identified as stroke patients as quickly as those who were hemiplegic. With time, this improved considerably. Real-time feedback was used whenever possible, a tool that has proved useful in other settings as well.[20]

Finally, the second group of patients who had long times were those with TIA. This was more difficult, because even though the state DPH mandated that TIA patients undergo the same steps as AIS patients, it was (and remains) illogical to emergency clinicians that a TIA patient has to have a neurologist paged at 3 a.m. or have a CT performed within 25 minutes. It remains illogical to this author, who tried to have the DPH rule modified, but one should not expect logic from a governmental agency. Even though TIA patients should be evaluated expeditiously, it does not need to be done within minutes. In this case, the committee educated the ED and neurology staff so that they understood that the state DPH mandated it to be so. Once the staff understood that (logical or not) the hospitals had to comply, these numbers improved as well.

# Practical tips for developing practice guidelines

Table 21.3 outlines the steps involved in developing a practice guideline.

First and foremost, choose subjects that matter. Select medical issues that are high-frequency (patients presenting with acute severe headache), high-risk (not missing SAH), and high-cost (avoiding expensive vascular imaging) over those that have the opposite profile, for example, diagnosis and treatment of Guillain–Barré syndrome. Not only will the former guideline

**Table 21.3** Steps in creating a practice guideline

| 1. Define an important topic | Is it:<br>A common problem with variable current practice?<br>One that has high-risk outcomes?<br>With potential cost savings or practice standardization? |
|---|---|
| 2. Keep it simple | **Have you:**<br>Ensured that its implementation is realistic locally?<br>Solicited input from key stakeholders in the ED?<br>Evaluated its impact on current workflow? |
| 3. Think administratively | **Have you:**<br>Vetted it with any external stakeholders outside the ED?<br>Incorporated easy-to-capture, meaningful metrics?<br>Evaluated impact on hospital economics? |
| 4. Implement, then measure | **Have you:**<br>Done ongoing quality assurance of outcomes?<br>Provided feedback to key individuals?<br>Made appropriate changes based on results? |

See text for details of each box.

have more impact, but the more that staff use it, the more familiar they will be with using it.

Defining the population that the policy includes is important. A policy about stroke might include "patients who have the abrupt onset of a focal neurological deficit within three hours." This is different from a policy that includes "patients whom the clinician thinks are having an acute ischemic stroke," and different still from one that includes "patients with acute neurological symptoms and a negative CT scan." Defining the patients to whom the policy refers is crucial, and sometimes difficult.

Make the practice guidelines that you use, whether locally produced or not, evidence-based. Both nurses and physicians will respond better to being "told what to do" if there is a rational basis for it in the medical literature. Some practitioners, especially those not trained in the technique, might rebel against having a practice guideline mandating an ultrasonographic approach for internal jugular central intravenous access. However, if the data show that it is clearly safer, which it did convincingly in one Italian study of nearly 2000 cases, physicians may accept it more willingly.[21]

Simplicity is another virtue in guidelines, although it does not ensure compliance. In fact, lack of compliance, even with simple scientifically valid guidelines, can be quite high. In a Canadian study of ED patients with TIA, even at a tertiary care hospital, fully 28% of the patients discharged did not receive an antiplatelet drug from the ED.[22] So although simplicity with guidelines does not ensure compliance, it certainly encourages it. It also makes staff education and measurement of results easier.

The issue of compliance with guidelines is an important one. Several studies have shown relatively good compliance,[23–25] whereas others have documented less than ideal compliance.[22,26–29] One Australian study documented that even good short-term compliance can drop off over time, partly due to staff turnover and partly due to other barriers.[30] Highly interactive implementation may help with compliance.[20,31] Placing information about the guidelines on the computer has shown mixed results in terms of increased compliance.[32,33]

Be realistic about how a given guideline impacts your individual ED. Some aspects of a given guideline may make perfect sense in a large hospital but not be feasible in a more peripheral setting. A guideline that includes magnetic resonance imaging (MRI) for stroke makes no sense in a hospital that does not have an MRI machine. This particular example becomes more germane since the American Academy of Neurology (AAN) recently published their guideline on MRI for acute ischemic stroke.[34] The evidence upon which it is based is quite correct – MRI is clearly superior to CT – but in a setting where MRI is not available or its hours are limited, then the recommendation is meaningless.

When you are either creating a practice guideline or implementing one, ED staff involvement is vital. While it may be obvious that nurses and doctors should be included, there are some occasions in which secretarial or technical staff should also be involved. Their perspective will necessarily be different but might be vitally important to proper implementation, perhaps in the way a patient is registered or in the transport of a blood sample to the lab. Be very specific about who is responsible for any given action within a guideline. If there is ambiguity, each person will naturally think that the responsibility falls to someone else.

Nurses and physicians in particular will have opinions about how a given guideline impacts their day-to-day workflow. Steps in a guideline that create new work (without adding new value) or that interfere with current workflow (without good reason) are more likely to fail if they are not vetted with the staff. There is a real danger of creating steps that make sense administratively but which take the clinician away from the patient. These steps can kill an otherwise perfectly good guideline. This is one important reason to discuss it first with the staff.

Some guidelines, if they are designed thoughtfully and implemented well, might even improve workflow or decrease documentation time. This is easier with an electronic medical record, but certainly is also true with paper. Decreasing workload gives the staff another incentive to use the guideline.

This is particularly true for the leader who does not work clinically in the ED. Not only will it ensure that you are not missing some important component, but it will also show your staff that you value their opinions and have the intelligence, foresight, and humility to research problems in an area in which you may not have specific expertise. For the same reasons, it is wise to vet the policy with the relevant staff both while it is being created and again when it is being implemented.

It is also important to solicit external feedback. Vetting the guideline with specialists from outside the ED (within the hospital) or specialty organizations outside of emergency medicine has value. This external vetting process is not for permission but to learn the issues that those outside groups see. Understanding how other specialties perceive the ED is useful politically. Some of their comments may have useful content of which the ED director might have been unaware. Some guidelines, for example for massive transfusion, require input from multiple departments.[20] A massive transfusion protocol is an ideal one for any ED that sees significant trauma, because there are moderately good clinical data to support it and it requires the close cooperation of at least traumatology, the blood bank, and the ED.[35–38]

When the ACEP Clinical Policies Committee writes a new policy, they routinely vet it with other relevant organizations, such as the AAN for a neurological policy or the AHA for a cardiovascular one. The same occurs in reverse: if the AAN or AHA is preparing a policy that relates to the practice of emergency medicine, they will send it to ACEP for review and possible endorsement.

Another tip is to create metrics that are easy to record (in the context of routine practice), important for patient care, and easy to abstract from the chart or the computer. There is an entire chapter on informatics (Chapter 18), but to the extent that one can capture data electronically, so much the better. This removes the responsibility for frontline staff to record it, improves the quality of the data, and allows for easier generation of reports.

Once the ED director implements a guideline, it is valuable if not imperative to review its impact on a regular basis. The most brilliant guideline will have difficulties that were unanticipated when it was created. Sometimes these are easily remedied and sometimes not, but either way one needs to be aware of them. Define a team from the various affected departments to meet regularly for as long as it takes to resolve ongoing issues. Aside from solving the inevitable problems, it gives the staff an outlet for any grumbling that results from the new guideline, as well as the sense that the leader has anticipated the problem(s), even if he or she has not anticipated the specific ones that arise. Regular review may also help improve compliance. It also supplies the fuel for revisions to the guideline based on actual experience.

A last but extremely important goal has to do with knowledge translation. In this case, even if the ED director is successful on all of the points above, including compliance, does using the guidelines actually improve the clinical outcomes in our patients? There are some studies that suggest that outcomes are improved: for example, reduced hospitalization for childhood asthma,[23] improved survival in sepsis,[24] and reduction in organ failure when massive transfusion protocols are used.[35]

---

**Case study 21.2.  Procedural sedation protocol**

Use of propofol for procedural sedation in the ED has been a contentious area. Many EDs are "not allowed" to use propofol for this indication by their institutional anesthesia departments. This stems from official anesthesiology's stance that propofol should not be used by non-anesthesiologists.[39] As reviewed in an ACEP Clinical Policy, however, the literature in fact shows that when used properly, propofol for procedural sedation in the ED is safe.[40]

In the author's experience and opinion, propofol is a far superior agent for procedural sedation, as compared to the most commonly used traditional agents such as midazolam. Successful implementation of institutional guidelines for propofol use must combine intelligent use of the safety and effectiveness data that exist, physician education, and ongoing quality assurance of cases. Using the ACEP Clinical Policy (and the references upon which it is based) goes a long way in terms of the first issue.

Physician education can be done in many ways. At one institution, the emergency physicians must take an online test that is administered every two years and which is written largely by anesthesiologists. Amongst the group of emergency physicians, there was initial resistance to this; however, the reality is that taking the test does ensure a baseline level of knowledge and helps with the issues of both knowledge retention and staff turnover. The propofol policy at most institutions includes regular audit of problem cases. At the outset, review of all cases is a good idea, although emergency physicians, not doctors from other departments, should perform the reviews. That said, the review must be honest and pay careful attention to making certain that the results at a given institution mirror those reported in the literature.

## Case study 21.3. Back pain protocol

This protocol was developed at a hospital after two ED patients with back pain due to spinal cord or cauda equina were initially misdiagnosed (Fig. 21.1). Back pain is an incredibly common chief complaint in the ED, and cord compression, though rare, is an important bad outcome to avoid. As well, reduction of expensive imaging (MRI) in patients who do not require it is another important goal. Thus, this guideline incorporates all the issues that make for a good practice guideline.

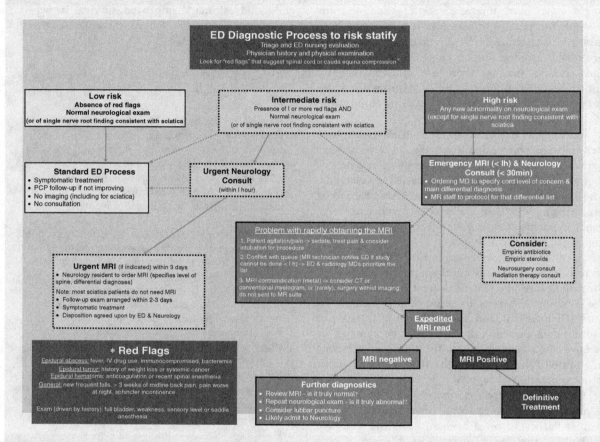

**Figure 21.1** Protocol for evaluation of patients with back pain.

The protocol was developed in concert with the departments of neurology, neurosurgery, radiology, and emergency medicine. The primary purpose was to facilitate rapid diagnosis, but a secondary purpose was to reduce unnecessary expensive imaging (see low-risk and standard ED process boxes on the left side of the protocol).

Notice that time frames are specified in the boxes containing "Neurology consult." This helps the emergency physician when consultants are responding more slowly than needed, as the emergency physician can simply pull out the guideline that the neurology departmental leadership agreed to and show it to the consultant who is responding slowly.

As well, there is a box in the center of the protocol titled "problem with rapidly obtaining the MRI." This box was added to the guideline later, after audit of a number of cases showed that patient inability to tolerate the scan (something under the control of the emergency department) and poor prioritization of patients (something under the control of the radiology department) were the two most common causes of delays. As in the stroke protocol example above (Case study 21.1), this process also helps individual clinicians from various departments to sit down together and work through a given issue, which has other dividends beyond the problem at hand.

# References

1. Agrawal P, Kosowsky JM. Clinical practice guidelines in the emergency department. *Emergency Medicine Clinics of North America* 2009; **27**: 555–67, vii.

2. Hacke W, Donnan G, Fieschi C, *et al.* Association of outcome with early stroke treatment: pooled analysis of ATLANTIS, ECASS, and NINDS rt-PA stroke trials. *Lancet* 2004; **363**: 768–74.

3. Hacke W, Kaste M, Bluhmki E, *et al.* Thrombolysis with alteplase 3 to 4.5 hours after acute ischemic stroke. *New England Journal of Medicine* 2008; **359**: 1317–29.

4. Wahlgren N, Ahmed N, Davalos A, *et al.* Thrombolysis with alteplase 3–4.5 h after acute ischaemic stroke (SITS-ISTR): an observational study. *Lancet* 2008; **372**: 1303–9.

5. Pollack CV, Roe MT, Peterson ED. 2002 update to the ACC/AHA guidelines for the management of patients with unstable angina and non-ST-segment elevation myocardial infarction: implications for emergency department practice. *Annals of Emergency Medicine* 2003; **41**: 355–69.

6. Yusuf S, Zhao F, Mehta SR, *et al.* Effects of clopidogrel in addition to aspirin in patients with acute coronary syndromes without ST-segment elevation. *New England Journal of Medicine* 2001; **345**: 494–502.

7. Bohan J. Guidelines in emergency medicine. In J Marx, R Hockberger, R Walls, eds., *Rosen's Emergency Medicine: Concepts and Clinical Practice*, 6th edn. Philadelphia, PA: Mosby Elsevier, 2006: 3034–45.

8. Grimshaw JM, Russell IT. Effect of clinical guidelines on medical practice: a systematic review of rigorous evaluations. *Lancet* 1993; **342**: 1317–22.

9. Jain S, Elon LK, Johnson BA, Frank G, Deguzman M. Physician practice variation in the pediatric emergency department and its impact on resource use and quality of care. *Pediatric Emergency Care* 2010; **26**: 902–8.

10. Stiell IG, Clement CM, Brison RJ, *et al.* Variation in management of recent-onset atrial fibrillation and flutter among academic hospital emergency departments. *Annals of Emergency Medicine* 2011; **57**: 13–21.

11. Chan EW, Taylor DM, Knott JC, Kong DC. Variation in the management of hypothetical cases of acute agitation in Australasian emergency departments. *Emergency Medicine Australasia* 2011; **23**: 23–32.

12. Calver LA, Downes MA, Page CB, Bryant JL, Isbister GK. The impact of a standardised intramuscular sedation protocol for acute behavioural disturbance in the emergency department. *BMC Emergency Medicine* 2010; **10**: 14.

13. Edlow JA, Panagos PD, Godwin SA, Thomas TL, Decker WW. Clinical policy: critical issues in the evaluation and management of adult patients presenting to the emergency department with acute headache. *Annals of Emergency Medicine* 2008; **52**: 407–36.

14. Morgenstern LB, Luna-Gonzales H, Huber JC, *et al.* Worst headache and subarachnoid hemorrhage: prospective, modern computed tomography and spinal fluid analysis. *Annals of Emergency Medicine* 1998; **32**: 297–304.

15. Savitz SI, Levitan EB, Wears R, Edlow JA. Pooled analysis of patients with thunderclap headache evaluated by CT and LP: is angiography necessary in patients with negative evaluations? *Journal of the Neurological Sciences* 2009; **276**: 123–5.

16. Edlow JA. What are the unintended consequences of changing the diagnostic paradigm for subarachnoid hemorrhage after brain computed tomography to computed tomographic angiography in place of lumbar puncture? *Academic Emergency Medicine* 2010; **17**: 991–7.

17. McCormack RF, Hutson A. Can computed tomography angiography of the brain replace lumbar puncture in the evaluation of acute-onset headache after a negative noncontrast cranial computed tomography scan? *Academic Emergency Medicine* 2010; **17**: 444–51.

18. Ransom SB, Studdert DM, Dombrowski MP, Mello MM, Brennan TA. Reduced medicolegal risk by compliance with obstetric clinical pathways: a case–control study. *Obstetrics and Gynecology* 2003; **101**: 751–5.

19. Hyams AL, Brandenburg JA, Lipsitz SR, Shapiro DW, Brennan TA. Practice guidelines and malpractice litigation: a two-way street. *Annals of Internal Medicine* 1995; **122**: 450–5.

20. Nunez TC, Young PP, Holcomb JB, Cotton BA. Creation, implementation, and maturation of a massive transfusion protocol for the exsanguinating trauma patient. *Journal of Trauma* 2010; **68**: 1498–505.

21. Cavanna L, Civardi G, Vallisa D, *et al.* Ultrasound-guided central venous catheterization in cancer patients improves the success rate of cannulation and reduces mechanical complications: A prospective observational study of 1,978 consecutive catheterizations. *World Journal of Surgical Oncology* 2010; **8**: 91.

22. Chang E, Holroyd BR, Kochanski P, *et al.* Adherence to practice guidelines for transient ischemic attacks in an emergency department. *Canadian Journal of Neurological Sciences* 2002; **29**: 358–63.

23. Hampers LC, Thompson DA, Bajaj L, Tseng BS, Rudolph JR. Febrile seizure: measuring adherence to AAP guidelines among community ED physicians. *Pediatric Emergency Care* 2006; **22**: 465–9.

24. Norton SP, Pusic MV, Taha F, Heathcote S, Carleton BC. Effect of a clinical pathway on the hospitalisation rates of children with asthma: a prospective study. *Archives of Disease in Childhood* 2007; **92**: 60–6.

25. Girardis M, Rinaldi L, Donno L, *et al*. Effects on management and outcome of severe sepsis and septic shock patients admitted to the intensive care unit after implementation of a sepsis program: a pilot study. *Critical Care* 2009; **13**: R143.

26. Heskestad B, Baardsen R, Helseth E, Ingebrigtsen T. Guideline compliance in management of minimal, mild, and moderate head injury: high frequency of noncompliance among individual physicians despite strong guideline support from clinical leaders. *Journal of Trauma* 2008; **65**: 1309–13.

27. Kane BG, Degutis LC, Sayward HK, D'Onofrio G. Compliance with the Centers for Disease Control and Prevention recommendations for the diagnosis and treatment of sexually transmitted diseases. *Academic Emergency Medicine* 2004; **11**: 371–7.

28. Krym VF, Crawford B, MacDonald RD. Compliance with guidelines for emergency management of asthma in adults: experience at a tertiary care teaching hospital. *CJEM* 2004; **6**: 321–6.

29. Lougheed MD, Olajos-Clow J, Szpiro K, *et al*. Multicentre evaluation of an emergency department asthma care pathway for adults. *CJEM* 2009; **11**: 215–29.

30. Brand C, Landgren F, Hutchinson A, *et al*. Clinical practice guidelines: barriers to durability after effective early implementation. *Internal Medicine Journal* 2005; **35**: 162–9.

31. Ratnapalan S, Schneeweiss S. Guidelines to practice: the process of planning and implementing a pediatric sedation program. *Pediatric Emergency Care* 2007; **23**: 262–6.

32. Melnick ER, Genes NG, Chawla NK, *et al*. Knowledge translation of the American College of Emergency Physicians' clinical policy on syncope using computerized clinical decision support. *International Journal of Emergency Medicine* 2010; **3**: 97–104.

33. Tierney WM, Overhage JM, Murray MD, *et al*. Can computer-generated evidence-based care suggestions enhance evidence-based management of asthma and chronic obstructive pulmonary disease? A randomized, controlled trial. *Health Services Research* 2005; **40**: 477–97.

34. Schellinger P, Bryan R, Caplan L, *et al*. Evidence-based guideline: The role of diffusion and perfusion MRI for the diagnosis of acute ischemic stroke: Report of the Therapeutics and Technology Subcomittee of the American Academy of Neurology. *Neurology* 2010; **75**: 177–85.

35. Cotton BA, Au BK, Nunez TC, *et al*. Predefined massive transfusion protocols are associated with a reduction in organ failure and postinjury complications. *Journal of Trauma* 2009; **66**: 41–9.

36. Dente CJ, Shaz BH, Nicholas JM, *et al*. Improvements in early mortality and coagulopathy are sustained better in patients with blunt trauma after institution of a massive transfusion protocol in a civilian level I trauma center.

*Journal of Trauma* 2009; **66**: 1616–24.

37. Milligan C, Higginson I, Smith JE. Emergency department staff knowledge of massive transfusion for trauma: the need for an evidence based protocol. *Emergency Medicine Journal* 2011; **28**: 870–2.

38. Schuster KM, Davis KA, Lui FY, Maerz LL, Kaplan LJ. The status of massive transfusion protocols in United States trauma centers: massive transfusion or massive confusion? *Transfusion* 2010; **50**: 1545–51.

39. American Society of Anesthesiologists Task Force on Sedation and Analgesia by Non-Anesthesiologists. Practice guidelines for sedation and analgesia by non-anesthesiologists. *Anesthesiology* 2002; **96**: 1004–17.

40. Godwin SA, Caro DA, Wolf SJ, *et al*. Clinical policy: procedural sedation and analgesia in the emergency department. *Annals of Emergency Medicine* 2005; **45**: 177–96.

## Further reading and resources

www.guideline.gov – a US-based national clearinghouse for guidelines from various societies that refers to hundreds of individual guidelines, although many do not impact emergency medicine. It also has other resources for creating guidelines, an archive of commentaries about various guidelines and other relevant information.

www.acep.org – ACEP's website. Under the "practice resources" tab, there is information about its clinical policies and also about policy statements. The former read more like practice guidelines while the latter read more like political statements. Both are useful. In addition, there is a great deal of other information relevant to the specialty.

www.nice.org.uk – the website of the UK's National Institute for Health and Care Excellence (NICE). NICE publishes numerous guidelines, some of which are relevant to emergency medicine. At the home page are many other links, including those about how to implement practice guidelines.

www.americanheart.org – another site that includes many professional guidelines dealing with cardiovascular and cerebrovascular diseases.

www.cochrane.org – the homepage of the Cochrane reviews. There are hundreds of reviews here all with exceptional methodology. Many of the guidelines at this site are directly relevant to emergency medicine. There is not a separate section for emergency medicine but as of February 2014 there were 505 cardiovascular reviews and 660 neurological ones.

Most other North American, European, and Australasian professional societies write guidelines and post them electronically on their websites. A partial list of these includes:

- Canadian Association of Emergency Physicians (www.caep.ca)
- European Society for Emergency Medicine (www.eusem.org)
- Société Française de Médecine d'Urgence (www.sfmu.org)
- Società Italiana Medicina d'Emergenza-Urgenza (www.simeu.it)
- Australasian Society for Emergency Medicine (www.asem.org.au)
- Sociedad Española de Medicina de Urgencias y Emergencias (www.semes.org)

Chapter

# 22

# Emergency department observation units

Christopher W. Baugh and J. Stephen Bohan

## Key learning points

- Define the purpose of an observation unit.
- Understand the practical logistics of establishing and operating an observation unit.
- Learn which patients are best suited for observation management, and the importance of protocol-driven care.
- Understand the benefits and drawbacks of fast-track units.

## Introduction

Currently half of all inpatient admissions to hospitals come from the emergency department (ED). The US Centers for Disease Control and Prevention (CDC) survey data from 2010 reveal that there are nearly 130 million visits annually to EDs in the United States, a number that is increasing at a rate of about 1% per year while inpatient capacity is static or declining,[1] a phenomenon also present in the UK and continental Europe. In Germany, for example, the patient volume in EDs grew by 8% in 2007 while the number of inpatients only rose by 2.1%, according to the Federal Statistical Office.[2] Some of these inpatient stays are short, leading funders to question if they are necessary at all. Many institutions, however, are now managing these patients as outpatients in short-stay "observation" units, most often operated by the ED. Such patients require either further treatment or diagnostics before being safely discharged from the ED, within less than 24 hours. Despite the historical, clinical, and business basis for the creation and growth of ED observation units (EDOUs) the conceptualization and implementation of such units remains elusive to many who could potentially benefit from their use. This chapter is intended to clarify the rationale for and operating characteristics of such units, and to provide support for their clinical, fiscal, and administrative benefits, including their contribution to patient safety.

## Strategic case for observation units

Today, acute-care hospitals are facing substantial pressure to increase patient access, safety, quality of care, and satisfaction without increasing costs. In this era of mounting scrutiny and transparency, few "win–win" initiatives exist that have the potential to lower costs while improving patient safety and satisfaction without adversely impacting access to care or the quality of care delivered. However, the increased use of the EDOU, for those hospitals with the volume of ED visits to justify one, has the potential to be one of those rare initiatives.

All stakeholders in the healthcare system benefit from EDOU use. Patients are more accurately diagnosed before leaving the ED and are discharged home faster, payers avoid costly inpatient admission charges, hospitals keep scarce inpatient bed capacity open for more appropriate patients, and providers deliver care in a setting that more appropriately matches patient needs to resources.[3] Since every aspect of care delivered in this setting is at least equivalent to, if not better than, the alternative of inpatient care, use of the observation unit can be considered a dominant strategy for managing eligible patients. A dominant strategy is one that does at least as well as every other strategy in all situations but does strictly better than every other strategy in at least one situation.[4] Emergency medicine and hospital leadership should be familiar with the concept of the EDOU and its importance not only to the ED but to the entire hospital.

---

## Logistics: planning an emergency department observation unit

### Bed capacity and patient flow considerations

Logistically, the EDOU is usually a discrete unit with 4–20 beds contained within or adjacent to the ED.[5] These units usually have the capacity to care for about 5–10% of the total ED volume, with an average EDOU stay of about 10 hours per patient.[3] Patients are admitted to the EDOU from the ED if they require additional diagnostics or therapies beyond their initial ED stay, but will likely be able to be discharged home within 24 hours. On average, about 80% of patients managed in the EDOU are able to be safely discharged home, while the remainder requires inpatient hospitalization.[3,6]

Historically, bed space in the ED specifically designated for patients requiring more time beyond the normal (4–6-hour) ED visit were called observation units, as observing the patient over time was a tried and true test for various acute pathologies such as appendicitis. Since the initiation of these units in the 1960s, diagnostic technology has improved dramatically, and in many cases – again, such as appendicitis – the "tincture of time" can be replaced by a picture. As a result of this evolving diagnostic role, these units have earned newer designations as *clinical decision units* or *rapid diagnostic units* – but for the purposes of this chapter we will use the term *emergency department observation unit*, or EDOU. The clinical utility of EDOUs was first established around the care of patients with chest pain in whom clinicians feared an impending heart attack. Asthma, kidney stones, skin infections, and allergic reactions were also soon recognized to be suitable for EDOU care. Numerous research studies have been published over the past two decades showing safe and effective protocols in a wide range of conditions.[7–11]

The implication for healthcare managers and administrators is that if sufficient patient volume exists in their institution to justify the expense of an EDOU, opening or enlarging one to maximize both clinical utility and profitability should be strongly considered. One can expect about 5–10% of ED volume to be managed in an observation unit.[3] Given a ratio of five patients managed per nurse in an EDOU, the minimum efficient size of a dedicated EDOU should be five beds, which translates into a minimum ED volume of about 30 000–50 000 annual visits, assuming average length of stay and bed turnover calculations discussed previously.

Administrators working in a hospital that contains an ED with a volume over 30 000 annual visits but does not have a dedicated observation unit should work with the clinicians staffing the ED to determine if adding this additional resource makes sound clinical and financial sense for that particular institution. The information below aims to provide the background necessary to perform the analysis to answer such questions. Such an analysis, of course, should calculate the expected return on investment over several years and compare an EDOU project to competing alternatives, such as expanding the acute-care ED space or adding additional inpatient capacity.

### Scope of emergency department observation units

While placing a patient in observation has become more common in EDs in Europe and Australasia, the business basis for the creation and growth of EDOUs remains unclear to many hospital administrators and even physicians. The American College of Emergency Physicians (ACEP) began to formalize the scope of observation medicine by creating the first observation unit guidelines in 1988.[3]

The growth of EDOUs over the past four decades has been fueled by the acknowledgment that emergency physicians should no longer be forced into a dichotomous decision between discharge home or inpatient admission, especially as patients become more medically complex and require more diagnostic testing and therapeutic interventions than can be expected from an average ED visit. In the United States, the recognition of the value conferred by observation resulted in federal government recognition of such units for payment purposes, initially for a few specific diagnoses but subsequently for any condition thought appropriate by the attending physician. It took several years until this development took form in continental Europe. Mostly due to the impact of a new reimbursement system for hospitals with bundled payments, the economic section of the German Society of Interdisciplinary Emergency Departments has recommended establishing an EDOU since 2009.[12]

### Staffing

The major fixed costs involved in maintaining an EDOU lie in the staffing. The number of EDOU patients that a single nurse can manage is higher than in the acute-care or inpatient areas of the hospital, usually around one nurse per five patients, and physician staffing tends to be minimal to care for these patients.[3] This ratio is safe because patients in observation have been selected as representing a low-acuity population amenable to simple care algorithms with a high likelihood of discharge home. In contrast, nursing ratios in the acute-care area of the ED can be as high as one nurse per patient (or even more, during a major trauma resuscitation, for example) but often average around one nurse per three or four patients, which is similar to most inpatient ratios.[13] Similar to the difference in nursing ratios, fewer medical assistants are needed to care for observation patients, since they tend to be much less active than acute care ED patients.

The use of physician extenders, such as nurse practitioners and physician assistants (discussed in more detail in the section on fast track, below), is also well established in the EDOU setting.[3] These providers offer a less expensive alternative to having a direct physician presence in the EDOU, in countries where these professions exist. Even with the use of a physician extender, a supervising physician should be ultimately responsible and available for each patient in observation. Critical decisions, such as the overall observation management plan and endpoints for successful discharge, are usually made by the supervising physician and subsequently managed by the physician extender. If a patient decompensates or if test results are concerning, the supervising physician is re-engaged by the physician extender to intervene. However, much of the hands-on work needed to care for observation patients can be safely handled by an experienced physician extender.

## Treatment algorithms and protocols

Adherence to evidence-based clinical protocols is an essential component of maintaining an efficient EDOU. The observation literature that has developed over the past two decades provides helpful guidelines for optimal patient selection and management in the observation setting. These studies include explicit inclusion criteria, which help to identify the patients most likely to be successfully managed in the EDOU and subsequently discharged home. Patient selection is a critical element of the observation process – patients who are too sick will swamp the more limited resources of the EDOU and ultimately need inpatient

management regardless. Patients who should have been sent home prior to the observation stay will crowd the EDOU needlessly and expose patients to the hazards of the hospital without any benefit. Finding the right observation candidate – one unsafe to send home after the initial ED evaluation, but also likely to avoid an inpatient stay if observed, can be difficult. Department leadership should work to develop protocols that remove much of the subjective nature of this decision by providing evidence-based tools. Explicit inclusion criteria, by diagnosis or complaint, can be incredibly valuable, especially to less experienced clinicians.

In addition, once a patient is deemed ideal for observation, the management plan for that patient should be evidence-based. Using the available literature, algorithms of care that consider the unique resources available in that specific hospital should be readily available. These are often included as part of the observation admission note (see example of chest pain observation protocol, Appendix 22.1). These treatment algorithms remove uncertainty from the evaluation and create efficiencies as staff become accustomed to the routine steps needed to manage a patient with a specific protocol in observation. Finally, the endpoints needed for discharge should be explicit from the outset. These can also be included as part of the standard observation discharge note. This helps prevent patients from spending too much time in observation, which is a real concern if the plan is unclear or not well communicated. More detail about protocol-driven care can be found in elsewhere in this book (see Chapter 21).

# Benefits

## The clinical case for observation units

The clinical benefits of observation medicine have been well established across a variety of clinical conditions. In most cases, observation units provide a venue for the execution of efficient diagnostic and treatment algorithms when applied to appropriately selected patients. The scientific literature in support of EDOUs was largely first built on the concept of chest pain centers designed to effectively rule out acute coronary syndromes in low-risk patients and provide subsequent risk stratification while avoiding costly hospital admission.[14–17] Subsequently, over 10 distinct clinical entities with demonstrated clinical diagnostic or therapeutic equivalence to inpatient admission were identified. Specifically, EDOU care has demonstrated clinical efficacy in the management of chest pain,[18] cocaine-associated chest pain,[19] asthma,[20] acute-onset atrial fibrillation,[21] transient ischemic attack,[22] acute decompensated heart failure,[11] and numerous other diagnoses.

### Impact on patient satisfaction

Several studies have demonstrated higher patient satisfaction with observation care versus routine inpatient care, specifically for asthma and chest pain.[23,24] In addition to providing care that patients prefer, this aspect of observation care may also have a broader impact. As the international focus on healthcare quality continues to shift toward more patient-centered metrics, patient satisfaction will likely play a prominent role with respect to pay-for-performance payments and publicly reported hospital quality data.[25]

---

**Case study 22.1. Falling**

A 79-year-old male presented to the ED, referred from his primary care doctor's office for "falling." His family had called the primary care physician in the morning and he was seen at 1 p.m. and directed to the ED, arriving in a room about 4 p.m.. He had a history of hypertension and benign prostatic hyperplasia (BPH) and no recent changes in medicines or recent hospitalizations. Other than falling and the bruises resulting he had no complaints, particularly no chest pain, no dyspnea, no syncope or pre-syncope, no leg swelling, no unilateral weakness, and no fever or chills. He was not on any anticoagulant. His vital signs showed BP 130/88, pulse 90 and regular, $O_2$ saturation 94% on room air at rest. Physical exam showed a conversant patient with multiple bruises and ecchymosis on extremities and trunk. There was no swelling of the face or scalp. He was able to move all four extremities and had no extremity deformity. There was no evidence of upper or lower extremity weakness. He could walk with light assistance, did not complain of dizziness, but did say he felt unsteady. He did not fall while walking in the ED.

ED evaluation included a normal ECG, chest x-ray, and CT scan of the brain. Blood alcohol level was zero. Neurology was consulted and an MRI was ordered. The patient was transferred to the EDOU pending MRI of the brain. Several hours later the MRI of the brain was completed and showed no mass or bleed, offering no hint as to the cause of the patient's

---

falling episodes. The neurology resident discussed the case with his attending, who suggested that it might be a proprioception problem and recommended imaging of the spinal cord. A spine MRI was performed and confirmed posterior column compression due to spinal stenosis.

By this time it was morning, and a physiotherapy consultation was obtained to test the patient with a walker. This proved successful, and the patient was discharged home at noon (20 hours after arrival) with appointments made for a home assessment for fall prevention by a visiting nurse and follow-up with neurology, primary care, and physiotherapy.

---

### Improved diagnostic sensitivity and specificity

Another way of conceptualizing the benefit of observation is that it increases both the specificity and the sensitivity of ED patient management. The additional time for diagnostics allows for more accurate diagnoses, and for the minority of patients who need additional care as an inpatient, they are more likely to be admitted to the correct service after an observation stay than after the initial emergency evaluation. Additionally, higher sensitivity is achieved through the use of observation. The best example of increased sensitivity is in the diagnosis of myocardial infarction (see Case study 22.2). Currently, it is very difficult to make a definitive diagnosis of myocardial ischemia upon presentation to the ED without a characteristic electrocardiogram. Serum cardiac biomarkers have greatly enhanced the clinician's ability to determine if a patient's chest pain represents a true heart attack, but a significant limitation of these markers is the well-known delay of many hours between the cardiac event and a positive blood test.[26] By keeping patients in the EDOU and checking serial cardiac biomarkers, fewer patients with an atypical presentation would be discharged home from the ED. Adding cardiac stress testing to this observation protocol can further increase the sensitivity for detecting clinically significant coronary artery disease.

---

**Case study 22.2. Low-risk chest pain**

A 57-year-old woman with a history of hypertension and obesity presented to the ED with two hours of severe, pressure-like non-radiating substernal chest pressure. She had no known personal or family history of coronary artery disease. On arrival her blood pressure was 165/88 mmHg and the rest of her

---

vitals were otherwise unremarkable. She was in mild distress, but her physical exam was non-focal. Her ECG was a normal sinus rhythm at 90 beats per minute, with no evidence of acute coronary ischemia. She was given aspirin and her pain resolved within the first 30 minutes in the ED. Initial serum cardiac biomarkers were within normal limits and the patient was admitted to the EDOU for a second set of cardiac biomarkers and an exercise tolerance test (ETT). Six hours after the initial set of markers was drawn, the second set was drawn, which was also normal. Repeat ECG at this time was unchanged. The patient did not have any recurrence of her chest pain while in the EDOU, and she underwent an ETT the morning after her admission, which showed she was low-risk. The patient was reassured that the underlying cause of her chest pain the day before was very unlikely to have been an acute coronary syndrome, given the results of serial cardiac markers, ECG, and ETT. While this complete evaluation took about 12 hours, a similar office-based evaluation would have likely taken several days, if not longer. This also assumes that the patient would have kept her follow-up appointments; one of the useful aspects of observation care is that the patient is already present, and the plan does not rely on all the uncertainties of multiple visits over time.

### Impact on patient safety

Finally, the impact of proper EDOU use on patient safety should not be underestimated. Patient safety can be improved if patients are admitted to the correct service after an observation stay, since changes in service after a patient has been admitted create not only unnecessary administrative work but, more importantly, additional opportunities for errors in communication via additional patient handoffs. Handoffs have been identified as a critical patient safety issue, and the ED is the unique setting of many handoffs to inpatient services prone to numerous communication and care transition errors.[27]

Patients managed in observation and then discharged home as an alternative to inpatient hospitalization have much less exposure to the hospital and its associated risks. These dangers include exposure to multi-drug-resistant bacteria, falls, medication errors, physical deconditioning. and many others that are well documented and harm thousands of patients every year.[28] The best way to treat these complications of hospitalization is to avoid them altogether, and an observation stay that keeps a patient in the hospital for a fraction of the time of a routine inpatient hospitalization is an effective strategy to minimize exposure to these risks and greatly impact patient safety.

## The business case for observation units

With ED and inpatient beds already in shortage, the EDOU needs to provide a compelling financial argument to senior hospital leadership to justify the expense of its initiation and maintenance.[29] The creation or expansion of observation units is usually compared to alternative competing capital projects such as expanding acute-care ED beds or inpatient beds in most hospital settings. Observation units are distinct from these two care settings because they use algorithm-driven care allowing for standardized, rapid treatment and evaluation within the 24-hour window required for observation stays. The ability for EDOUs to deliver care and provide additional risk stratification through efficient resource use and shorter hospital stay centers on a business model that has proven quite profitable to date.

An EDOU creates a third disposition option that more accurately matches healthcare resources to patient needs. Accordingly, the first and foremost goal of the EDOU is to augment the clinical capacity of the ED. In support of this goal is the EDOU's ability to maximize ED efficiency (as well as inpatient efficiency by freeing up beds) and profitability. Additionally, another financial benefit arises from patients who are discharged home from an EDOU. Some countries have payers that audit short-stay inpatient admissions and re-collect payments for those that are deemed inappropriate. Especially in these countries, a benefit is derived from the avoidance of a short-stay inpatient admission that would otherwise have potentially resulted in a loss for the hospital, if payment were subsequently denied via such an audit process. Additionally, for every patient managed in observation and sent home who would have otherwise been admitted, an inpatient bed can be filled by a patient that is more profitable for the hospital. Chest pain is the most common EDOU diagnosis and provides the best example of this phenomenon.[30,31] In certain countries, the inpatient and observation payments may actually be similar, but the cost to manage a patient in the observation setting is much lower. Prior studies have shown that the higher fixed costs and longer length of stay associated with inpatient care can create a loss for the hospital,

**Table 22.1** Advantages of observation care versus inpatient care

| | Observation unit | Examples/rationale | Inpatient unit | Examples/rationale |
|---|---|---|---|---|
| **Costs** | | | | |
| Average length of stay | ~ 10 hours | Protocol-driven care with minimal variability | ~ 2 days | More diagnostic variability |
| Patient-to-nurse ratio | Up to 5:1 | Limited number of diagnostic and treatment protocols | Usually 3:1 or 4:1 | More heterogeneous mix of patients requires higher ratios of nurse staffing |
| Room size requirements and fixed costs | Flexible rooms, use of curtains | Patients preselected as low risk/acuity with low nursing needs, rooms can be smaller with less equipment | Minimum standards limit flexibility | More heterogeneous mix of patients requires more fixed resources; trend toward private rooms |
| **Payments** | | | | |
| Revenue | Fee for service | Discrete payments for diagnostics (e.g., ECG, chest x-ray, stress test) and therapeutics (e.g., medications) | Bundled | Inpatient payments bundle all diagnostic and therapeutic services |
| Risk of denial and/or audit | Low | Payers have less incentive to investigate lower cost encounters | High | Patients with short inpatient stays (i.e., 1–2 days) are targeted by payers as possibly inappropriate |

Inpatient length of stay estimate assumes patient would have been candidate for ED observation care.[2,31]

whereas management of the same patient in an EDOU would have generated a profit.[31] Table 22.1 summarizes the most striking cost and payment differences between observation and inpatient care.

## Measures of observation care

Emergency physicians have recognized that longer observation stays require structured diagnostic and treatment algorithms in order to efficiently facilitate patient disposition. As a result, many departments use structured observation medicine protocols for all patients designated as "observation status," including patients who, for lack of a bed, may not physically be in an EDOU, but rather receive observation care in the acute-care area of the ED. This "virtual" observation unit carries the advantage of not requiring the significant fixed costs of creating a distinct unit, particularly in hospitals with notable space or budget limitations. However, the highest potential for cost savings, patient comfort, and hospital bed utilization efficiency lies in dedicating a physical space to observation. The placement of the unit at a significant distance from the ED does not change the internal dynamic but results in a loss of efficiency in physician

coverage, transport, and communication. As a result, understanding the financing of an EDOU is critical to justify its creation.[32–34]

Moving beyond the sources of payments and costs, an essential component of a profitable EDOU is operational efficiency. Maximum efficiency in the EDOU, and subsequently profitability, requires optimizing three main operational variables: the occupancy rate, duration of observation, and discharge-home rate. Pushing more patient volume through the EDOU creates a more robust disposition option from the ED while also diverting patients away from inpatient services, thus mitigating both ED and inpatient crowding. Additionally, maximizing the number of patients seen in the EDOU enables the ED to capture many additional observation payments, if available, which in turn may help finance less profitable services. The more patients cared for in the EDOU, the more bed capacity is created on the inpatient side.

The EDOU operational metrics of occupancy rate, length of stay, and discharge-home rate are intertwined, as illustrated in the triangle in Figure 22.1. When one of these variables is significantly changed, the two others are also affected. Ultimately, the task of

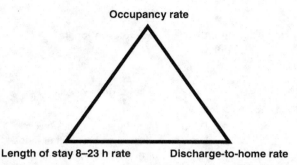

**Figure 22.1** Key operational variables of observation unit care: the interrelationship between three key operational variables in the observation unit.

patient selection for observation is the critical task of the clinician, and proper patient selection will optimize these variables as well as the care of the patient. Managers of observation units need to provide patient selection support in the form of well-constructed and applied inclusion and exclusion criteria in addition to well-established diagnostic and treatment algorithms. Finally, while profit and efficiency maximization are important considerations of EDOU management, one must always caution against letting payment parameters dictate clinical management. Payment rules will remain in constant flux, and at the end of the day focus must be centered on providing the right care to all patients in the right place at the right time.

### Occupancy rate

Since it is impossible to exactly match patient arrivals to departures (time needed for bed turnover, daily variation, etc.), the maximum occupancy rate will always be less than 100%. However, an optimal occupancy rate approaching maximum capacity is obviously beneficial for a dedicated EDOU with fixed resources (e.g., number of beds, nursing staff).

### Duration of observation

The duration of observation should be at least eight hours for every patient, in order to justify the added expense of operating the EDOU. Two important considerations define the lower limit for observation: the minimum time needed for meaningful observation interventions and payer rules, which vary by country but usually require a minimum stay for additional observation payments. The maximum length of stay should also be less than 24 hours, as stays longer than one day are an inefficient use of the EDOU. Thus, to maximize EDOU volume, the maximum

number of patients can be cared for in the EDOU if every patient stays just over eight hours, but never less. This is in addition to time spent in the ED.

### Discharge-home rate

Assuming a maximum occupancy rate near 90%, and optimal length of stay between 8 and 24 hours for all EDOU patients, the discharge-to-home rate remains the elusive variable to optimize. Clearly, the ideal rate would approach 100%, as long as the unintended consequence of increasing short-stay (< 24-hour) inpatient admissions was avoided. Additionally, inpatient admission after an observation stay, while sometimes necessary, represents inefficient use of resources. Even in idealized clinical trial settings, however, around 20% of patients evaluated in the EDOU require admission, and this may represent a more realistic outcome, given the clinical uncertainty surrounding these patients.

The available scientific literature shows that larger-scale recent studies on EDOU utilization for diagnoses such as chest pain, atrial fibrillation, transient ischemic attack, and cocaine-associated chest pain all reveal discharge rates between 80% and 100%.[10,22,35–37] Notably, one study reports lower discharge rates for patients admitted to the EDOU for congestive heart failure exacerbations (73%).[38] In addition, Brillman *et al.* suggest that units with a discharge-home rate less than 70% should question their guidelines for observation.[39] Finally, self-reported rates provide additional support for benchmarks. The text *Observation Medicine: the Healthcare System's Tincture of Time* by Graff contains many self-reported discharge-home rates from different observation units throughout the USA, all of which appear to cluster around 80%.[3]

## Fast-track units

On the opposite side of the spectrum of observation care is fast-track care. Patients with very straightforward needs who can be rapidly assessed and discharged are best suited for the fast track. Most fast-track care is delivered in a distinct area of the ED, often staffed by physician extenders, such as nurse practitioners or physician assistants. These professionals, who are frequently used in the United States and sometimes also called mid-level practitioners, have special training to function autonomously in many clinical settings, including a fast track.

Common complaints managed in this area include minor sports injuries, rashes, minor wounds, cold symptoms, and others that require minimal time and resources to expedite patient throughput in the department.

Benefits of a dedicated fast track are the following: (1) efficiencies of equipment location close to the patients who need it most (e.g., a slit lamp for eye exams); (2) smaller room size due to lower-acuity complaints; (3) more patients per nurse due to lower frequency of nursing interventions; and (4) shorter waits and faster throughput time for patients with minor complaints, since they are not competing for the same resources as more ill or complicated patients.

Drawbacks to a dedicated fast track include the following: (1) provider dissatisfaction with caring for a narrow spectrum of ED patients; (2) providers who never work fast-track shifts may lose important emergency practice skills (e.g., casting) due to lack of exposure to common low-acuity conditions; and (3) potential for inefficient use of space if there is not sufficient volume of low-acuity patients during hours of operation to continuously fill fast-track rooms with new patients as others complete their visit.

The literature suggests that implementation of a dedicated fast track has the potential to significantly decrease waiting time to see a caregiver, overall length of stay, complaints, and the return visit rate for low-acuity patients suited for care in this setting.[40] While these potential gains clearly benefit patients, some departments struggle with balancing the job satisfaction and educational commitments to staff (especially in relation to trainees, such as resident physicians), and choose to integrate low-acuity patients with all others throughout the department, doing away with the dedicated fast-track concept. Which model to pursue should be carefully considered in the context of these competing interests.

## Conclusions

There are two compelling arguments for observation: improved clinical decision making, with the resultant increased patient safety, and financial benefits. Observation units can convert previously unprofitable hospital admissions into profitable observation stays, while still delivering appropriate evaluation, treatment, and risk stratification to patients. Furthermore, moving patients to an EDOU frees up costly and overcrowded ED resources, such as acute-care treatment rooms, for undifferentiated patients in the waiting room who may be in need of urgent medical attention. The current literature basis for patient management in the observation setting is strongest in several specific conditions. However, future research will likely expand the scope of patients that can be safely managed in the EDOU, which will create more opportunities to divert patients out of the ED and also away from inpatient beds, thus acting as a mitigating force against both ED and hospital overcrowding. In this era of increasing pressure to practice high-quality medicine at lower cost without sacrificing key aspects of care such as patient access or satisfaction, the ED observation unit provides a valuable resource that helps clinicians and administrators meet these challenges.

## References

1. Pitts SR, Niska RW, Xu J, Burt CW. National hospital ambulatory medical care survey: 2006 emergency department summary. *National Health Statistics Reports* 2008; **7**: 1–39.

2. Hogan B, Brachmann M. In-hospital emergency care grows even as the specialty faces staunch political opposition. *Emergency Physicians International* 2010; **02**: 25–6.

3. Graff LG. *Observation Medicine: the Healthcare System's Tincture of Time*. American College of Emergency Physicians. https://acep.org/Physician-Resources/Practice-Resources/Administration/Observation-Medicine (accessed January 2014).

4. Dixit AK, Nalebuff BJ. *Thinking Strategically: the Competitive Edge in Business, Politics, and Everyday Life*. New York, NY: Norton, 1993.

5. Brillman JC, Tandberg D. Observation unit impact on ED admission for asthma. *American Journal of Emergency Medicine* 1994; **12**: 11–14.

6. Baugh CW, Bohan JS. Estimating observation unit profitability with options modeling. *Academic Emergency Medicine* 2008; **15**: 445–52.

7. Schneider EC, Lieberman T. Publicly disclosed information about the quality of health care: response of the US public. *Quality in Health Care* 2001; **10**: 96–103.

8. Radosevich DM. A framework for selecting outcome measures for ambulatory care research. *Journal of Ambulatory Care Management* 1997; **20**: 1–9.

9. Berwick DM, Enthoven A, Bunker JP. Quality management

in the NHS: the doctor's role, I. *BMJ* 1992; **304**: 235–9.

10. Berwick DM, Enthoven A, Bunker JP. Quality management in the NHS: the doctor's role, II. *BMJ* 1992; **304**: 304–8.

11. Peacock WF, Young J, Collins S, Diercks D, Emerman C. Heart failure observation units: optimizing care. *Annals of Emergency Medicine* 2006; **47**: 22–33.

12. Brachmann M, Geppert R, Niehues C, Petersen PF, Sobotta R. Oekonomische Aspekte der klinischen Notfallversorgung. http://www.dgina.de/media/veroeffent/20090729_Positionspapier_2009_07_08_MB_F.pdf (accessed January 2014).

13. Greene J. Nurse groups, administrators battle over mandatory nursing ratios: California law debated on national stage. *Annals of Emergency Medicine* 2009; **54** (3): 31–3.

14. Greenhalgh J, Long AF, Brettle AJ, Grant MJ. Reviewing and selecting outcome measures for use in routine practice. *Journal of Evaluation in Clinical Practice* 1998; **4**: 339–50.

15. McGlynn EA. Introduction and overview of the conceptual framework for a national quality measurement and reporting system. *Medical Care* 2003; **41** (1 Suppl): I1–7.

16. Goddard M, Davies HT, Dawson D, Mannion R, McInnes F. Clinical performance measurement. Part 2: avoiding the pitfalls. *Journal of the Royal Society of Medicine* 2002; **95**: 549–51.

17. Zalenski RJ, McCarren M, Roberts R, *et al.* An evaluation of a chest pain diagnostic protocol to exclude acute cardiac ischemia in the emergency department. *Archives of Internal Medicine* 1997; **157**: 1085–91.

18. Graff L. Chest pain observation units. *Emergency Medicine Journal* 2001; **18**: 148.

19. Cunningham R, Walton MA, Weber JE, *et al.* One-year medical outcomes and emergency department recidivism after emergency department observation for cocaine-associated chest pain. *Annals of Emergency Medicine* 2009; **53**: 310–20.

20. Rydman RJ, Isola ML, Roberts RR, *et al.* Emergency department observation unit versus hospital inpatient care for a chronic asthmatic population: a randomized trial of health status outcome and cost. *Medical Care* 1998; **36**: 599–609.

21. Decker WW, Smars PA, Vaidyanathan L, *et al.* A prospective, randomized trial of an emergency department observation unit for acute onset atrial fibrillation. *Annals of Emergency Medicine* 2008; **52**: 322–8.

22. Ross MA, Compton S, Medado P, *et al.* An emergency department diagnostic protocol for patients with transient ischemic attack: a randomized controlled trial. *Annals of Emergency Medicine* 2007; **50**: 109–19.

23. Rydman RJ, Zalenski RJ, Roberts RR, *et al.* Patient satisfaction with an emergency department chest pain observation unit. *Annals of Emergency Medicine* 1997; **29**: 109–15.

24. Rydman RJ, Roberts RR, Albrecht GL, Zalenski RJ, McDermott M. Patient satisfaction with an emergency department asthma observation unit. *Academic Emergency Medicine* 1999; **6**: 178–83.

25. Barr JK, Giannotti TE, Sofaer S, *et al.* Using public reports of patient satisfaction for hospital quality improvement. *Health Services Research* 2006; **41**: 663–82.

26. Jaffe AS, Babuin L, Apple FS. Biomarkers in acute cardiac disease: the present and the future. *Journal of the American College of Cardiology* 2006; **48**: 1–11.

27. Cheung DS, Kelly JJ, Beach C, *et al.* Improving handoffs in the emergency department. *Annals of Emergency Medicine* 2010; **55**: 171–80.

28. Baker GR, Norton PG, Flintoft V, *et al.* The Canadian adverse events study: the incidence of adverse events among hospital patients in Canada. *CMAJ* 2004; **170**: 1678–86.

29. Roberts R, Graff LG. Economic issues in observation unit medicine. *Emergency Medicine Clinics of North America* 2001; **19**: 19–33.

30. Graff L. *Observation Medicine.* Stroneham: Andover, 1993.

31. Sieck S. Cost effectiveness of chest pain units. *Cardiology Clinics* 2005; **23**: 589–99.

32. Lied TR. Performance measures and batting averages. *Health Affairs (Millwood)* 1999; **18**: 260–1.

33. The President's Advisory Commission on Consumer Protection and Quality in the Health Care Industry: report synopsis. *Caring* 1998; 17: 22–41.

34. Finarelli M. Observation units can improve outcomes, financial performance. *Health Care Strategic Management* 2003; **21** (8): 10–12.

35. McGlynn EA. Selecting common measures of quality and system performance. *Medical Care* 2003; **41** (1 Suppl): I39–47.

36. Siu AL, McGlynn EA, Morgenstern H, *et al.* Choosing quality of care measures based on the expected impact of improved care on health. *Health Services Research* 1992; **27**: 619–50.

37. Bolmey AL. Outcome measures in the health-care industry:

an elusive goal. *Obesity Research* 2002; **10** (Suppl 1): 10S–13S.

38. Nelson EC, Mohr JJ, Batalden PB, Plume SK. Improving health care, part 1: the clinical value compass. *Joint Commission Journal on Quality Improvement* 1996; **22**: 243–58.

39. Brillman J, Mathers-Dunbar L, Graff L, *et al.* Management of observation units. American College of Emergency Physicians.

*Annals of Emergency Medicine* 1995; **25**: 823–30.

40. Wiler JL, Gentle C, Halfpenny JM, *et al.* Optimizing emergency department front-end operations. *Annals of Emergency Medicine* 2010; **55**: 142–61.

## Further reading

Graff LG. *Observation Medicine: the Healthcare System's Tincture of Time*. American College of Emergency Physicians. https://acep.

org/Physician-Resources/Practice-Resources/Administration/Observation-Medicine (accessed January 2014).

# Appendix 22.1. Chest pain observation protocol

I. Exclusion criteria:

  A. Ischemic ECG changes

  B. Troponin or CKMB percentage newly positive

  C. Probability of discharge home within 24 hours < 80%

II. Typical EDOU interventions:

  A. Monitor vital signs q4 hours

  B. Telemetry

  C. Serial ECGs and cardiac markers at 6 hours from initial set

  D. Provocative testing (i.e., ETT, MIBI, ECHO) or coronary CTA at attending discretion

III. Disposition criteria:

  A. Home

    1. ED attending does not suspect cardiac ischemia

    2. Results of any imaging or provocative testing reviewed

  B. Hospital

    1. Ischemia suspected

    2. Any diagnosis requiring further inpatient hospitalization

IV. Time frame:

  8–24 hour observation

| EMERGENCY DEPARTMENT OBSERVATION UNIT<br><br>*PLEASE SIGN & DATE EACH ENTRY* | ADHERE PATIENT IDENTIFICATION HERE |
|---|---|

## ED OBSERVATION ADMIT NOTE

PROTOCOL: **CHEST PAIN**

RELEVANT HISTORY AND PHYSICAL EXAM FINDINGS:

| ☐ CAD risk factors: | ☐ Previous stress test and/or cath results: | ☐ ECG: |
|---|---|---|
| Family history: | ☐ Reviewed and non-contributory ☐ Other | |
| Social history: | ☐ Reviewed and non-contributory ☐ Other | |

OBS INTERVENTIONS:

☐ Monitor vital signs q4 hours ☐ Telemetry ☐ EKG at 6 hours ☐ Cardiac markers at 6 hours

Provocative Testing: ☐ Standard ETT ☐ MIBI ☐ Stress Echo ☐ Other
☐ Coronary CTA ☐ No provocative testing (explain rationale):

MEDICAL DECISION MAKING/GOAL OF OBSERVATION PERIOD:

HOW OFTEN WILL PATIENT BE EVALUATED BY MD/PA: ☐ Q4H ☐ Q6H ☐ Q8H ☐ Q shift

MORNING/DISCHARGE PLAN:

| PCP contacted:<br>☐ Yes ☐ No | PCP name: |
|---|---|
| ☐ Resident ☐ PA | Print name: |

Resident/PA signature: _____ Time & date: _____

### THIS SECTION TO BE COMPLETED ONLY BY THE ATTENDING PHYSICIAN

☐ I have interviewed and examined this patient and I agree with the observation and admission and plan of care as described above. Please see ED visit record for further detail.

Signature of Attending: _____ Date & time: _____

Printed name: _____ Provider ID #: _____

| EMERGENCY DEPARTMENT<br>OBSERVATION UNIT<br><br>*PLEASE SIGN & DATE EACH ENTRY* | ADHERE PATIENT IDENTIFICATION HERE |
|---|---|

## ED OBSERVATION DISCHARGE NOTE

**PRESENTING COMPLAINT:**

**OBSERVATION COURSE:**

☐ EKGs reviewed ☐ Cardiac markers reviewed ☐ Imaging reviewed

☐ Relevant physical exam and VS reviewed
☐ Provocative test or CTA results, if obtained:

Comments:

**DISPOSITION:**

**DISCHARGE DIAGNOSIS:**

**DISCHARGE AND FOLLOW-UP PLAN:**

DISCHARGE INSTRUCTIONS GIVEN: ☐ Yes ☐ No

| Check one: | ☐ Resident ☐ PA | Signature: | Date & time: |
|---|---|---|---|
| PCP Contacted: | ☐ Yes ☐ No | PCP name : | |

### THIS SECTION TO BE COMPLETED ONLY BY THE ATTENDING PHYSICIAN

☐ I have interviewed and examined this patient and participated in the discharge from observation. I agree with the discharge arrangements above.

Signature of Attending: _____ Date & Time: _____

Print name: _____ Provider ID #: _____

☐ Optional: Please see my dictated note on this patient. Dictation #: _____

Chapter

# 23

# Optimizing patient flow through the emergency department

Kirk Jensen and Jody Crane

## Key learning points

- The benefits that improving flow in your emergency department can provide.
- How tools developed in industry can help an emergency department manage and improve flow.
- How an emergency department can implement the necessary methods to optimize patient flow.

## Introduction

One of the most important ways you can improve how well your emergency department (ED) works involves using a concept not limited to healthcare settings, in fact one commonly encountered by businesses of all kinds: flow. We can define *flow* in this sense as the movement of customers through a business operation. In the case of the ED, it is specifically the movement of patients through the department as they are evaluated, treated, and released or admitted to the hospital (Fig. 23.1). At certain points, small changes in the flow of patients can lead to long delays. But small changes you in turn make in managing that flow can also lead to dramatic cuts in the time patients spend in the ED. Making the movement of those patients more effective can thus pay big dividends in improving their satisfaction – and the quality of their care – as well as improving the satisfaction of your staff correspondingly. And this in turn can result in improved financial success for the hospital. In this chapter we will look at some ways to go about improving flow.

## The big picture: a strategic view of flow improvement

Businesses have for years used service operations theory and management principles to understand and manage flow. The key concepts are demand and capacity, queuing, variation, the psychology of waiting, and constraints. They are often interrelated, so understanding all of them helps to give an overall picture of movement within a complex system – as an ED is.

Improving flow will require you to analyze the current processes in your department and then implement some new procedures (Fig. 23.2). Before you begin, though, understanding these theories is a necessary and enlightening first step.

## Matching demand and capacity

In simple terms, *demand* is how many of your resources are being used at a particular moment, and *capacity* is how many resources you have in relation to the number of patients. Matching demand to capacity is an important component of optimizing flow. When demand exceeds capacity, waiting times grow longer and patient frustration increases. Physicians, nurses, and technicians become stressed. When capacity exceeds demand, your resources – human and otherwise – are not being used effectively; in fact, they are being wasted. Patients coming into your department are unscheduled, the number fluctuating randomly, so matching the demand for services to the resources that provide them may seem a hopeless challenge. In fact, however, we have learned that the number of patients who will come to your ED *is predictable*. The arrival of patients, plotted over time, follows a mathematical pattern known as a Poisson arrival pattern. Though specific numbers vary, this pattern holds generally for EDs everywhere.

Because we know what the pattern is, we can implement steps to match the capacity to the demand. Essentially there are two approaches: "smoothing" patient demand, or managing your resources to

*Emergency Department Leadership and Management*, ed. Stephanie Kayden, *et al.* Published by Cambridge University Press.
© Cambridge University Press 2015.

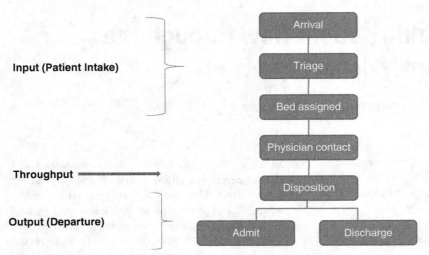

**Figure 23.1** The life cycle of a patient visit. The various stages of a visit to the ED constitute input, throughput, and output. How effectively a patient goes through the stages is flow – smooth or not.

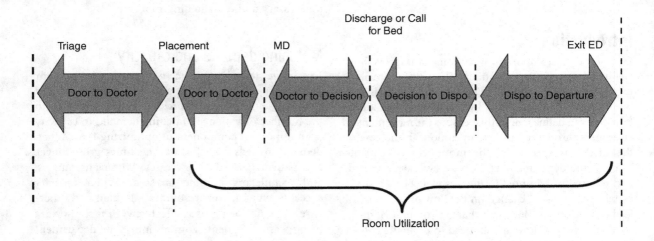

*There are opportunities for performance improvement within each sub-cycle: 4 major intervals and 5 Ds*

**Figure 23.2** The components of patient flow: door to doctor, doctor to decision, decision to disposition, disposition to discharge. Breaking an ED visit into its components and then analyzing the processes in each component presents opportunities to improve those processes and thereby improve flow.

meet that demand. In matching capacity to demand, successful businesses such as McDonald's make use of queuing theory.

## Queuing

The system that patients move through involves a series or network of queues. If you have more than one patient waiting for a service, you have a queue (even one person waiting is technically a queue, but one person waiting usually does not result in problems in the ED). Queuing theory is the mathematical study of waiting lines, developed by engineers to provide models for predicting how systems that serve random arrivals rather than constant or scheduled

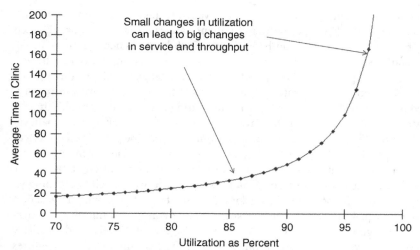

**Figure 23.3** Queue behavior as a function of utilization. Delays start increasing exponentially once usage reaches around 85% of capacity.

Courtesy Chuck Noon, PhD, UT PEMBA

arrivals behave. The first work on queuing theory, which studied telephone traffic congestion causing delays that led to customers hanging up without being served, was published more than a century ago, so the phenomenon is well understood by this point.[1]

An important implication of queuing theory is that as the use of service providers increases, the waiting increases. The problem is that it does not increase proportionally, but exponentially. In other words, when queuing systems with high degrees of variation reach high rates of use, they tend to go bad fast. At usage rates above about 85% of capacity, waiting times take off like a rocket lifting off from the earth (Fig. 23.3).

By those same mathematical principles, however, making small changes that affect the usage rate so that it drops below the takeoff point can have a dramatic impact on waiting times. When you act to match capacity to demand, you reduce the likelihood that queuing will reach that point.

## Variation

We see variation all the time in the ED: patients have different illnesses or injuries requiring different levels of resources and amounts of time to assess and treat; healthcare providers have different levels of skill, training, and experience and take different amounts of time to perform similar actions. Variation can also cause an exponential increase in waiting times: if several patients arrive requiring extensive resources, delays can accumulate for other patients, and again a point is reached where waiting times take off.

The more variation can be smoothed, the more efficient the flow of patients will be. Some of the ways we will look at for matching demand to capacity also help manage variation.

## The psychology of waiting

When waiting is inevitable, businesses have developed methods based on the psychology of waiting to manage those delays. These are built on several observations researchers have made about people waiting.[2] Actions that make waiting *seem* shorter to patients include keeping them occupied, starting the process quickly, calming their anxiety, telling them how long their waiting will likely be, explaining why they are waiting, treating patients equitably in making them wait compared with other patients, and letting them wait with friends or family rather than alone. Another point to keep in mind is that people are more willing to wait when they perceive the service they are waiting for to be valuable. If we consider these actions, frequent communication clearly becomes a key. So does continual monitoring of waiting areas.

## Constraints

We mentioned earlier that the patient's experience in the ED involves a series of queues. When patients enter the ED, their experience consists of a series of interactions with healthcare workers – possibly as many as 20 queuing interfaces. To improve the interactions within this network of queues, you must understand the theory of *constraints*. A management theory introduced by Eliyahu Goldratt about 25 years ago, it defines a constraint as any resource, mindset, or policy that prevents an organization from moving closer to its goal.[3] It classifies a system's resources as "bottlenecks" and "non-bottlenecks" based on the demand placed on them and their capacity. A bottleneck resource has a capacity less than the demand placed on it. In the ED, for instance, triage often forms a bottleneck, when too many patients arrive for the triage nurse to effectively segment without queues forming. A physician is similarly frequently a bottleneck, when more patients appear than that doctor can diagnose and treat efficiently enough to handle the volume. A non-bottleneck resource, on the other hand, has a capacity equal to or greater than the demand placed on it. Changing processes to improve a non-bottleneck resource may make them more efficient but will not improve throughput time in the ED; a hospital, for example, might add a patient care coordinator in the ED – often an effective step. But if adding a coordinator does not improve throughput time as a whole in a particular ED, then the lack of one was not a bottleneck in that ED. Working on bottleneck resources and improving them so that their capacity can meet the demand is the only way to move an organization closer to its goal. Working on non-bottleneck resources does not improve flow – from a patient flow perspective it is a waste of time.

To manage constraints, an ED needs to repeatedly remove or reduce the constraint constituting the greatest relative bottleneck. In the queuing framework, managing bottlenecks means moving critical constraints from high states of utilization to lower states of utilization, thus realizing the exponential benefits in flow achieved by optimizing the performance and capacity of the scarcest resources.

## The operational details: how to manage flow

Once you understand the principles that underlie flow management, you can put into practice procedures based on them. Because the concepts are interrelated, the procedures often are as well; using a method to match capacity with demand, for example, can affect variation as well. In this section we examine a number of specific ways to improve flow in your ED.

### Measuring patient demand

To match your capacity to the demand requires measuring patient demand and then developing a system

to meet it. You want the answers to these questions: How many patients are coming into your ED each month? Each day? Each hour? When are they coming during the day? As the Poisson pattern indicates, these numbers are predictable. To obtain them, track data in your ED over time and analyze the pattern, then match your staffing coverage at particular times – of the day, of the week, of the year – to the pattern. Determine not only the numbers but what services these patients will require at various times; plot use of lab and radiology services at different times, for instance, and plan your service capacity accordingly.

In tracking the data, break the patient arrivals into categories such as chief complaint, number of emergency service arrivals, severity levels, and ancillary utilization. Knowing the patterns in these categories enables you to predict specific numbers for your department. Also predictable is that variation will occur, so in addition to matching service capacity to patient demand in advance by tracking the data, develop a plan for how you will respond when the demand rises unexpectedly. An ED can, for example, arrange for patients who need beds and are going to be admitted to board in hallways of inpatient units rather than in the ED, and for patient overflow during peak hours it can arrange to use the vacated space of units that operate only during daytime hours. Training staff to perform some functions of another position if necessary is another method that can alleviate high demand – having technicians start intravenous administration, or having a triage nurse who does not have any patients at the moment help discharge patients from the nearby fast track – and track variation in detail to discern patterns in it as well, for they do occur even in random variation. For a more detailed discussion on predicting demand and handling it, see Mayer and Jensen's work on flow.[4]

### Shaping demand

You may think you can do nothing to affect patient demand, and that all your efforts to improve flow should be directed toward managing service capacity. In fact, though, you can take some steps to shape demand. One is to introduce and publicize scheduled appointments for less acute complaints. Another is to promote vaccination for the flu among your patients and in your community. Decreasing the number of people likely to come down with an illness shapes the resulting demand for your department's services.

## Segmenting patient flow

Dividing patients into segments or streams based on the severity of their condition allows you to effectively handle multiple patients simultaneously, and to smooth flow. In emergency medicine, there are three basic streams of patients based on their condition – low acuity, mid acuity, and high acuity. A system based on the Emergency Severity Index (ESI), which provides five levels in which to sort patients, further refines the streams.[5] (Other five-level triage systems are equally effective for segmenting patient flow by severity and resource needs: see Chapter 19.) By segmenting streams of patients, you create unique pathways customized for each particular stream and can design individual processes for each. Patients in one stream follow the same basic steps throughout their visit. The basic streams may divide further: for instance, the high-acuity stream may subdivide into substreams of acute heart attack, acute stroke, acute traumatic injury, and acute life-threatening infection with end-organ compromise. Each of these substreams would have a well-defined process with separate steps.

Patients who fall into the two least severe categories (4 and 5 in the ESI segmentation model), and many in the middle category (3), can be fast-tracked. Fast track, we emphasize, is something you *do*, not somewhere you put patients (for more on this concept, see Jensen and colleagues' work on flow[6]). Your fast-track process should enable you to quickly and efficiently assess and treat patients whose complaints are not severe. You should make sure you have appropriate fast-track staff to meet demand, particularly in the hours when you know the demand will be highest.

## Triage: removing a potential bottleneck

Look closely at your triage process, because it can easily become a bottleneck to patient flow. As with fast track, triage is something you *do* and not somewhere you put patients. Consider whether some aspects of triage would fit more effectively at another stage in the process. Triage should be brief: gather information sufficient to direct the patient into a segment based on severity of condition.

EDs traditionally have had four different queues that all patients enter: triage, physician assessment, treatment, and discharge. Each queue makes the patient wait. An alternative approach is to use a one-queue process, in which patients receive assessment, treatment, and discharge in one series of steps,

without additional waiting times. Team triage is an effective way to implement this process.[7] The team consists of several providers, including nurses and doctor, as well as mid-level providers, such as physician assistants or nurse practitioners, who can diagnose and treat patients more fully than a nurse can but not as fully as a physician can, and lab and radiology technicians, who quickly assess and register patients, then send them to a treatment area or a results-waiting area (both nearby). The least severe and the most severe streams can be efficiently sorted into the proper channel for treatment, either the fast track or a bed. The mid-level patients can be treated in the team triage area and discharged. This is one process that helps prevent a bottleneck from forming in triage.

## Optimizing your resources

If you want to improve flow in your ED (Fig. 23.4), having the right staff, the right staff mix, and the appropriate amount of staffing to meet projected demand is critical. Hiring and motivating excellent staff is the beginning point. As we noted in regard to triage, forming an effective team from physicians, nurses, mid-level providers, and technicians is equally important. And as we emphasized in regard to the fast track and predicting demand in general in the ED, so is having enough resources in place to handle that demand and provide high-quality care. Fast-tracking patients is one of the most effective actions you can take to improve flow – but the fast-track process must include sufficient staff, space, and resources.

The results waiting area is where patients who do not need beds can stay while awaiting results of lab work or tests. Monitor this area closely and keep in mind the practices emphasized in our discussion of the psychology of waiting. Providing magazines or televisions, for example, helps keep patients occupied and reduces anxiety.

We mentioned the importance of sorting patients into the right channel. Determining who needs a bed is a key component. Not all patients in the ED need beds. You should consider beds as scarce resources, and directing patients who do not need one into the fast track, or to results waiting, or for treatment in team triage rather than into a bed is a means of avoiding bottlenecks. To borrow from business again, we can point to restaurants and the concept of turning over tables. The more you turn over beds,

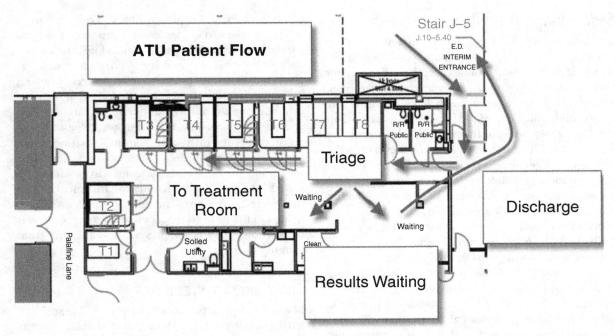

**Figure 23.4** Streamlined front-end ED patient flow. Layout of your ED affects flow. ATU, advanced treatment unit.

the more patients you can treat with the same high level of care – you are increasing capacity without adding any resources. We like to use the phrase "keep your vertical patients vertical" – in other words, patients with less acute needs should keep moving without occupying beds. Make sure you have processes established with specific criteria for who needs a bed and who does not.

Obviously, your staff members are critical resources. To optimize their effectiveness, they should concentrate on carrying out only the tasks that they are best suited to perform. Doctors, in other words, should not be carrying out activities that secretaries or scribes can do. Nurses should not be entering data on computers. In addition, persons in these roles should constantly perform those functions they are suited for and intended to perform. Physicians should be kept busy seeing patients.

---

**Case study 23.1.   The virtual bed**

Responding to a nearly limitless volume of patients in its urban setting, the ED staff at Metropolitan Hospital implemented the concept of a physician in triage, starting a shift from 11 a.m. to 7 p.m. consisting of a physician, a technician, and a nurse in a project known as "Virtual Bed." The team operated directly behind triage, and instead of placing the

---

patient back in the waiting room the triage nurses would move the patient to the treatment area. There, the physician would perform a brief exam, order the necessary diagnostic tests, and begin any basic treatment that could be initiated at that point. The patient would then be sent back out to the waiting area where the lab and radiology would begin the necessary tests, placed in a set of rooms labeled "Virtual Beds." When the testing was complete, the patients would be moved to the back and discharged by a treating physician.

The benefits of this system were undeniable. The patient would be seen by a physician within minutes of arrival, was quickly made "in-process," and had pain or other pressing issues addressed promptly. The waiting time had turned into "results waiting" time and the patient length of stay dropped.

## Keeping track of your patients

Tracking arrival patterns is not the only type of data collection you should do. Keep track of patients' progress through the system while they are moving through it. A real-time dashboard enables you to accomplish this goal, either a simple whiteboard with patients listed along with where they are in the process or a more complex computer system with clearly visible monitors showing these details and more. A patient-care team should monitor progress and results; a secretary or technician should physically accompany patients to their next location in the process when results are available.

Tracking patients as they flow through the system allows you to tell quickly when bottlenecks begin to occur, so that you can act to reduce them before backlogs cause demand to reach the takeoff point. It also helps you predict your future needs for service capacity.

## Facilitating admissions

One cause of delays in the ED is the admission process to the hospital for those patients who need to enter. To address this issue, keep track of times from the decision to admit a patient to when he or she actually is admitted and record the reasons for the delays. Having this information will help you understand why delays are occurring, and it also helps you predict how many patients will need admission and what units they will go to (since this flow of patients also follows a Poisson pattern). Use the results of your tracking to communicate in advance likely numbers of patients who will be admitted, and the times of admission, to the hospital staff members responsible for placing patients.

If your ED is boarding significant numbers of patients, then flow can be impaired seriously. Taking steps to reduce this boarding is one of the most effective actions you can take to improve flow. Improving the admission process as we just discussed is one way. Another is to convince the hospital to implement a process whereby patients waiting for rooms can be moved to the hallways of the units where they will be admitted rather than remaining in the ED.

## Collaborating with ancillary services

Improving flow means working not only with your team in the treatment area but also with ancillary services such as the radiology department, the lab, the pharmacy, and even housekeeping. Cutting delays even by just a little with each step can reduce bottlenecks. For example, having an x-ray technician note visibly with a card attached to a patient's chart "x-ray back" and putting the chart in the ED doctor's inbox can reduce waiting time for that patient. Cumulatively, such reductions in waiting time can cut overall delays in the department significantly.

Work with housekeeping in admitting patients. Housekeeping staff should be kept involved in the

projection of likely admissions and in identifying empty beds as soon as they are available. Effective communication and coordination in this aspect of operations can have a significant impact on boarding in the ED and thus is one way to reduce bottlenecks and improve flow noticeably.

Examine the current processes for interaction between the ED and these other sections and try to identify similar steps, even small ones, that can improve flow and reduce delays by adjusting processes.

---

**Case study 23.2. Super track, super results**

The fast track in the ED at Acme Medical Center was typical of many in that if the main area of the ED was overrun, sick patients would overflow into the fast track, and the flow of lower-acuity patients would essentially cease. The average length of stay of low-acuity patients at the time was over two and a half hours. A flow-improvement team designed a new super track, moving supplies it needed out of the supply storage system and into a cart in the area and moving critical equipment such as printers and computers to the area to virtually eliminate the need for the providers to leave. The team assessed the arrival rates and service rates and projected length of stay to arrive at the right combination of physician assistants, nurses, and beds based on the time available to see patients. Team members ran several pilots of the new concept and proved quickly that they could see 60% more patients with 33% less staff and 75% fewer beds. The team was able to reduce the length of stay of ESI Level 4 and 5 patients from an average of two and a half hours to about 50 minutes.

---

## Putting the theories and methods to work

In implementing methods to improve flow, you will find that using an established system of operational management will help you do so more effectively. A number of such systems exist, such as Lean management, Six Sigma, and total quality management. Health care recently has seen Lean management adapted for its specific needs.

## Lean management

Lean management is an approach to operations management resulting from an intensive study of why Toyota has been so successful for the last half-century. The approach focuses on processes and on developing people. Its implementation into health care started in aspects that were direct crossovers from manufacturing, such as inventory management. More recently, it has become more prevalent in clinical operations such as EDs and operating rooms. Lean management is characterized by several key components: creating patient value, eliminating waste, promoting flow, making continuous improvement, and developing people.

We noted in our discussion of segmenting patient flow that patients in one stream should follow the same steps. This idea incorporates the Lean principles of creating patient value and eliminating waste. All of the activities in a patient process can be classified as value-added or non-value-added. Value-added activities are those steps that move the patient closer to wellness, services that patients desire, services done right the first time. Physician examination is a good example of a value-added step. This is, after all, the main reason a patient comes to the ED in the first place. Other examples would be use of labs and radiographs – but only if they change the management of the patient's course through the system for the better or otherwise enhance the patient's well-being – the psychological well-being, for example, of knowing he or she does not have a fracture. Non-value-added activities are those steps that do not create patient value and that patients do not want. "Traditional" triage is a classic example of a non-value-added activity. No patient comes to the ED to be interviewed by a nurse in order to determine how long the patient can wait. At the extreme, triaging a patient when there are idle physicians and available beds is an obvious example of a wasteful step.

The Lean concept of waste addresses how to manage non-value-added activities. The goal is to eliminate as much waste as possible (you cannot eliminate it entirely). Lean management identifies a number of forms of waste; in healthcare settings, these translate to such actions as:

- Moving equipment back and forth through the ED.
- Keeping patients in remote areas of the ED or running around the department looking for supplies or equipment.
- Keeping inventory that is not in use.
- Waiting, the most obvious form of waste in healthcare, which permeates the entire patient experience in just about any healthcare setting.

- Overprocessing or doing more than the patient needs, such as multiple providers asking redundant questions or insisting on triage protocols rather than getting the patient in front of the provider and ordering only what is necessary.
- Overproduction, such as generating reports that go unread.
- Not doing an activity right the first time (known as defects), resulting in having to go back and ask the patient a question again because a provider did not document the encounter as it occurred, or having to order a test or medication because the wrong one was ordered initially.
- Not using your human resources to actively engage in problem solving and process improvement.

The goal of improvement efforts under Lean management is to create value and eliminate waste within processes, continually increasing the amount of value-added activity relative to the amount of non-value-added activity, and thus increasing the *value-added ratio*.

Organizations using Lean management place frontline employees in control of improving the system, as these people are the ones who will have the best answers. Such organizations empower these staff members by teaching them tools to help them improve their workplace. These organizations typically implement over 90% of employee improvement suggestions, and continually examine and improve processes.

For more information on the development and implementation of Lean management, see the work of Womack *et al.* and Spear.[8,9] For its specific implementation in health care, see the white paper on the subject from the Institute for Healthcare Improvement.[10]

## Plan–do–study–act cycles

Improvement efforts, to succeed, require tests of their effectiveness and subsequent adjustment. The "plan–do–study–act" (PDSA) cycle is a key component of your process to improve flow.[11] You should run small testing cycles often rather than large ones infrequently. Under the PDSA process, you propose one change and test it for a short time.

The "plan" phase involves defining the objective and diagramming how it should be attained; specifically, what do you want to do in this cycle, who should do it, and where and when should it be carried out? Consider what you are trying to learn from the test.

The "do" phase involves implementing the plan, during which you should document any problems and observations. You organize the data you have collected during the test and start to analyze them. "Study" means analyzing fully what you learned in the test and summarizing the lessons. "Act" means deciding what changes you need to make in this plan if you are going to implement it permanently.

You then repeat the cycle, testing your change on a wider scale and assessing any adjustments, and develop new ideas to test. This process helps ensure that ideas that seem promising actually work to improve flow; testing them on a small scale and continuing to test and adjust as a result of what you learn will lead to changes that actually are effective in improving flow. Such a process helps keep your staff engaged in the improvement efforts and active in examining processes and seeking better ways to operate your ED.

## Hiring and staffing

As we have emphasized, the team of healthcare professionals you put in place in your department is critical in improving flow. Getting the right team for the ED begins with focusing on hiring the right people. Once they are in place, making sure they receive the training they need, evaluating their performance, and coaching them for better performance are key actions. If people are what make organizational change effective, having the right people is crucial. Having motivated staff members empowered to examine processes, suggest changes, and help implement and test those changes will go a long way toward achieving your goals for improving flow.

---

**Case study 23.3. Building in flow**

Nightingale Hospital opened a new facility 10 miles from its main facility. During the design process, administrators asked the ED team to review the ED design in the new facility. Experienced at implementing projects to improve flow, the team was able to architecturally hardwire the principles it had developed at the main site, making flow in the new department more efficient by complementing the operational design with the layout. It contains twice as many triage rooms as originally planned, and an internal waiting room was added between the intake area and the main ED to facilitate keeping vertical patients vertical. In addition, the rooms were stocked with all of the supplies to treat most patients. The new facility was budgeted to see about 25 000 annual patient visits, but immediately handled volumes amounting to about 40 000 annual visits. The average time from arrival to seeing a doctor is 30 minutes. Length of stay averages a little over two hours, and the walk-out rate has been less than 1% every month since it opened. Patient satisfaction is usually above the 90th percentile. Carts replaced specialized rooms, so that any procedure could be done in any room.

## The impact of smoothing flow

Improving flow brings multiple benefits to your ED. It creates a more pleasant environment for both patients and staff, increasing customer satisfaction and employee fulfillment. In doing so, it provides a safer department and enables your staff to consistently provide high-quality care.[12–14] Achieving improved flow allows you to increase service capacity without necessarily adding new resources, by making existing resources more effective, adding value to the steps in your processes, and reducing waste in your system. All of these improvements also, on a practical level, will increase the profitability of your hospital.[4,6,15–17]

---

## References

1. Erlang AK. The theory of probabilities and telephone conversations. *Nyt Tidsskrift for Matematik* 1909; **20B**: 33–9.

2. Maister DH. The psychology of waiting lines. In JA Czepiel *et al.*, eds. *The Service Encounter: Managing Employee/Customer Interaction in Service Business*. Lexington, MA, Lexington Books, 1985; 113–23.

3. Goldratt E. *The Goal*. Great Barrington, MA: North River Press, 1986.

4. Mayer T, Jensen K. *Hardwiring Flow: Systems and Processes for Seamless Patient Flow*. Gulf Breeze, FL: Fire Starter, 2009.

5. Gilboy N, Tanabe P, Travers D, Rosenau A, Eitel DR. *Emergency Severity Index, Version 4: Implementation Handbook*. AHRQ Publication No. 05–0046–2. Rockville, MD: Agency for Healthcare Research and Quality,

2005. http://www.ahrq.gov/research/esi (accessed January 2014).

6. Jensen K, Mayer TA, Welch SJ, Haradan C. *Leadership for Smooth Patient Flow*. ACHE Management Series. Chicago, IL: Health Administration Press, 2007.

7. Patel PB, Vinson DR. Team assignment system: expediting emergency department care. *Annals of Emergency Medicine* 2005; **46**: 499–506.

8. Womack J, Jones DT, Roos D. *The Machine That Changed the World: the Story of Lean Production*. New York, NY: Free Press, 1990.

9. Spear SJ. *Chasing the Rabbit: How Market Leaders Outdistance the Competition*. New York, NY: McGraw-Hill, 2009.

10. Institute for Healthcare Improvement. *Going Lean in Health Care*. IHI Innovation Series white paper. Cambridge, MA: IHI, 2005. http://www.ihi.org/resources/Pages/IHIWhitePapers/GoingLeaninHealthCare.aspx (accessed January 2014).

11. Langley J, Nolan K, Nolan T, Norman C, Provost L. *The Improvement Guide*. San Francisco, CA: Jossey-Bass, 1996.

12. Institute of Medicine. *To Err is Human: Building a Safer Health System*. Washington, DC, National Academies Press, 2000.

13. Leape LL, Berwick DM. Five years after To Err Is Human: what have we learned? *JAMA* 2005; **293**: 2384–90.

14. Wears RL, Vincent CA. The history of safety in healthcare. In P Croskerry, KS Cosby, SM Schenkel, RL Wears, eds., *Patient Safety in Emergency Medicine*. Philadelphia, PA: Lippincott Williams & Wilkins, 2009; 8–11.

15. Leatherman S, Berwick D, Iles D, *et al*. The business case for quality: case studies and an analysis. *Health Affairs (Millwood)* 2009; **22**(2): 17–30.

16. Martin LA, Neumann CW, Mountford J, Bisognano M, Nolan TW. *Increasing Efficiency and Enhancing Value in Health Care: Ways to Achieve Savings in Operating Costs per Year*. IHI Innovation Series white paper. Cambridge, MA: IHI, 2005. http://www.ihi.org/IHI/Results/WhitePapers/IncreasingEfficiencyEnhancingValueinHealthCareWhitePaper.htm (accessed January 2014).

17. Nolan T, Bisognano M. Finding the balance between quality and cost. *Healthcare Financial Management* 2006; **60** (4): 66–72.

Chapter

# 24

# Emergency department overcrowding

Venkataraman Anantharaman and Puneet Seth

## Key learning points

- Emergency department overcrowding is multifactorial.
- Emergency department overcrowding can have a negative impact on the patient, the staff, and the entire organization.
- Solutions to emergency department overcrowding focus on patient input, throughput, and output.

## Introduction

Emergency department (ED) overcrowding is a common phenomenon in most countries across the world. It is characterized by patients waiting for hours before being seen by a doctor, spending many hours in an ED before definite disposition decisions are made, and/or staying for hours or days before being transferred to an inpatient hospital bed. In all these circumstances there is overwhelming of ED resources in the absence of a disaster or a mass casualty incident. Its consequences include impaired quality of care, endangered patients' safety, impaired staff morale, and increased costs.

## Definitions

There have been previous attempts to define over-crowding in EDs. Some are based on waiting times for initial consultation.[1] Some consider overcrowding a result of lengthy ED management processes. Many regard the presence of patients in the ED awaiting placement in the inpatient wards (ED boarding or access block) as an indicator that the ED is over-crowded. Overcrowding would be seen when all or some of those three situations occur. Some available definitions include:

- a situation where patients in the ED requiring inpatient care are unable to gain access to appropriate hospital beds within a reasonable time frame[2]
- a situation where the demand for ED services exceeds the ability to provide care within a reasonable time[3]
- a situation in which the identified need for emergency services outstrips available ED resources[4]

ED overcrowding has got to do with critical numbers of patients whose initial care process gets interrupted and cannot proceed promptly owing to a holdup in one or more hospital areas. The critical number depends on the size of the institution and the discomfort threshold of that community for waiting in the ED. The term "overcrowding" reflects the symptom rather than the cause of care processes that go far beyond the hospital, in terms of either large ED patient "input" or moving patients through for prompt reversion to ambulatory management. Telltale signs suggesting ED overcrowding include:[4]

- patients being treated in hallways
- hospitals sending away/diverting ambulances
- patients stuck in EDs owing to lack of inpatient beds
- patient care not meeting the community's quality standards

## Consequences of ED overcrowding

The ED is a place of immense unpredictability. A surge in patient numbers, with accompanying anxious family members or friends, results in many negative effects.

---

*Emergency Department Leadership and Management*, ed. Stephanie Kayden, *et al.* Published by Cambridge University Press.
© Cambridge University Press 2015.

## Consequences for the patient

The individual patient may be affected in multiple ways:

- **Patients may leave without being seen**, resulting in delay in consultation and care. Their symptoms may carry graver diagnoses than initial presentation suggests.
- **Prolonged stay of critically ill patients** leads to worse outcomes.[5] This is particularly true for patients needing intensive care.
- **Longer waiting times** until first consultation with the ED physician lead to inordinate delays in appropriate treatment. Some aspects deserve special attention:[5]

  (a) Delay in pain relief. The longer consult times naturally result in later administration of appropriate analgesics.

  (b) Delay in time-critical interventions. This includes entities such as percutaneous coronary interventions for acute myocardial infarction,[6] thrombolysis for acute stroke, craniotomy for extradural hemorrhage, laparotomy for perforated viscus, etc. Outcomes for all these instances are likely to be worse with such delays.

  (c) Patient dissatisfaction and more frequent complaints. Patients are likely to experience unhappiness and dissatisfaction when their suffering is prolonged. This translates into negative vocal and written feedback, flaring of tempers, and a general deterioration of the ED atmosphere.

  (d) Risk of infectious disease. Prolonged presence of a large number of people in a limited floor area such as the ED has grave implications for the spread of infectious diseases. A patient with an airborne infection risks infecting others in a crowded ED. This constitutes a serious public health challenge.

  (e) Compromise of patient privacy. Patient privacy is more likely to be compromised, in varying degrees, when overcrowding occurs.[7] Patients being treated in hallways are often not in a position to be mindful of their state of dress. Doctors unable to find satisfactory examination space might be tempted to take short cuts to expedite assessment and treatment.

Patients requiring unplanned admissions are most affected by access block. Affected groups include the elderly, those with chronic and complex conditions, nursing-home patients whose conditions are exacerbated by cold weather, and children. Access block for these patients leads to a greater incidence of medical errors, adverse events, delays in medical treatment, reduced access to diagnostic and sometimes therapeutic facilities, and inefficient case management.

## Consequences for the organization (the hospital and the community)

- **Increased ambulance diversions** result in longer run times, reduced availability of emergency vehicles, and increased potential for poor outcomes for their emergency patients.[8] This places an unnecessary burden on the ambulance service:

  (a) It becomes less productive, because more ambulances are "busy" at any point in time.

  (b) The number of ambulances available for individual or mass casualty calls is compromised.

  (c) There is no clear evidence that ambulance diversions actually help ameliorate ED overcrowding. Diverting ambulances may temporarily lessen the patient load in the index ED, but, in addition to delaying the care of patients, many of whom may require transfer back to the index department at the patient's parent hospital, the increased workload on the receiving EDs, the negative feelings generated amongst ED colleagues, and the impact on their overcrowding are often not appreciated. A ban on ambulance diversions in Massachusetts, USA, in 2009 did not worsen ED wait times. Moreover, an Oregon Health & Science University study demonstrated that each hour spent on diversions resulted in US$1086 in forgone hospital revenues.[9] With an increase in staffed ICU beds from 47 to 67, diversions decreased from 307 to 114 hours monthly, with US$175 000 in additional monthly revenues from ambulance patients.

  (d) Some communities have developed policies to ensure control measures are in place before going on diversion.[10] In practice, the ease of diverting ambulances versus implementing strict in-hospital patient flow discipline has meant that lip service is usually paid to these policies, and ambulance diversions have become the norm in many communities.

- **Long ED length of stay (LOS).** This would not reflect well on the efficiency of ED patient flow. In societies that publish wait times and length of stay, the need to maintain a good reputation for prompt care delivery is crucial to ensure continuous support from hospital and community.

- **Prolonged inpatient LOS.** This leads to increased cost of inpatient care. Bill size comparisons do not augur well for hospitals whose EDs have a major crowding problem.

- **Increased inpatient mortality.** Access block contributes significantly to increased inpatient mortality, especially at 10 days.[11]

- **Increased medical errors.** With the same number of nurses serving more patients within the ED, medical errors become more likely.[5,12] This has medicolegal implications for the hospital.

## Consequences for ED staff

- **Increased stress among nurses.** EDs that experience routine overcrowding are likely to have nurses who are "burnt out" or fatigued.[13]

- **Nurse recruitment or retention.** Nurses often leave for other departments or vocations because of unreasonable workloads. This poses problems and challenges with recruitment, and with retention of a limited pool of skilled nurses and other ancillary staff.

- **Provider stress and dissatisfaction.** ED doctors also report high levels of dissatisfaction when constantly exposed to overcrowding. In spite of high expectations from patients, there is an ever-rising risk of litigation because decisions made under duress and inappropriate work environments are more likely to be erroneous.[14] This leads to lower quality of care and/or flight of talent.

- **Negative impact on teaching and research.** ED physicians are under constant pressure to attend to the critically ill and "clear the queue." In such circumstances, research projects and teaching of students and residents are compromised.

- **Confrontations among patients, family, ED staff.** When the number of individuals being served far exceeds service capability, tempers are likely to flare. These confrontations worsen patient satisfaction and staff morale.

- **Friction between disciplines.** The pressure to get a disposition plan, coupled with lack of inpatient beds, often leads to confrontations between ED physicians and inpatient colleagues.[14]

## Misconceptions about ED overcrowding

Over the years many myths about the causes and effects of overcrowding have been perpetuated by those refusing to recognize this as a health-service-wide issue. Some of these myths include:[15]

- **"Primary care patients are the main cause of ED overcrowding."** It is the relative unavailability of primary care physicians on nights and weekends that contributes to their increased ED visits. A US literature review published in 2008 revealed the following:[16]

  (a) Uninsured patients are no more likely to make a non-urgent ED visit than those with private insurance, and they are under-represented in the ED for primary-care-type visits compared with their population profile. This may be owing to unwillingness to seek ED care, given its cost.

  (b) Private family physicians' clinics have seen a significant decrease in uninsured patients. As a result, ED visits for conditions that could have been prevented with adequate primary care have increased.

Constant attention to primary care as the cause of ED overcrowding results in less time and resources to focus on the real issues that result in overcrowding, and persistence of this belief is detrimental to finding real solutions.[17] Removing one-fifth of such patients would be expected to reduce ED workload by less than 5%, and would therefore have only a marginal impact on overcrowding.[18]

- **"Arrangements with other health centers can be activated when the ED is overcrowded to transfer some patients there."** The logistics required for such transfers are massive, and numbers transferred are usually inadequate to improve the ED situation.

- **"Get more doctors and nurses to manage the additional patients waiting for beds."** This ignores the fact that ED overcrowding is a daily affair. Hardly any society in the world has spare doctors able to drop tools and work in overcrowded EDs where they are likely not familiar with departmental procedures, further adding to the confusion.
- **"Cancel elective procedures in the hospital or reschedule these when the ED is overcrowded."** This is usually to the detriment of the hospital. Such cancellations and rescheduling lead to unhappy elective patients and longer times to elective surgery. The effort and cost involved is high and should not be underestimated.
- **"Once admitted, the same level of care is provided regardless of patient location."** Admitted patients are generally managed more promptly if they are close to their dedicated discipline's ward. The ED, being usually fairly far away from such dedicated wards, is not the best environment to carry out all the various aspects of management by non-ED-based doctors.
- **"The ED should solve its own overcrowding problem. There is nothing my department can do about it."** This point of view fails to take into consideration that access block is a major cause of ED overcrowding, and that patient flow through inpatient services and access to urgent and emergent procedures have a significant impact on ED overcrowding.

## Causes of ED overcrowding
### "Input" of patients to the ED

**Case study 24.1**

A prime example of many primary care patients contributing to ED numbers occurred in Singapore in the early 1980s.[19] Sustained public education measures and a number of social interventions decreased such ED visits significantly. This effort also involved ensuring easy access to primary care and encouraging the setting up of 24-hour primary care clinics in various parts of the country. As a result, pure primary care attendance at EDs decreased from nearly 50% to below 10%. Whether such measures will work similarly in another community would be conjecture.

Instances of primary care patients frequenting EDs can be seen in many communities around the world, with local variations. There are a number of common reasons why such patients present to the ED:

- **Lack of easy access to primary care.**[20] Though a common contributor to increased ED census, it is hardly the main factor in overcrowding. In communities with inappropriately limited access to primary care, the ED functions as a safety net and allows access to those denied such services.
- **Use of the ED for access to specialist physicians.** Many EDs tend to have arrangements with outpatient clinics for priority in terms of the waiting times to consult other specialists. This arrangement may be taken advantage of by patients or primary care physicians.
- **Use of ED by uninsured, non-urgent patients.** Most countries have legislation that mandates EDs to attend to all emergencies regardless of ability to pay. In some, where ED services are free, people tend to present with non-urgent complaints to avoid the inconvenience of visiting primary care clinics. In societies where charges for ED care are significantly higher than at primary care, the family physician may be a lower-cost alternative.
- **A high-acuity patient population in the community.** This includes areas with large numbers of elderly people or industrial areas with higher likelihood of work accidents. High-acuity patients are a valid group to be seen at EDs. The presence of large numbers of such patients begets the need to ensure adequate staffing and facility resources for appropriate care.

### Patient flow through the ED

**Case study 24.2**

There are 60 persons in an ED waiting area, of whom 20 have no seating space. They are waiting to be seen, or for physician's repeat review, procedures for minor injuries, radiology, appointment letters, discharge prescriptions, or the pharmacy. Some are relatives of patients. The critical care and resuscitation areas have 10 patients, each with acute potentially life-threatening problems and some of whom are being jointly reviewed with colleagues from other medical disciplines. A total of nine ED nurses and five ED doctors are on duty. A process review report of that ED has just been released and shows a patient consultation process with 11 stages, four of which may be unnecessary. Nurse staffing is only at 60% of budgeted strength. There is also no dedicated area for ED observation care. The ED chief is at wit's end as to how to use the report to improve patient flow.

Positive and negative approaches to ED patient flow are possible:

- **Shortage of medical and nursing staff to manage inflow of patients**. This can easily become the rate-limiting step in the processing of clinical workload, despite best efforts by ED staff to prioritize the tasks at hand.[21] What constitutes adequate medical staffing for an ED will depend on case mix, care processes, and time taken for each of these. Some EDs have determined staffing–patient ratios required for optimal patient care, considering these factors and matching staff deployment with patient arrivals.
- **Inefficient ED processes, with patients spending the bulk of their ED time waiting for definitive procedures**. ED processes need critical review, preferably by a workgroup comprising both ED and non-ED personnel. Redundant processes might hamper quick patient disposition. Examples of poor processes include serial conduct of many steps in the ED care regimen, poor signage for patients looking for radiology, toilets, pharmacy, etc., failure to match manpower with patient flow intensity, and lack of guidelines and protocols for junior doctors dealing with common emergencies and other hospital departments, resulting in unnecessary lateral referrals.
- **Shortage of floor space, resulting in the available area becoming overwhelmed with patients quickly and frequently**. Many EDs have been designed to accommodate patient loads anticipated at the time of planning of the hospital, and based on unrealistically short process times.[22] When these process times do not become reality, crowding becomes the norm. Increasingly, EDs must undertake innovative approaches to manage patients in smaller floor areas. The space crunch also affects patient privacy, which may be crucial in some cultures. Lack of ED floor space often, then, becomes a bottleneck in patient flow and management (see Chapter 17).

- **Increasing age, complexity, and acuity of patients presenting to the ED**.[22] With rising healthcare standards, people live longer despite complex medical conditions. This, combined with rising expectations, places an additional burden on the ED. Frequently, such patients resuscitated in the ED spend hours waiting for an ICU bed, thus clogging up the resuscitation area and keeping the nurses busy. Even for those not requiring acute resuscitation, it takes longer to manage a patient with multiple medical issues compared to, for example, one with angina pectoris.

## "Output" of patients from the ED

> **Case study 24.3**
>
> By 2:30 p.m. at Central City Hospital the ED has seen 112 patients. Nearly 30 have been admitted. Another 24 are awaiting bed allocation. After accommodating 15 patients in the ED observation unit (EDOU), another nine are on trolleys along the main ED corridor. There are only 12 discharges from the inpatient wards that morning and another three hours are required for their out-processing. Some patients in the observation unit are feeling unwell and repeatedly pressing the nurse call-bell without receiving prompt attention. One patient is screaming and threatening to sue the hospital. Another is crying in pain. An elderly gentleman wants a urinal. Nurses are trying to complete treatment orders, serve food, and provide bedpans. Some of them yell back at patients to wait a little longer.
>
> The chairman of the hospital just opened a transit admissions ward an hour earlier. By 3:15 p.m., all nine corridor patients are cleared and 12 of the 15 lodgers in the EDOU have been moved to the new ward. The nurses have just completed attending to the two needy patients. The nurse in charge has not seen a quieter EDOU for some time.

Perhaps the most frustrating aspect of overcrowding is having to cope with patients who have been seen, and require inpatient care, but are physically still in the ED. Common causes of this are as follows:

- **Lack of inpatient beds for admitted ED patients**. Most hospitals regard an occupancy rate of 85% at 23:59 hours as the maximum level for efficiency and a threshold for declaration of full house.[23] Some even report more than 90% occupancy. Inpatient bed occupancy rates above 85%, rather than increased numbers of low-acuity patients in the ED, is the commonest cause of overcrowding Most communities cope well with large numbers of low-acuity patients. Systems fail when access block sends the numbers of boarders skyrocketing in the ED. Sometimes the issue is specifically a lack of intensive care beds. Some communities have seen sharp declines in the number of total inpatient beds over the last two decades, in spite of increasing proportions of high-acuity patients requiring critical care presenting to their EDs. In the United States, for example, total inpatient beds decreased by 39% between 1981 and 1999 because of managed-care hospital cost-containment strategies, while ED requirements for inpatient beds increased.[24] In Canada the five years between 1995 and 2000 saw a 40% reduction in hospital beds.[25] The planned decreases did not, apparently, take into consideration overall community needs for inpatient beds, but purely hospital-based financial perspectives. In Australia, inpatient beds were reduced from 2.65 (1998/99) to 2.4 per 1000 population (2002), resulting in very ill patients remaining in the ED for long periods and taking up resources for other new patients being admitted.[26] For intubated blunt trauma patients, the risk of pneumonia is increased by approximately 20% for every additional one-hour ED stay.[27] A modest decrease in hospital occupancy can lead to significant reductions in waiting time for inpatient beds.[28]

- **Inpatient residents vetting of senior emergency specialists' admission decisions at the** ED. The prevalent system of residents from various disciplines screening ED admissions already vetted by senior ED physicians results in delaying transfers for additional hours, carrying out of routine inpatient procedures in the ED, and unnecessarily competing for consultation and treatment rooms there. A practice of a bygone era when ED doctors were the most junior in the hospital, this process has become entrenched into many mindsets within the inpatient environment. Many hospital residents clerk their admissions in the ED, whose staff then initiate what would generally be routine inpatient procedures. This results in ED staff having to divide their time between fresh arrivals

and boarders. Though this is obviously a major factor hampering patient flow, it is hardly being addressed.

- **Inpatient patient care processes that unnecessarily prolong average length of stay in the wards**. These include delays in making arrangements for laboratory and radiological investigations, and poor discharge planning resulting in families being relatively unprepared to take their loved ones home.[29] Patients being admitted for elective inpatient procedures are sometimes not offered current concepts of same-day surgery and pre-admission testing.
- **Lack of community convalescent facilities, with difficulty in freeing up beds in acute-care hospitals**. This results in stable geriatric and convalescent patients taking up many beds in acute hospitals. This is compounded by difficulties in transferring patients to community facilities owing to restrictive screening practices by convalescent facilities and lack of adequately staffed transport resources. A decline in nursing-home capacity over the years, owing to lack of community planning in recognizing the need for such homes and allocating and training manpower for them, has also contributed.[30]
- **Seasonal variations in ED overcrowding**. Seasonal variations have occurred because some hospitals close their general wards temporarily during holiday periods to allow for staff welfare, creating congestion at the ED.[31] General ward staff who do not see the congestion in the ED are oblivious to the impact of such closures on general patient care. During the winter large numbers of geriatric patients seek care for chronic cardiorespiratory conditions, increasing the demand for inpatient beds. The ED then bears the brunt of the congestion.

## Whose problem is it?

Traditionally, ED overcrowding has been regarded as an emergency medicine problem. Hospital administrators, senior colleagues in other areas of the hospital who seldom visit the ED and see the congestion there, and community healthcare administrators have, for many years, taken ED chiefs to task over their inability to resolve overcrowding problems. It is increasingly recognized, however, that the ED component of the overcrowding is relatively small.[18]

It is also not enough to state that ED overcrowding is the hospital's problem and then expect the hospital administration to fix it. Often, ED overcrowding is beyond the capability of an individual hospital to completely resolve. It is a system-based problem requiring a response that addresses the issue of patient flow through the whole healthcare continuum and that recognizes that kinks and blocks downstream have severe repercussions on the quality of care in the earlier phases of disease management. While preventive strategies are important for long-term health planning in any community, and must be one of the cornerstones of the healthcare planning process, resource availability and reducing systemic blocks in a timely manner are crucial to achieving cost efficiencies in the provision of health care.

From a holistic perspective, ED overcrowding is everyone's problem. All levels of the hospital, as well as the community health coordinator, need to be involved in ensuring that the various stages of patient flow are well managed.

## Emergency department staff

The ED needs to address departmental processes that contribute to overcrowding. Taking ownership of ED processes is crucial to establish credibility with other hospital departments. Getting buy-in from the various grades of ED staff is critical for success. This will allow them to actively participate in implementing ED patient flow initiatives. It involves asking tough questions of departmental processes, reviewing them, and then championing the process of change from within.

## Hospital management

Senior management support is essential to address patient flow processes. Senior hospital management must interact with all areas of the hospital that impact patient flow, advocate the need to minimize waiting by patients, and strive for more seamless and hassle-free processes. Senior management also demonstrates support by addressing roadblocks in the move to smoother patient flow.

The various clinical departments in the hospital hold the inpatients. Their role in moving towards efficient inpatient care processes, in communicating with their staff on measures needed to streamline these processes, and in reviewing their patient discharge practices will be important. These would also apply to support departments such as nursing, radiology, and laboratory services.

Over the years the tendency to regard each clinical department in a hospital as a separate business unit, although it has generated more consciousness of cost efficiency and financial bottom lines, has also unwittingly led to a greater departmental silo mentality. As a result, pressures to ensyure good fiscal performance, keep direct revenue-generating processes alive, and give up those that appear to result in greater cost without apparent direct revenue generation have become more common. Often such practices do not consider the impact on the patients waiting in the ED or on discharge efficiency.

Sometimes, senior management needs to demonstrate its seriousness in wanting to tackle the problem of overcrowding. In our institution the chief executive officer sanctioned and created the space for the setting up and staffing of a transit admissions ward – which almost immediately resulted in a decrease in ED boarders and a boost to staff morale.

## Public health authorities

When local, state, or provincial health authorities take ownership of the ED overcrowding problem, they are better able to influence the creation, allocation, and availability of resources and adjust local regulations for a healthcare system with smoother patient flow. These agencies bring different perspectives to the issue of overcrowding and access block, such as addressing public communication and educational needs that facilitate initiatives for better distribution of healthcare resources.

## Measuring ED overcrowding

Common international measures to indicate magnitude of overcrowding are lacking. Disagreements and differences in types of data usually collected lessen the quality of efforts to quantify the problem and its impact on the health of the community. There is a need for an Utstein-style format to quantify the problem and measure the impact of interventions.

The Canadian Agency for Drugs and Technologies in Health (CADTH) listed 10 popular data-collection elements among ED officials documenting departmental overcrowding.[32] These, ranked in descending order of popularity, are as follows:

(1) Percentage of ED occupied by inpatients. Percentage of ED patients admitted, but not yet transferred to ward owing to lack of beds.

(2) Total ED patients. Number of patients in ED, including on stretchers, on chairs, in hallways, and in waiting room.

(3) Overall bed occupancy. Proportion of acute-care beds occupied by patients (indicated daily).

(4) Total time in ED (ED LOS). From first triage assessment to leaving department (to admissions floor or discharge).

(5) Percentage of time ED at or above stated capacity. Percentage of time of day that ED has more patients than stated bed capacity.

(6) Time from bed request to bed assignment. Time taken from admission decision to bed assignment (admitted patients only).

(7) Time from triage to emergency physician (EP). Time from assignment of triage category to examination by EP.

(8) MD satisfaction. Assessment of EPs' satisfaction working in ED and their perception of impact of ED overcrowding on care provided.

(9) Time from bed ready to transfer to ward. Time taken from bed assignment to leaving department (admitted patients only).

(10) Number of staffed acute-care beds. Active beds staffed and "open" in hospital (does not relate to capacity to expand).

Other measures have also been attempted to quantify ED overcrowding. Two quantification systems that use emergency providers' perceptions as outcome variables are the NEDOCS (National ED Overcrowding Study) scale and the EDWIN (ED Work Index) model.[33] Two other known indices are the Real-time Analysis of Demand Indicators (READI) and the Emergency Department Crowding Scale (EDCS). New Zealand has its Emergency Department Cardiac Analogy Model (EDCAM).[34] These measures or others may be starting points for use by communities in an effort to standardize data collection and provide the basis for allocation of resources and interventions to alleviate one of the most pressing problems facing EDs worldwide. The predictive abilities of these different scales vary widely. As of yet there is no unified scoring system for measurement of ED overcrowding.[34] Many EDs use time indicators (usually four hours in the UK and eight hours in Australia). Others, such as those in the USA, Canada, and Singapore, use the concept of reasonable time frame.

## Solutions

The multifactorial etiology of ED overcrowding means solutions that work in one community may not necessarily work equally well elsewhere. Solutions will need to be tailored to the location, the community, and the culture.

## ED input solutions

Attempts to reduce the primary care workload in EDs are popular in many communities, and some are listed here:

- **Advice telephone lines to divert patients from EDs**. The United Kingdom has tried diverting ED attendances through the use of telephone help lines.[1] Patients suspecting a condition requiring acute care may call a help line for advice. While this may result in some being diverted from EDs to primary healthcare facilities, the impact on patient safety, time to definitive care, and cost to the healthcare system is unclear. Advice lines have not demonstrated any impact on ED overcrowding or access block.

- **Public education to reduce ED visits**. The measures discussed in the section on input causes of overcrowding should be considered for communities where primary care access is suboptimal.

- **Triaging patients out of the ED**. Some EDs have tried to divert non-urgent visits either to general practice clinics or to specially set-up walk-in clinics within hospitals.[35] Primary care physicians have concerns if their patients are diverted to other primary care clinics, or if hospitals set up clinics that compete directly with them. The additional resources employed to achieve such diversions, the unhappiness of patients at being diverted after taking the trouble to present themselves to the ED, and the complaints generated have made such practices unpopular. The identification of "inappropriate" ED visits is fraught with inaccuracies when made at the front end of the department, before a careful assessment can be conducted.

- **Increased reliance on home-based care and community outreach programs**. Some hospitals try to manage a growing number of clinical conditions in the community setting. The National University Hospital Singapore uses its outreach program teams (consisting of trained nurses, social workers, and respiratory therapists) to manage patients with chronic obstructive pulmonary disease (COPD) exacerbation at home, thus cutting down inpatient admissions. The United Kingdom has pioneered the use of emergency care practitioners (ECPs) who assist in family clinic surgeries, conduct home and community visits, provide care in minor injury units, deliver after-hours services, and facilitate referrals to other services.[36] These have been shown to reduce the need for subsequent emergency referrals and unscheduled hospital admissions.

## ED throughput solutions

ED throughput solutions are important to decrease overall length of ED stay and improve decision making regarding inpatient admission or discharge.[37] These interventions may be made at many stages from triage to final ED disposition.

- **Co-locating primary care physicians and facilities within EDs**. These have not adequately addressed how such primary care patients are processed within the ED and the differing standards of care and due diligence exercised by primary care physicians and emergency physicians. They have not been able to demonstrate significant reductions in ED waiting times or alleviation of access blocks.[38]
- **Early identification of complex patients**. Specific patient groups at risk for developing long-term medical conditions, and those with complex comorbidities, need to be identified early, with strategies for better ambulatory management to minimize likelihood of repeat ED visits or long hospital stays. The elderly, and patients with chronic heart, renal, or other metabolic conditions, if identified early, may be initially managed within ED short-stay units or even admitted as inpatients for short periods and then planned for discharge with family education and ambulatory home care management. Such strategies can result in reduced ED visits by

groups who would otherwise occupy inpatient beds, sometimes for prolonged periods. There is potential for ED-based comprehensive geriatric assessments to improve health outcomes of high-risk elderly patients and reduce unplanned ED visits and in-hospital stays.[39]

- **Decreasing alcohol-related presentations**. Better methods of screening for alcohol-related presentations have led to appropriate referrals to alcohol management clinics, with reduction of ethanol-related illness and injury and reduction in ED visits and inpatient admissions of this cohort.[40]
- **Bedside registration after initial triage, rather than registration in series before or after triage**. This decreases door-to-doctor time and ED length of stay by placing the patient registration process in parallel with other ED-visit-related activities, instead of the traditional in-series process that registration counter staff and business office personnel are more comfortable with.[1,41]
- **Application of management principles** previously used in manufacturing can help streamline patient flow throughout the hospital. Application of Lean principles and queuing theory can result in streamlined triage, including senior physician triage,[42] team triage systems (see Chapter 19), and simpler registration systems, and can minimize unnecessary administrative procedures that usually burden nurses. Identifying major bottlenecks would be crucial, if these affect patient flow. Application of these principles can send a clear signal that change is possible.
- **ED observation units**. The use of EDOUs to treat a variety of common conditions that traditionally would have led to a hospital stay of an average of 2–3 days has helped reduce inpatient admissions and hence ED boarders and access block in a number of institutions (see Chapter 22). EDOUs can be a major tool employed by EDs to help reduce hospital bed occupancy rates, ED overcrowding, and healthcare costs, not to mention to enhance patient satisfaction and reduce the risk of nosocomial infections for such patients. These units cannot be used for boarding ED patients who require longer -term stay in hospital wards. The principles of rapid diagnosis, very frequent reviews, and aggressive management protocols used in EDOUs can potentially be used

in general medical and surgical wards to decrease length of stay there, resulting in freeing up even more hospital beds for those who truly require a longer hospital stay.

## ED output solutions (how to solve the access block)

ED output solutions potentially have the greatest impact on ED overcrowding and patient dissatisfaction, as access block is its most significant contributor.[43]

- **Creating institutional awareness of ED overcrowding and its adverse effects**. If part of the overall educational process for all hospital staff, this can create better cultural awareness between departments that they are dealing with a shared problem, and will help to minimize the silo mentality. Such sharing will have multiplier effects, enhance efforts of the entire healthcare institution in attempting to solve the problem, and lead to other process improvements including more coordinated scheduling of elective patients and surgical procedures.[5] This also eliminates delays in patient transfers from nursing handing/ taking over or bed preparation for the next patient and changes the culture of "lock-out" times when transfers cannot occur.

- **Direct admission rights for ED physicians**. In most institutions throughout the world, ED physicians are not given direct admission rights. Colleagues from various clinical disciplines review admitted patients in the ED, resulting in prolonged stay for additional hours in the ED, even if inpatient beds are available. Removal of the admission vetting procedure by multidisciplinary colleagues, especially if senior ED physicians have already completed this, can result in tremendous time savings, reducing congestion in the ED,[44] and would not significantly lead to unnecessary hospital admissions. There is a need to change the mindset of clinicians from various disciplines that they have to protect their inpatient beds and act as supervisors and gatekeepers for admissions coming through the ED.

- **Decreasing hospital occupancy rates**. A historical control observational study demonstrated that reducing access block by achieving decreased hospital occupancy significantly reduced ED

waiting times and ED overcrowding.[28] This requires aggressive discharge planning, which is usually given lip service. Medical and nursing leadership is needed to ensure that care management plans are the basis for provision of medical treatment, with appropriate modifications along the way and constant communication with families to enhance early hospital discharge while ensuring adequate patient management. "Hospital at home" concepts, sometimes called "early supported discharge," have been employed in Scotland, where they have contributed towards earlier discharges for some people, with increased patient satisfaction, reductions in hospital lengths of stay, increases in the number of patients still at home six months after discharge, greater community reintegration, improvement of health-related quality of life, and reductions in costs per patient.[45]

- **Hospitalist teams**. Teams consisting of medical specialists, case managers, and medical social workers can be formed to proactively manage patients and liaise with families and other institutions to ensure expedited discharge from hospital wards.[46] The principles of employment of hospitalists working closely with case managers would be similar to the principles of rapid, frequent assessment employed in the EDOUs described earlier. The employment of specialist nursing personnel for identified medical conditions, such as deep vein thrombosis, heart failure, and chronic bronchitis, in inpatient units has been demonstrated to reduce early readmissions after initial hospital discharge.[1]

- **Increasing bed capacity in the healthcare system**. The pattern of diseases presenting to hospitals with more older patients with multiple comorbidities requiring inpatient care results in an increase in average length of hospital stay and an increased need for beds at all levels of the healthcare system.[47] This includes not just acute and ICU beds, but more importantly additional ED, observation, and convalescent beds. Simplifying and streamlining procedures for transferring those requiring long-term bed care and rehabilitation to community nursing homes or ambulatory facilities does help. The pace of this change is slow in many communities, however. Senior leadership is essential in recognizing and setting into motion the processes to hasten this.

- **Additional beds in inpatient hallways.** In some countries, such as Israel, placing of additional beds in inpatient hallways has had a significant effect in decreasing ED boarding and crowding.[48] Inpatient staff, seeing patients in their hallways, then use measures to expedite patient care and patient discharge from their wards. The numbers of patients that are lodged in inpatient ward hallways do not ever come anywhere near the numbers typically boarded in the ED. Yet hospital administrators balk at implementing these procedures, not realizing that by doing so they are compromising the care of large numbers of patients who will eventually end up in the inpatient wards. Hospital staff who do not see patients in their hallways do not appreciate the dire situation of their near-future patients. The "out-of-sight, out-of-mind" approach has not worked. Hospital administrators have the potential to significantly impact ED overcrowding and improve patient care and safety by sanctioning additional beds in inpatient hallways.
- **Flexible surge management strategies.** Hospitals have been trying to develop surge capacity strategies for disaster situations. Use of these on a modest scale to manage overcrowding situations may be worth the while.[49,50] The surge capacity development cannot just be for EDs, but will need to involve the whole hospital, and sometimes the local healthcare community. Operating on the disaster mode for day-to-day operations may better enable healthcare institutions to develop the discipline and realize the benefits of more efficient resource management, without compromising quality of care for their patients. Practice and prolonged exercises are needed to learn the art of extended disaster-mode resource management.

## Conclusions

Interventions at a variety of levels have been attempted over the years to address the issue of ED overcrowding. It is clear today that ED overcrowding is a symptom of a healthcare system that is sick and needs multidisciplinary and multidimensional care remedies across the whole patient care spectrum. Healthcare leaders need to address this in unison and across existing silos in order to ensure the best level of emergency care for our patients through efficient processes. ED overcrowding is a reflection of the current inefficiency of the healthcare system in managing its workload at multiple levels. A number of interventions have generated modest improvements in specific environments. More carefully thought-through interventions that address all three aspects of the overcrowding spectrum – input, throughout, and output – will be likely to demonstrate lasting benefits.

## References

1. Forero R, Hillman K. *Access Block and Overcrowding: a Literature Review. Prepared for the Australasian College for Emergency Medicine.* Sydney: Simpson Centre for Health Services Research, UNSW, 2008.

2. Forero R, Moshin M, Bauman AE, *et al.* Access block in NSW hospitals, 1999–2001: does the definition matter? *Medical Journal of Australia* 2004; **180**: 67–70.

3. Canadian Association of Emergency Physicians, National Emergency Nurses Affiliation. Joint position statement: access to acute care in the setting of emergency department overcrowding. *CJEM* 2003; **5**: 81–6.

4. American College of Emergency Physicians, Crowding Resources Task Force. *Responding to Emergency Department Crowding: a Guidebook for Chapters.* Dallas, TX: ACEP, 2002. www.acep.org/library/pdf/edCrowdingReport.pdf (accessed January 29, 2011).

5. Cowan RM, Trzeciak S. Clinical review: Emergency department overcrowding and the potential impact on the critically ill. *Critical Care* 2005; **9**: 291–5.

6. Sabbah S, on behalf of the McGill Emergency Residents, PGY-5, McGill Emergency Medicine Program. McGill Emergency Residents' Position Statement on Hospital Overcrowding, 2008. http://www.mcgill.ca/files/emergency/ Resident_overcrowding_pos_statement.pdf (accessed January 29, 2011).

7. Mah R. Emergency department overcrowding as a threat to patient dignity. *CJEM* 2009; **11**: 365–9.

8. Schull MJ, Morrison LJ, Vermeulen M, Redelmeier DA. Emergency department overcrowding and ambulance transport delays for patients with chest pain. *CMAJ* 2003; **168**: 277–83.

9. McConnell KJ, Richards CF, Daya M, *et al.* Effect of increased ICU capacity on emergency department length of stay and ambulance diversion. *Annals of Emergency Medicine* 2005; **45**: 471–8.

10. Brennan J. Guidelines for ambulance diversion. *Annals of Emergency Medicine* 2000; **36**: 376–7.

11. Richardson DB. Increase in patient mortality at 10 days associated with emergency department overcrowding. *Medical Journal of Australia* 2006; **184** (5): 213–16.

12. Weissman JS, Rothschild JM, Bendavid E, *et al.* Hospital workload and adverse events. *Medical Care* 2007; **45**: 448–55.

13. Kilcoyne M, Dowling M. Working in an overcrowded accident and emergency department: nurses' narratives. *Australian Journal of Advanced Nursing* 2008; **25** (2): 21–7.

14. Rondeau KV, Francescutti LH. Emergency department overcrowding: the impact of resource scarcity on physician job satisfaction. *Journal of Healthcare Management* 2005; **50**: 327–40.

15. Physician Hospital Care Committee, Ontario Hospital Association, Ontario Medical Association, Ontario Ministry of Health and Long-Term Care. *Improving Access to Emergency Care: Addressing System Issues.* Toronto: OHA, 2006: 39–42.

16. Newton MF, Keirns CC, Cunningham R, Hayward RA, Stanley R. Uninsured adults presenting to US emergency departments: assumptions vs data. *JAMA* 2008; **300**: 1914–24.

17. Richardson DB, Mountain D. Myths versus facts in emergency department overcrowding and hospital access block. *Medical Journal of Australia* 2009; **189**: 369–74.

18. Stone K. *Excellence in Healthcare: Analysis of Patient Demographics for Patients Presenting to Rotorua Hospital Emergency Department in August 2008.* Unpublished report prepared for Lakes DHB by Rotorua Area Primary Health Services, 2008.

19. Anantharaman V. Impact of health care system interventions on emergency department utilization and overcrowding in Singapore. *International Journal of Emergency Medicine* 2008; **1**: 11–20.

20. United States Government Accountability Office. *Hospital Emergency Departments: Crowding Continues to Occur, and some patients wait longer than Recommended Time Frames.* GAO-09-347. 2009.

21. Jayaprakash N, O'Sullivan R, Bey T, Ahmed SS, Lotfipour S. Crowding and delivery of healthcare in emergency departments: the European perspective. *Western Journal of Emergency Medicine* 2009; **10**: 233–9.

22. Wallis LA, Twomey M. Workload and case mix in Cape Town emergency departments. *South African Medical Journal* 2007; **97**: 1276–80.

23. Lucas R, Farley H, Twanmoh J, *et al.* Emergency department patient flow: the influence of hospital census variables on emergency department length of stay. *Academic Emergency Medicine* 2009; **16**: 597–602.

24. Trzeciak S, Rivers EP. Emergency department overcrowding in the United States: an emerging threat to patient safety and public health. *Emergency Medicine Journal* 2003; **20**: 402–5.

25. Guo B, Harstall C. *Strategies to Reduce Emergency Department Overcrowding.* Health Technology Assessment Report 38. *Alberta Heritage Foundation for Medical Research*, 2006; **38**.

26. Fatovich DM, Hughes G, McCarthy SM. Access block: it's all about available beds. *Medical Journal of Australia* 2009; **190**: 362–3.

27. Carr BG, Kaye AJ, Wiebe DJ, *et al.* Emergency department length of stay: a major risk factor for pneumonia in intubated blunt trauma patients. *Jounal of Trauma* 2007; **63**: 9–12.

28. Dunn R. Reduced access block causes shorter emergency department waiting times: an historical control observational study. *Emergency Medicine Journal* 2003; **15**: 232–8.

29. Derlet R., Richards J., Kravitz R. Frequent overcrowding in U.S. emergency departments. *Academic Emergency Medicine* 2001; **8**: 151–5.

30. Wong HJ, Wu RC, Caesar M, Abrams H, Morra D. Smoothing inpatient discharges decreases emergency department congestion: a system dynamics simulation model. *Emergency Medicine Journal* 2010; **27**: 593–8.

31. Thomas J, Cheng N. Effect of a holiday service reduction period on a hospital's emergency department access block. *Emergency Medicine Australasia* 2007; **19**: 136–42.

32. Ospina MB, Bond K, Schull M, *et al. Measuring Overcrowding in Emergency Departments: A call for Standardization.* Technology Report No. 67.1. Canadian Agency for Drugs and Technologies in Health, 2006.

33. Jones SS, Allen TL, Flottemesch TJ, Welch SJ. An independent evaluation of four quantitative emergency department crowding scales. *Academic Emergency Medicine* 2006; **13**: 1204–11.

34. Richardson SK, Ardagh K, Gee P. Emergency department overcrowding: The emergency department cardiac analogy model (EDCAM). *Accident and Emergency Nursing* 2005; **13**: 18–23.

35. Murphy AW, Bury G, Plunkett PK, *et al.* Randomised controlled trial of general practitioner versus usual medical care in an urban accident and emergency department: process, outcome, and comparative cost. *BMJ* 1996; **312**: 1135–41.

36. Mason S, O'Keeffe C, Coleman P, Edlin R, Nicholl J. Effectiveness of emergency care practitioners working within existing emergency service models of care. *Emergency Medicine Journal* 2007; **24**: 239–43.

37. Pennsylvania Patient Safety Advisory. Managing patient access and flow in the emergency department to improve patient safety. *Pennsylvania Patient Safety Advisory* 2010; **7** (4): 123–34.

38. Wilson H. Co-locating primary care facilities within emergency departments: brilliant innovation or unwelcome intervention into clinical care? *New Zealand Medical Journal* 2005; **118** (1221): U1633.

39. Graf CE, Zekry D, Giannelli S, Michel JP, Chevalley T. Comprehensive Geriatric assessment in the Emergency Department. *Journal of the American Geriatrics Society* 2010; **58**: 2032–3.

40. McDonald AJ, Wang N, Camargo CA. US emergency department visits for alcohol-related diseases and injuries between 1992 and 2000. *Archives of Internal Medicine* 2004; **164**: 531–7.

41. Johnson N. Building the clockwork emergency department: a process improvement project. Poster, Emergency Nurses Association Conference 2009. http://www.nursinglibrary.org/Portal/main.aspx?pageid=4024&pid=21463 (accessed January 30, 2011).

42. Travers JP, Lee FC. Avoiding prolonged waiting time during busy periods in the emergency department: is there a role for the senior emergency physician in triage? *European Journal of Emergency Medicine* 2006; **13**: 342–8.

43. Solberg LI, Asplin BR, Weinick RM, *et al.* Emergency department crowding: consensus development of potential measures. *Annals of Emergency Medicine* 2003; **42**: 824–34.

44. Howell EE, Bessman ES, Rubin HR. Hospitalists and an Innovative Emergency Department Admission Process. *Journal of General Internal Medicine* 2004; **19**: 266–72.

45. Langhorne P, Taylor G, Murray G, *et al.* Early supported discharge for stroke patients: a meta-analysis of individual patients' data. *Lancet* 2005; **365**: 501–6.

46. Alpesh A. Value of hospital medicine in the inpatient management of community-acquired pneumonia. *Infectious Diseases in Clinical Practice (Supplement)*. 2004; **12**: S3–5.

47. Schneider S, Zwemer F, Doniger A, *et al.* Rochester, New York: a decade of emergency department overcrowding. *Academic Emergency Medicine* 2001; **8**: 1044–50.

48. Siegel B, Wilson MJ, Sickler D. Enhancing work flow to reduce crowding. *Joint Commission Journal on Quality and Patient Safety* 2007; **33** (Suppl): 57–67.

49. Ong MEH, Ho KK, Tan TP, *et al.* Using demand analysis and system status management for predicting ED attendances and rostering. *American Journal of Emergency Medicine* 2009; **27**: 16–22.

50. Green LV. Capacity planning and management in hospitals. In ML Brandeau, F Sainfort, WP Pierskalla, eds., *Operations Research and Health Care: a Handbook of Methods and Applications*. London: Kluwer, 2004.

Chapter

# 25

# Practice management models in emergency medicine

Robert E. Suter and Chet Schrader

### Key learning points

- Discuss the influence of a nation's healthcare financing and payment policies on the available choices of emergency medicine practice models.
- List the types of emergency medicine practice models that are used worldwide, and the relative advantages and/or disadvantages of each.
- Describe models of collaborative practice between emergency physicians that can improve patient care.

## Introduction

In most developed countries, the practice of assigning physicians to staff the emergency department (ED) became common in the twentieth century.[1] Originally staffed by young physicians-in-training and/or nurses, only in the past 40–50 years has the ED begun to be staffed by attending medical staff – most recently by trained emergency medicine specialists – with continued development of this trend globally.[1–6]

Since the birth of emergency medicine as a specialty, there have been dynamic changes in staffing and practice models in the ED that reflect the increasing professionalism and sophistication of emergency medicine practice. This has led to the continued expansion and refinement of practices, and the exploration of diverse scopes of ownership and control similar to that found in other specialties.

While expansion of roles is occurring, emergency physicians are for the most part characterized by their clinical practice in the hospital ED. Globally, in any individual hospital the type of emergency medicine practice model used is ultimately a function of the variables of the specific practice setting. These variables include hospital type, available reimbursement mechanisms, and local laws concerning the practice of medicine and nursing. All of these factors contribute to significant diversity in emergency medicine practice management models.

Worldwide, the biggest factor limiting the choice of emergency physician practice management models is the healthcare delivery and reimbursement system used in a particular country. In nations with national government dominance in healthcare provision and restrictions on private practice or reimbursement mechanisms, despite a growing market of private hospital systems, a majority of emergency care is provided using public funds, and usually in public facilities.[7] Even in countries with private delivery and reimbursement systems, such as the USA, emergency care continues to be provided in government-owned facilities.

With this in mind, hospitals can be characterized by two major groupings: private or public (local or national government) ownership, and teaching or non-teaching status. The combination of these factors can describe any specific hospital, and will determine the feasibility of using a particular practice management model, or the likelihood that it will be used, in the ED (Table 25.1). The model used by a particular hospital ED is further influenced by the details of national or regional policies for the provision and payment of health care in general, and emergency care specifically, in the country in which it is located.

## Payment/reimbursement models

Since global emergency medicine practice models are so hospital-dependent, and the types of hospitals available to practice in is defined by their funding

---

*Emergency Department Leadership and Management*, ed. Stephanie Kayden, *et al.* Published by Cambridge University Press.
© Cambridge University Press 2015.

**Table 25.1** Hospital types and common practice models

| Hospital type | Practice model | | | | |
|---|---|---|---|---|---|
| | Public employee | Hospital employee | Group employee | Contract contractor | Government assigned |
| Private: community | | X | X | X | |
| Private: teaching | | X | X | X | |
| Public: community | X | | * | * | X |
| Public: teaching | X | | * | * | X |

X Common association between practice model and hospital type.
* Occasional association between practice model and hospital type.

sources, it is important to first discuss reimbursement for emergency medicine. "Following the money" reveals why emergency care payment models and structure vary around the world.

In most countries, the government manages the healthcare system and controls the healthcare budget. The level of control over health care may be monopolistic, or may allow for some forms of private practice. Payments to physicians may be manifest in whole or in part by direct payments from the controlling government body to public hospitals. In these settings, accepting some form of government employment is often the only realistic physician practice option.

Even in countries that allow for private medical practice, it is frequently limited to physicians running private offices or clinics. Payment for private clinic services is negotiated as a cash transaction by those who can afford to pay. Major hospital services, including the types of major resuscitations that define emergency medicine, are relatively expensive, making this type of cash-only business model prohibitive or unrealistic for emergency physicians, leaving the provision of emergency care overwhelmingly public in these countries.

Increasing worldwide expenditures on health care have put pressure on government funding of health care. This has led to a renaissance of interest by wealthy citizens in supporting private health care in countries with national public healthcare delivery systems. Where this has occurred, it has allowed for the establishment of private hospitals, and theoretically for the establishment of private EDs. Given the economics of making an ED profitable, to run

a private ED in a country with a predominantly national healthcare system realistically requires that sufficient numbers of patients in the hospital's catchment area have some form of private or public insurance support similar to that found in countries with more available private healthcare delivery or payment.

In countries with more complex healthcare systems that include both public and private delivery and payments, such as the United States, payment systems are often more complicated. In private models, the predominant payment system is some form of fee-for-service. This is where a patient pays in advance or is billed in expectation of payment. Fee-for-service can occur by negotiation or by some form of a fee schedule. It may or may not be based on a standardized system that drives payment schedules, and these may exist with or without provisions for collecting the balance between public or insurance payments and the billed charge, or "balance billing."

In the USA the predominant standardized system that drives payments for physician services is the relative value unit (RVU). This "value" is assigned to a particular physician service in comparison to others. RVU-based methods of compensation have been developed, and they can offer hospitals, groups, and individual physicians a transparent means of reimbursement that is directly tied to a standardized measure of productivity. Physician salaries or other forms of payment can be paid based on the RVUs that physician billed or collected during a given time period.

There are several ways to enhance and reward productivity. One would be to just loosely review and refer to productivity as part of annual negotiations of a set physician salary. Additionally, if productivity exceeds certain benchmarks, an ED leader could offer varying incentives such as a financial bonus or other recognition. Alternatively, overall productivity could be used much more strictly, with each payment made to a physician based on his or her productivity during the period that the payment covers, causing a monthly variation in income. The greater a physician's work productivity, the higher the physician's financial reimbursement. This type of system theoretically evens out the differences between how hard different physicians work when on duty, and prevents groups or employers using these systems from "playing favorites" with regards to physician payments. On a practical basis, in a busy ED with multiple physicians on duty, a strictly productivity-based reimbursement system may breed unintended consequences. Physicians might compete to see the patients who are deemed sicker, or those needing higher reimbursed procedures performed. Depending on the specifics of the system, it might also encourage the performance of unnecessary tests or procedures.

Additional payment models in private health delivery systems may include contracted or non-standard rates. These occur when the provider agrees to a specific payment for services lower than his or her usual and customary charges, based on the anticipation that the payer will refer more patients, generating higher revenues by means of a higher volume of work performed. In emergency medicine, this type of negotiation assumes that it is possible to influence the behavior of emergency patients, often a difficult task. Agreement to contracted rates can also result from pressure from the hospital on the emergency physicians to have these contracts with payers that the hospital already has a contract with for hospital services.

Within private systems, a managed care organization (MCO) is analogous to a government healthcare delivery system. Instead of paying taxes, patients pay for healthcare insurance in the form of a subscription to services provided by a specific private delivery system. Classically, this means that employees or exclusive contractors of a specific healthcare provider deliver all needed services including emergency services and hospitalization in MCO-owned facilities. The benchmark example of this is Kaiser Permanente, the original MCO in the USA. When the MCO delivery system performs some or all services by contracting with providers who do not work for the MCO, the classic payment model used is "capitation." Capitation is one prorated "lump sum" payment that is made based on the anticipated use by subscribers each month, and providers agree to deliver all care needed by assigned MCO patients for that period. All of these services are considered to be covered by the capitation payment.

By increasing efficiency and reducing overall utilization, the MCO will attempt to lower overall costs, although this may be difficult to achieve while maintaining quality when emergency providers are not employed by the MCO. In these settings, emergency physicians are not incentivized to provide additional physician services to MCO patients, which may or may not be in the patient's interest.

## Collaborative practice issues

While emergency physicians are considered leaders of the ED team, they could not practice without a strong cast of supporting personnel. Globally, the most recognized supporting professional is the nurse. In some EDs, it is not uncommon that these two professions are the only ones represented.

In larger EDs, there is frequently additional support for both physicians and nursing staff. Commonly, an emergency specialist's role may be supplemented by general practice physicians or non-physician "mid-level providers" who are specially trained nurses or physician assistants who can evaluate patients with some form of oversight by specialist emergency physicians. Additionally, emergency physicians may be assisted by other physician support personnel such as "physician scribes." Scribes are employees who follow physicians in the ED and document in medical records while the physician is undertaking patient care, making the emergency physician more efficient.[8] Other support staff in the ED include medical assistants, emergency technicians, respiratory therapists (specially trained individuals who aid in assessment and treatment of respiratory disorders), social workers, and clerical personnel.

Legal restrictions on nurses and other non-physician practitioners may prevent the degree of collaborative practice found in some hospitals located in countries with less restrictive laws governing these areas. Hospitals in those countries that allow advanced practice may differ in terms of whether and how they use physician extenders, nurses, technicians, and other personnel, and the degree of delegation allowed and professional collaboration between them.

## Emergency physician practice models

The degree of government role in healthcare delivery and financing, and the relative market share of private health care, will determine the relative predominance and availability of any specific practice model for emergency physicians. That said, from the physician's contractual perspective, all models can be broadly categorized in one of three types: (1) national government-managed practice, (2) hospital-managed practice, or (3) group-managed practice.

## National government-managed practice
### National government employee

Globally, it is believed that emergency care is predominantly provided in healthcare systems that are owned and operated by national governments. In this setting, nearly all emergency care is provided by national government employees. In the context of this chapter, we refer to government employees who are ultimately managed by a government agency located in the national capital, not those that might be employed in local government practice models.

National government employees may be civilians, or may be engaged in some form of military service. Non-military national government civil service employees usually have fewer restrictions on their lifestyles, and may be comparatively exempt from involuntary changes in work schedule or location compared to the military, or even counterparts working in other sectors. While in some countries national "civil service" employees make less money than colleagues practicing under other arrangements, they may also have more job security and better retirement or other benefits.

Since its modern roots are often traced to wartime triage and treatment, emergency medicine is often a well-regarded member of the military medical corps. In the USA, emergency medicine specialists practice in the Army, Navy, and Air Force, as well as the uniformed commissioned corps of the Public Health Service.[9] Although salaries in the military are often significantly lower than those obtainable in private practice, emergency physicians may accept military roles in exchange for medical school loan forgiveness or other incentive programs, as well as for other intangible reasons.

National government employees, whether military or civilian, may be subject to specific assignments in different locales. For example, a government employee might be mandated to practice in an assigned location in the country, or even designated for an assignment overseas.

### Individual contracted provider

While unusual, the demand for emergency care in national government hospitals may be such that it may attempt to supplement its employed emergency physicians with individual contract providers. Contracts with individuals are most common when only a few specialists are needed for a defined period of time. When there is a need for larger numbers of physicians, or for a more sustained period of time, it is likely that the government will seek to contract with a group; this type of practice is discussed later under *group-managed practice*.

Emergency physicians who work directly for the government as individual contractors are essentially vendors of their services, and the contracts are sometimes termed "personal services contracts." These contract physicians typically enjoy higher compensation than they would have otherwise received as employees. They also have fewer obligations and restrictions on their lifestyle or on the types of benefits they may obtain – such as health/life insurance, retirement savings, etc. – since they will be able to do so in the free market. The trade-off is less job security and the need to become more involved in managing financial issues surrounding obtaining benefits (such as private life and disability insurance, health insurance, and child care), which may be expensive to obtain as an individual.

## Hospital-managed practice
### Assignment of on-call medical staff

The earliest means to staff hospital EDs was to rotate these duties among house-staff physicians in training, or, in non-teaching hospitals, the general medical staff. In academic medical centers this left junior physicians who were in training alone without oversight in the ED. In the USA the National Academy of Sciences put forth an influential paper in

1966 – *Accidental Death and Disability: the Neglected Disease of Modern Society* – which drew attention to the substandard treatment of accidental death and injury.[10] This critical review facilitated the development of the specialty of emergency medicine, facilitated its global development, and is slowly eliminating this practice in most urban settings around the world. Medical staff rotation may persist for some time in very rural, low-volume EDs that cannot afford other options, but is increasingly being replaced by trained and dedicated emergency providers.

### Public employee

Worldwide, most hospitals that provide emergency care are public or government-owned, even those hospitals not owned by national governments. Therefore, even in hospital-based practices, the most likely means of paying emergency physicians is as some form of government employee.

Many emergency medicine residencies are at public hospitals, and many emergency physicians are employed by public hospitals. Often these are managed at the individual hospital level even if they are owned by the government at the national or regional, as well as the local, level.

An example of this in the USA is the Veterans Administration (VA) healthcare system, which is owned by the federal government but essentially managed at the local level. Throughout the United States, the Department of Veterans Affairs has 140 medical facilities with 134 EDs or urgent care centers. Physicians who work in the VA are managed at the local level but participate in a national pay and benefits system that is potentially transferrable if the physician chooses to relocate. While there are many potential advantages to local management of federal facilities, the credentials of emergency physicians is not currently one of them. In spite of recently having an emergency specialist as the national CEO, as of October 2010 only 16% of physicians working in VA EDs were board certified by the American Board of Emergency Medicine.[11]

Local public hospital district employees will be limited to one local jurisdiction, although it may include multiple EDs. They work for a standard scale or negotiated wages, and may have less autonomy in their practice compared to other models. In return, they may have comparatively better retirement and health insurance benefits.

### Hospital employment

Even outside of the public sector, many emergency physicians have continued to enter into a direct employer–employee relationship with the hospital. A negotiated rate is the basic method of compensation and allows physicians to know exactly what they will earn.

In this model, several benefits exist to the practitioner. There is little-to-no overhead or financial obligation to the hospital. The physician does not need to spend time working on benefits packages or complicated accounting. Administrative tasks such as billing, coding, collections, and insurance are all performed by the hospital. Instead, the practitioner just has to show up to work and is often reimbursed at a negotiated wage.

There are several shortcomings to direct hospital employment as well. While these employees often enjoy the lack of responsibility in administrative tasks, they do not recuperate additional profits that may be generated from services that are billed and collected by the hospital. The physician, being a hospital employee, is subject to the decisions of the hospital in his or her practice. In the long run a set negotiated wage may encourage minimum effort in the workplace, as physicians have little financial incentive to work harder. Some hospitals have dealt with this latter problem by adding a bonus structure on top of salary in order to distinguish those who are harder workers from those who are not, to incentivize those who expend more effort. When doing this, hospitals need to be careful how they measure effort since, for example, the RVU system incentivizes increased patient resource utilization that could actually increase the hospital's operational expenses under many reimbursement systems.

### Case study 25.1.   Night hawks

An ED medical director of a public hospital has six physicians on staff, all of whom have different practice patterns. Some, in the twilight of their careers, have sought to work fewer nights. Some, naturally, are faster than their partners.

In this practice, younger members of the medical staff are rapidly becoming discouraged as they are working more and more nights to cover for their peers, often stressing family obligations and their personal well-being. The discontent becomes obvious when cooperation between practitioners ceases to exist.

As each practitioner is paid a set salary, with little variation between them, the medical director seeks ways that he might incentivize each member of his group who takes on the extra burden of night shifts; additionally, he also seeks to reward members of his staff who see patients more efficiently.

While the salary structure is already set, the ED manager decides to have the group meet together. He expresses knowledge of their discontent, and different solutions are proposed. One younger physician is agreeable to working as a "night hawk," or that he will work only night shifts for the group. In return, he does not have to work weekend nights, and is allowed to work two fewer shifts than the rest of the group. Another physician agrees to pick up a majority of the weekend nights, but he also gets a shift reduction and priority in scheduling the rest of his shifts.

Finally, in an attempt to encourage productivity, the group decides that the providers who see patients most efficiently will be awarded preference in holiday scheduling and the choice of a funded trip to an educational conference.

Morale increases as workers who had been burdened by extra night shifts now feel rewarded for their sacrifice. Additionally, a healthy competition soon begins to see patients at a quicker pace.

### Individual contracted provider

While unusual, hospitals may choose to individually contract with non-employee providers and then take responsibility to manage them. Since physicians are perceived as difficult to manage, hospitals often want to avoid this, and usually contract out the management responsibility for anyone they do not want to employ (see *group-managed practice*).

Theoretically, direct contracting offers some legal and financial advantages to hospitals that are willing to assume the management task. From a physician standpoint, this situation is similar to being a hospital employee, with possible tax advantages or the flexibility of being an independent contractor, as has been discussed earlier in this chapter.

## Group-managed practice

### Academic group employee or contractor

Even before the full recognition of emergency medicine as a distinct specialty in the United States, there have been training programs in place to train emergency physicians. Most academic groups either are controlled by a university or medical school or have an exclusive provider agreement with a single university, medical school, or community teaching hospital or system. Irrespective of employment status, these academic emergency physicians would then provide care to contracted academic EDs while training new physicians in the practice of emergency medicine.

Academic careers allow for specific concentrations for continued involvement beyond clinical care and administration. Academic groups, with the ability to focus on education and research, have helped to further develop continued growth in ED ultrasound, toxicology, emergency medical services (EMS), medical simulation, and international medicine, to name a few.

### Entrepreneurial academic groups

Entrepreneurial academic groups, or departments within academic hospitals, may expand beyond their primary resident training institution and decide to staff the EDs of satellite hospitals. This is often a way of enhancing the collections of an academic ED, for instance through transfers and referrals from the satellite hospitals. An entrepreneurial approach offers two distinct benefits. First, academic centers are often located in areas with a significantly uninsured or underinsured population and may require hospital subsidies to be able to operate. By pursuing private hospital contracts in areas that have higher insurability or a higher proportion of privately insured patients, academic groups can begin to operate at a profit, thus requiring less in hospital subsidies and strengthening their hold on the hospital contract. Additionally, by having a satellite hospital contract that is free of resident training, academicians are also afforded an opportunity to practice independently.

**Academic group employee.** While not common in most countries, emergency physicians may be employed directly by a single specialty or multispecialty academic practice group contracted with a training institution or medical school. Many of the same risks and benefits exist for physicians as when they enter into a direct employee agreement with a hospital owned by a medical school. Providers still operate at a negotiated rate, while understanding there are specific limits in reimbursement and autonomy in their practice. University systems often consist of public, state-funded universities. When they create and manage groups, the academicians who work for them are also public employees.

**Academic group contractor.** Academic emergency physicians may also practice as independent contractors within a group. In contrast to academic employee status, the physician has all of the same advantages and disadvantages discussed previously. Contractor status is most likely to be offered by more entrepreneurial academic EDs.

## Physician-owned group employee or contractor

While it is commonplace for emergency physicians to work for a hospital, government, or academic entity, physician-owned groups have developed in those countries where private practice is feasible. In a few countries where legal conditions exist to support it, physicians who want autonomy in their practice environment and financial incentives for physician productivity have developed physician-owned groups that contract with private hospitals to provide staffing for emergency services.

These physician-owned groups could take many forms. The first is a single-owner group, where one physician-owner contracts with a hospital to provide staffing of EDs. This owner has physician-employees or contractors that he or she pays at a negotiated rate to practice in the ED. This allows the physician-owner to maintain control of the practice environment while recuperating the financial incentive when physician productivity is enhanced. However, the physician-owner is also responsible for billing, collections, and compliance for the ED staff.

As a physician-employee in a single-owner model, there is greater flexibility in negotiating salary rates while working with leadership that understands the complexities of practicing emergency medicine. However, the financial incentive of independent contracted practice can be limited to those who own the practice.

Physician-led groups may develop into a business-like structure, be it incorporating, or forming a partnership or democratic group. This enables physicians to have ownership in their practices with the responsibility of managing the clinical and operational aspects of their business. Concerns such as insurance, billing, coding, and reimbursement will all need to be answered by the ownership group.

### Physician-owned group with support from a practice management organization

While emergency providers can be strong clinicians, few are familiar with all of the necessary business concerns of emergency medicine contracts. To supplement ED group ownership, independent group practice management organizations have been started. These group management organizations serve to augment ED practice by consulting on or providing administrative services, such as billing and information technology, for a fee, while allowing the ownership group or hospital to maintain overall control.

Group management organizations do not seek to own individual ED contracts. Rather, they offer consultation and training to physician groups who seek to advance to ownership in their practice environment. Specific services include assistance in proposal development and contract negotiation, with the expectation that they will continue to be employed for administrative needs after contract acquisition.

While seeking to continue within specific roles in a contract group, group management organizations do offer physicians an opportunity to develop ED ownership.

### Contract management organization employee or contractor

The tremendous growth in emergency medicine, coupled with the success of emergency medicine practice groups, has led to the inevitable development of corporate-based contract management service organizations in those countries that allow a free-market approach to medical care. These companies, which may be investor-owned, often operate as a "one stop shop," seeking to offer hospitals services in addition to ED staffing.[12] These groups often will develop their own billing and coding, risk management and insurance, or prehospital service companies.

While physicians are hired as independent contractors or employees and hold leadership positions within the group, the company's primary obligation is to achieve profitable status and report to shareholders in the company. In countries where they exist, such as the United States, a corporate-based contract management service organization is often a large regional or national group.

Although superficially similar to direct hospital employees, physicians who work as part of a large contract management group may see an emphasis on quality and satisfaction in the ED, as a result of concerted efforts to reduce costs while seeking to improve the customer (patient) experience.

**Contract group employee.** Normally, contract group employment results from the legal structure of the country, region, or state that the group is operating in, since it is rarely the first choice of any contract group, because of the complexities of employment law. When employed, physicians may or may not benefit from a simplified benefits package compared to their contracted counterparts. They do benefit from some additional legal protections compared to a contracted status. At the same time, usually, the total financial outlay is identical to what would have been paid to a contractor.

**Contract group contractor.** Most contract groups prefer to be in a contractor relationship with physicians, if given the choice. This avoids laws protecting employees, and allows the physician to benefit from the tax advantages that often correspond to this relationship.

## Special situation: total staffing

In some circumstances, hospitals have contracted with groups to provide all staffing to EDs. This includes physicians, as well as nurses, technicians, clerical staff, and housekeeping. This is analogous to a physician leasing space for an office in a clinic building. These "turn-key" operations create a situation where all members of the ED team are employed by the same emergency-services-focused operation.

Physicians, as well as the auxiliary staff, often are very satisfied with their work environment, as there is usually a common expectation of all employees by the contract groups. Additionally, global efforts in quality and patient satisfaction are usually supported universally.

Paradoxically, in this situation happiness in the ED can lead to conflict if a well-functioning independent ED brings light to operational or human resources problems in other parts of the hospital. Significant disconnects can occur between the ED staff and the rest of the hospital, and if these make the hospital administration look bad, the competing interests can lead to contract termination. For example, a hospital and staffing group may disagree about who is responsible for specific quality measures, or a better nursing compensation package in the ED than the hospital offers to intensive care unit (ICU) nurses may lead to competing goals that ultimately result in the hospital choosing not to renew the contract, in support of overall goals, in spite of stellar performance in the ED.

---

**Case study 25.2. Different teams**

A not-for-profit hospital with multiple ED sites was unhappy with the productivity and performance of its hospital-employed medical staff. These physician employees included several ex-medical directors who had negative attitudes toward nearly all change initiatives.

The hospital CEO used the excuse of a new affiliation with another hospital system to contract with that system's physician group. The physicians in this group were not hospital employees, but rather were independent contractors for the group that had a contract with the hospital system to provide emergency physicians.

Initially, the hospital agreed to complete replacement of the employees, with the option of the employees becoming part of the new group. Just before the contract was to take effect, however, under pressure from nurses and medical staff, the hospital reneged on this agreement and told the employed physicians that they could remain employed, with the new group just providing leadership and any new emergency physicians.

The new chief of emergency services started the position with the ED significantly understaffed, and a handful of members of his group rotating into the hospital to help out from their usual hospitals. The employed physicians staged an active resistance, refusing to join the new group and attempting to recruit nursing staff and other hospital employees to resist the leadership of the new group,

Active physician recruitment continued, and the ED was eventually brought up to full staffing by heroic recruiting efforts of the new group. Performance measures moved forward, but the nursing staff was still divided by the continued efforts to sow unrest by some prior medical directors who remained as hospital-employed physicians.

Eventually the hospital system merger that prompted the initial change disintegrated, and the hospital changed to another group that promised full partnership to all physicians, and was therefore able to win over the hospital employees.

This case illustrates that mixing physician practice models in one facility is fraught with conflict and problems, and is probably a bad idea. While the hospital ultimately ended up with an outcome that it was satisfied with, it endured two years of conflict and pain that distracted everyone from the business of providing quality patient care and improving the ED and the hospital.

---

# References

1. Curry C. A perspective on developing emergency medicine as a specialty. *International Journal of Emergency Medicine* 2008; **1**: 163–7.

2. American Academy of Emergency Medicine Board of Directors, European Society for Emergency Medicine Council. Position statement on the role of government in securing emergency medical care. *European Journal of Emergency Medicine* 2002; **9**: 3–4.

3. Ciottone G, Old A, Nicholas S, Anderson P. Implementation of an emergency and disaster medical response training network in the Commonwealth of Independent States. *Journal of Emergency Medicine* 2005; **29**: 221–9.

4. Hsu E, Dey C, Scheulen J, Bledsoe G, VanRooyen M. Development of emergency medicine administration in the People's Republic of China. *Journal of Emergency Medicine* 2005; **28**: 231–6.

5. Edlich R. My revolutionary adventures in the development of modern emergency medical systems in our country. *Journal of Emergency Medicine* 2008; **34**: 359–65.

6. Hsia R, Razzak J, Tsai AC, Hirshon JM. Placing emergency care on the global agenda. *Annals of Emergency Medicine* 2010; **56**: 142–9.

7. Platz E, Bey T, Walter F. International report: current state and development of health insurance and emergency medicine in Germany. The influence of health insurance laws on the practice of emergency medicine in a European country. *Journal of Emergency Medicine* 2003; **25**: 203–10.

8. Scheck A. The next big thing: medical scribes. Scribes push emergency medicine closer to adoption of electronic medical records. *Emergency Medicine News* 2009; **31** (2): **13**, 16.

9. Lai MW, Lewin MR. *Emergency physicians in the United States military: a primer. Annals of Emergency Medicine* 2003; **42**: 100–9.

10. Division of Medical Sciences, Committee on Trauma and Committee on Shock. *Accidental Death and Disability: the Neglected Disease of Modern Society.* Washington, DC: National Academy of Sciences, National Research Council, 1966.

11. Kessler C, Chen J, Dill C, Tyndall G, Olszyk MD. State of affairs of emergency medicine in the Veterans Health Administration. *American Journal of Emergency Medicine* 2010; **28**: 947–51.

12. Flynn G. A clash of practice models: debate roils around mega-group medicine. *Annals of Emergency Medicine* 2006; **47**: 347–50.

# Further reading

Schlicher N. *Emergency Medicine Advocacy Handbook.* Irving, TX: Emergency Medicine Residents Association, 2009.

Wolper L. *Physician Practice Management Essential Operational and Financial Knowledge.* Sudbury, MA: Jones & Bartlett Learning, 2004.

Zink B. *Anyone, Anything, Anytime: a History of Emergency Medicine.* Philadelphia, PA: Mosby Elsevier, 2005.

# Emergency nursing

Shelley Calder and Kirsten Boyd

## Key learning points

- Define the role of the emergency nurse.
- Discuss the role of the charge nurse in the ED, and the importance of collaboration between nurse and physician leadership.
- Define the role of the advanced practice nurse in the emergency department.

## Introduction

Healthcare systems in the twenty-first century are challenged to provide increased services with fewer resources. Emergency departments (EDs) for many have become the interim solution to a larger health-care crisis. The challenges of our current healthcare system create barriers for providers in the clinical setting. Emergency nurses and physicians have joined forces to maintain standards of safe patient care. This partnership is important to move initiatives forward, grow volume, and provide patient-centered care.

As the landscape of health care evolves, collaborative partnerships in emergency care are critical, both within and beyond the institution.

## Emergency nurse
### Role of the emergency nurse

The emergency nurse is a uniquely skilled individual who is able to provide excellent patient care in organized chaos. Emergency nursing is a recognized specialty within the nursing profession of many countries. Unlike other specialties that focus on a particular disease process, clinical setting, or age group, the emergency nurse's specialty is his/her ability to care for a wide range of patients across the lifespan that require stabilization or resuscitation. Emergency

nursing care is episodic, primary, typically acute, and it can occur in a variety of settings.[1,2]

## Evolution of the emergency nurse specialty

While the specialty designation of emergency nursing is quite new, the literature suggests that something resembling emergency nursing existed in practice from as early as the days of Florence Nightingale. The specialty earned its official designation in 1970, championed by two nurses, Anita Dorr and Judith Keller. Dorr and Keller recognized the dedication and specialized nursing skills required to care for patients in the acute phase of illness. Following in the footsteps of physician colleagues, who had established the American College of Emergency Physicians (ACEP) in 1968, the Emergency Nurses Association (ENA) was officially launched in 1970.[3]

The ENA is an international organization that now represents emergency nurses in 32 countries around the globe. The ENA is committed to the advancement of emergency nurses and provides visionary leadership for emergency nursing and emergency care.[3]

### Qualifications

The required qualifications of the emergency nurse are variable, depending on institutional preferences. The preferred provider is a registered nurse with specialty training in emergency nursing. Specialty training and certifications available but not required for emergency nurses include the Trauma Nurse Core Course (TNCC), Emergency Nursing Pediatric Course (ENPC), and Core Advanced Trauma Nursing (CATN). These certifications are offered by the ENA in the USA and internationally. Basic Life Saving (BLS), Advanced Cardiac Life Support (ACLS), and Pediatric Advanced Life Support (PALS)

---

*Emergency Department Leadership and Management*, ed. Stephanie Kayden, *et al.* Published by Cambridge University Press.
© Cambridge University Press 2015.

are also highly recommended certifications for healthcare providers who either direct or participate in the resuscitation of a patient.[4]

Emergency nurses also have the opportunity to complete a Certification in Emergency Nursing (CEN). This certification is available in Canada, the USA, and 18 other countries. CEN certification is met by completion of a written exam measuring emergency nursing knowledge.[5] The CEN expires every four years.

## Standards of emergency nursing

Emergency nursing standards are the recommended goals, guidelines, and education unique to the specialty as defined by the ENA. The ENA has expanded the basic nursing process to include detailed standards and competencies specific to emergency nursing. The ENA also serves as a source of best practice, as well as a leader in a variety of areas that impact EDs around the globe.

## Scope of emergency nursing practice

The scope of emergency nursing practice is continually expanding, as is the role in the clinical setting. Emergency nurses have attempted to bridge the gaps in clinical care that are caused by crowding etc. by increasing their productivity and scope of practice. Treatments that typically in recent years would not have been considered in the ED have now become part of daily practice – for instance, invasive hemodynamic monitoring.

Emergency nurses specialize in assessing, intervening in, and stabilizing a variety of illnesses or injuries with minimal time, resources, or information. Because of the range of medical conditions that may require urgent treatment and care, they must be knowledgeable about general as well as specific health issues. The ENA identifies the following unique characteristics and core educational requirements of the emergency nurse:[6]

- knowledgeable in all disciplines: pediatrics, obstetrics, medicine, cardiology, trauma, orthopedics, oncology, infectious disease, psychiatry, and others
- knowledgeable in nursing care for all age groups
- delivers pediatric and adult trauma care
- knowledgeable in emergency preparedness

- demonstrates competence in the use of emergency equipment and technology
- functions efficiently and safely in high-stress situations
- adapts to unexpected increase in workload, while maintaining standards of practice
- works effectively as a team player
- skillfully practices triage of patients
- provides crisis intervention for patients and family
- proficient in public relation and customer care
- advocates and assists patients in accessing health care
- participates as a resource for medical instruction
- works collaboratively with prehospital care providers

Emergency nursing leaders would benefit from using these core competencies and educational requirements in the development of job descriptions and ongoing evaluation processes.

## Practice settings

The role of emergency nurses and their scope of practice are often defined by the environment in which they practice. Emergency nurses predominately are found in EDs. However, emergency nursing skills and services have been successfully used in the prehospital setting, health clinics, urgent care centers, schools, industry, and correctional facilities.[1]

## Charge nurse

EDs that experience overcrowding and high volumes require strong frontline leaders to manage daily operations. Implementation of a charge or resource nursing role will provide the continuous clinical leadership that is required seven days per week, 24 hours per day in the ED.

## Responsibilities

The charge nurse role may be described as the air traffic controller of the ED. The charge nurse, in collaboration with the ED attending physician, ensures smooth clinical operations and delivery of safe and efficient patient care. Ideally this individual should not carry a patient assignment, but if department volume is low this may be feasible. Charge nurse responsibilities may include: oversight of patient placement and flow, triage, chart review, nursing operations including staffing, problem solving, management of patient, family, physician or staffing complaints, clinical liaison for communication with inpatient services and outside facilities, in addition to acting as a general nursing resource. These individuals are also expected to champion process improvements and professional development in the department.

## Qualifications

When considering the qualifications of a charge nurse it is imperative for the nurse leaders to recognize that the charge nurse is an extension of nursing leadership. Potential candidates for the charge nurse position should possess similar decision-making and leadership capabilities to your core leadership team. Leary and Allen describe 12 qualities of an effective charge nurse:[7]

(1) competent and capable leader
(2) on the journey to self-awareness
(3) skilled at delegation
(4) utilizes available resources
(5) always clarifying expectations
(6) a change agent
(7) master at working through conflict
(8) patient satisfaction and service recovery expert
(9) patient safety and error prevention specialist
(10) mentor to those who follow
(11) an inspirational and resilient person
(12) mission-focused

These individuals should also be knowledgeable of departmental and facility-specific policies, procedures, and protocols. Nurses oriented to the charge nurse role should be current in all required departmental competencies of the staff nurse and triage nurse in addition to the departmental required certifications (e.g., BLS, ACLS, PALS).

## Training

Training for the charge nurse position should include both didactic and clinical components. The didactic portion of the training should focus on core charge nurse responsibilities and leadership development. Leadership development should include exploration of leadership styles, decision making, operations improvement, listening techniques, and conflict resolution.

Clinical training is the final piece of charge nurse orientation and can be used to ease the transition of the staff nurse to the charge position. Support from charge nurse mentors and staff colleagues is critical in the success and growth of the new charge nurse.

## Case management and care coordinators
### Roles and responsibilities

EDs are the access point for many patients who may not have sufficient support at home, who lack knowledge of how to navigate the healthcare system, who are homeless or have substance abuse issues, or who are aging with chronic conditions and simply can no longer manage at home. Hospitals are the most expensive form of health care.[8] Case managers or care coordinators can play an important role in facilitating services at point of entry to support the needs of the patient while maximizing the resources needed to safely provide care to patients.

Case managers, also referred to as care coordinators, are specialized nurses who are essential members of the ED care team. Case managers participate collaboratively in the assessment, planning, implementation, coordination, and monitoring of ED patients. In conjunction with the nursing process, case managers evaluate options and services to meet an individual's healthcare needs while examining the available resources to promote quality and cost-effective outcomes.[8]

In 1997 Brewer and Jackson completed a pilot study of utilizing case management in the ED.[9] Their findings suggested that a nurse case manager in the ED reduces discharge risk, improves patient and family after-hours access, facilitates appropriate use of community resources, improves communication with payers, provides a mechanism to make cost-effective disposition decisions, and improves overall patient outcomes.

Case managers can provide an important link with community resources and referring physicians. The education and training background of this role is that of an experienced nursing professional who receives additional education in community resources and insurance coverage plans. The partnership of the nurse case manager with the physicians, as well as with the nurses, is critical.[8] Physicians play an important role in consulting with case managers for those patients who do not meet admission criteria but have social or care needs that can be met in the home setting – again, allowing for cost-effective patient-centered care.

According to Brewer and Jackson, patients who will benefit most from case management coordination and services are those who require or would benefit from:[9]

- care monitoring
- education in skills that assist in managing chronic illness effectively
- assistance in connecting with community resources available
- a clinical advocate to help manage within the healthcare system
- assistance in managing between primary, acute, and long-term healthcare options

In the ED setting, case managers in the department can begin to assist those patients who do not medically require admission but have social needs or safety risks at home. They are also very important in the care of those patients who are being admitted, in anticipating their needs at home once they can be discharged. Family members of elderly patients who are being discharged from the ED to home often feel they need a lot of support to have home services set up for the needs that they are unable to manage themselves. These services are essential for many patients to reside in their home.

When patients are ready to leave the hospital, but are not safe to return home because of care needs, nurse case managers play an instrumental role in connecting families with the resources available to them. Conversations about long-term care facilities led by the nurse case manager will provide a source of knowledge for patients and families when returning home is not safe for the patient.[9]

Nurse case managers in the ED will see those patients identified by physicians or nursing staff who meet established criteria of risk. It is often not necessary for the case manager to see every patient, but it is therefore important to establish guidelines on who the case manager will see, or be notified about, if care needs are to be met and resources utilized appropriately. As physicians and nurses become more comfortable with the role of case manager, the partnership will develop and strengthen. Patients who visit your ED will be offered a service that is unique in

preventing medically unnecessary admissions and promoting use of community services.

## Triage

Triage, a process unique to emergency nursing, is the separation, sorting or selection of patients based on acuity. In the twenty-first century, triage has evolved from a rapid sorting mechanism to a dynamic process incorporating patient acuity, resource utilization, patient flow, quality, and patient satisfaction.

## Qualifications

The ENA and ACEP recommend the use of a clinical nurse with a minimum of six months of emergency experience.[10] Alternatively, paramedics, physicians, and physician extenders (healthcare providers who can practice under the supervision of physicians in certain countries) have been identified as potential options to perform triage in the ED.

### Triage standards and competencies

Please see Chapter 19 for details.

## Training

A combined didactic and clinical orientation to triage will provide a practice framework for the skilled practitioner. Fortunately many of the five-level systems developed in recent years provide training tools and guidelines for implementation. Institution-specific policies, clinical pathways, and a briefing on disaster management should also be included in the curriculum.

## Collaboration between nurse and physician leadership

Leadership between the nurse leader/administrator and the physician chief of the ED is a critical component in building a care team. The partnership demonstrated and lived daily by the leaders of the department will provide a role model of the desired relationship and enable all care teams to achieve excellent patient care.[11]

The position of the ENA is in support of collaborative and interdisciplinary work involving all members of the care team (e.g., nurses, physicians, technicians, and care coordinators).[11] There are many aspects of a patient encounter in the ED that depend on all care-team members performing duties that complement each other, as well as on standards of care that interconnect.

Nursing- and physician-led partnerships on clinical pathways, operational changes, and policy/procedure development are instrumental in a collaborative model.[12] One way to start to build these partnerships is to engage key leaders within the department by scheduling team meetings, co-chaired by the chief physician and nurse leader. Agendas should cover aspects of clinical care, operations, and relationship building.[13] A multidisciplinary forum for discussions as well as decision making provides a powerful demonstration of partnership and the engagement of the team. Ownership and accountability for all parties will grow as the message from these forums reaches the frontline staff and physicians as they care for the patients.

---

**Case study 26.1. Triggers in the ED: identification of patients with abnormal vital signs**

The ED leadership at an academic ED sought to improve critically ill medical patients' time to doctor and therapeutic intervention, including antibiotics, by use of a "trigger system." When any of the criteria listed below were met by a patient, an overhead call would alert the attending physician, the nurse in charge, and the assigned care team to respond to the patient's room immediately. The "trigger" could be called at the triage area upon initial intake, or if the patient experienced any changes during his or her stay in the ED. In a collaborative initiative, physician and nursing teams identified the following triggers:

- heart rate < 40 or > 130 beats per minute
- systolic blood pressure < 90 mmHg
- respiratory rate < 8 or > 30 per minute
- oxygen saturation < 90% on room air
- acute changes in mental status
- all patients allocated an Emergency Severity Index (ESI) of 1
- stroke, sepsis, and major trauma
- marked nursing concern regarding the patient's condition

Prior to implementing the new trigger program, a retrospective chart review was performed in order to determine the feasibility of this approach, and it was found that 71 out of 2165 patients would have met the above-defined trigger criteria. The average time to initial physician evaluation was 20 minutes, with time to therapeutic intervention 60 minutes and time to antibiotics 114 minutes.

Following the implementation of the trigger program the department saw considerable improvements in all of the variables: the time to initial physician evaluation decreased to 11 minutes, the time to therapeutic intervention to 24 minutes, and the time to antibiotics to 63 minutes (Fig. 26.1). In conclusion, the implementation of an ED trigger program allowed for more rapid time to doctor, therapeutic intervention, and antibiotics.

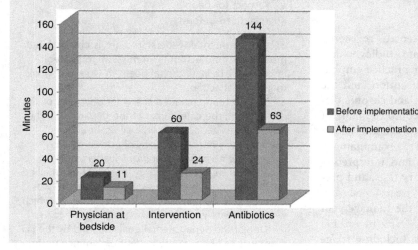

**Figure 26.1** Emergency department triggers. Time to intervention, before and after implementation of an ED trigger program.

## Advanced practice nurses

In emergency medicine, the term advanced practice nurse (APN) is used to describe the advanced practice roles of clinical nurse specialist (CNS) and nurse practitioner (NP). The ENA defines an APN as a registered nurse who has completed a graduate degree in a specialty area of nursing and has a direct and/or indirect clinical practice in the specialty area.[14]

## Clinical nurse specialist

The CNS in the ED is a licensed registered nurse who has completed graduate studies in nursing as a clinical nurse specialist. The ED CNS is an expert in clinical practice and standards of care, and has advanced knowledge specific to emergency nursing. The CNS influences direct client care, nurses, and nursing practice, as well as organizational policy and practice.[15]

In addition to providing direct patient care, the CNS impacts care outcomes by providing expert consultation for nursing staff and by implementing improvements in healthcare delivery systems. CNS practice integrates nursing practice, which focuses on assisting patients in the prevention or management of illness, with medical diagnosis and treatment of disease, injury, and disability.[15,16]

A CNS frequently partners with physicians, nurse managers, and other staff to improve patient care. The development of clinical pathways and guidelines is an example of the type of collaborative process improvement that a CNS frequently leads or participates in as a team member.

## Nurse practitioner

Nurse practitioners (NPs) are licensed registered nurses who have completed graduate studies within a nurse practitioner program. Their practice emphasizes health promotion, disease prevention, and the diagnosis and management of acute and chronic diseases.[17] The NPs in the ED setting complete many of the typically physician-driven tasks, including taking histories, conducting physical examinations, ordering, supervising, performing, and interpreting appropriate diagnostic and laboratory tests, and prescribing pharmacological agents, treatments, and non-pharmacological therapies for the management of the conditions they diagnose.[17] NPs in an ED can be used in a variety of settings, including triage and fast track.

## Conclusions

The nurse's role in the ED is a dynamic one that touches all levels of patient care. The education and training for each nursing role shares the common thread of nursing education with specializations to provide excellence in ED settings.

The partnership between the physician and the nurse is essential, and improves the care of the patient. True patient-centered care is dependent on partnership involving all care-team members. As we look to improve systems and be fiscally responsible, each member of the team plays an important role. The outcome will be a patient receiving the right care, at the right time, in the right setting.

---

**Case study 26.2.  Department of Emergency Medicine annual operating plan**

An academic medical center recently embarked on the journey of creating an annual operating plan (AOP). The AOP is guided by the hospital mission to provide extraordinary clinical care, where the patient comes first, supported by world-class education and research. One of the institutional goals identified on the AOP was to strengthen efforts to achieve excellence in clinical quality, safety, and the patient experience. The institution identified the following foundational supports required to achieve these goals:

- quality and safety
- patient experience
- financial sustainability
- continuous improvement
- respect for people
- healthcare reform

Each departmental leadership team is charged with making the connection from mission, to strategic imperatives, to institutional goals, to work unit goals, to individual actions.

The ED team included the chief physician of the department, the chief nurse of the department, the physician residency director, a clinical nurse specialist, the nurse manager, physician quality leaders, the physician operations leaders, and non-clinical supervisors with responsibilities for allied health members in the department. The team was charged with defining departmental initiatives which would ultimately roll up to the institutional goals.

One of the departmental goals defined by the ED team was to improve the patient experience in the

ED. Pre-intervention patient satisfaction was measured by an outside vendor using a standardized tool. The information collected was non-specific and the number of survey responses limited (3%). Together, ED leadership and staff developed an electronic patient survey tool. The survey consisted of 10 questions and would be completed prior to patient discharge. Within the first quarter the information collected and the number of surveys completed improved dramatically (18%). The information collected from this survey assisted the team in identifying patient satisfaction drivers, providing feedback to all disciplines and initiating relevant departmental improvements. The department continues to use outcomes and data collection for collaborative intervention and strategies.

The result of this work is a concise ED AOP that is a partnership between the nursing and physician leaders directly linked to the organizational fiscal-year goals. The champions of each initiative report out on a routine basis to the department management committee, where all leaders in the department have a seat. The purpose of the "reporting out" is to keep these initiatives moving forward to improve care, operations, and growth of the department. The results of this work are then shared with frontline staff (nurses, technicians, secretaries, and registrars) to align the goals and efforts and create a united team. It has proven effective to organize the team and promote partnerships amongst nursing and physician leaders.

# References

1. Newberry L, ed. Sheehy's Emergency Nursing: Principles and Practice, 5thedn. St. Louis, MO: Mosby, 1998: 3–5.

2. Howard PK, Steinmann RA, eds. *Sheehy's Emergency Nursing: Principles and Practice*, 6th edn. St. Louis, MO: Mosby Elsevier, 2009.

3. Emergency Nurses Association. *History of ENA*. http://www.ena.org/about/Pages/Default.aspx (accessed January 2011).

4. American Heart Association. *Advanced Cardiovascular Life Support Provider Manual*. Dallas, TX: AHA, 2006.

5. Emergency Nurses Association. *CEN FAQs*. 2011 http://www.ena.org/bcen/certified/CEN/Pages/CENFAQ.aspx (accessed January 2011).

6. Emergency Nurses Association. *Scope of Emergency Nursing Practice*. Des Plaines, IL: ENA, 1999.

7. Leary C, Allen SJ. Navigating the path of leadership: 12 qualities of an effective charge nurse. *Nurse Leader* 2006 **4** (6), 22–3.

8. Walsh K. ED case managers: one large teaching hospital's experience. *Journal of Emergency Nursing* 1999; **25**: 17–20.

9. Brewer B, Jackson L. A case management model for the emergency department. *Journal of Emergency Nursing* 1997; **23**: 618–21.

10. Emergency Nurses Association. *Triage: Meeting the Challenge*. Des Plaines, IL: ENA. 1998

11. Emergency Nurses Association. Position statement: collaborative and interdisciplinary research. *Journal of Emergency Nursing* 2006; **32**: 385–7.

12. Kotter JP. What leaders really do. *Harvard Business Review* 1990; **68** (3): 103–11.

13. Zavotsky KE. Developing and ED training program: how to "grow your own" ED. *Journal of Emergency Nursing* 2000; **26**: 504–6.

14. Emergency Nurses Association. Position statement: advanced practice in emergency nursing.

Des Plaines, IL: ENA, 2007. http://www.ena.org/SiteCollectionDocuments/Position%20Statements/AdvPracticeERNursing.pdf (accessed January 2011).

15. Emergency Nurses Association. Position statement: scope of practice for clinical nurse specialists in emergency care. Des Plaines, IL: ENA, 2010. http://www.ena.org/IQSIP/NursingPractice/Documents/ENACNSScope.pdf accessed January 2011).

16. Emergency Nurses Association. Competencies for clinical nurse specialists in emergency care. Des Plaines, IL: ENA, 2010. http://www.ena.org/practice-research/Practice/Quality/Documents/CNSCompetencies.pdf (accessed January 2011).

17. Emergency Nurses Association. Scope of practice for the nurse practitioner in the emergency care setting. Des Plaines, IL: ENA, 2009. http://www.ena.org/IQSIP/NursingPractice/scopes/Documents/NPScope.pdf (accessed January 2011).

# Disaster operations management

David Callaway

## Key learning points

- Emergency physicians are uniquely suited to leadership positions in disaster operations and are central to planning for disasters at local, national, and international levels.
- Certain key concepts – the disaster cycle, hazard, risk, and vulnerability – provide the framework for effectively understanding, preparing for, and managing disasters.
- Use of an incident command system (ICS) clarifies roles and communications among disaster response leaders and allows for a streamlined, effective response.

## Introduction and history

Between 1970 and 2010, disasters resulting from natural hazards cost the lives of more than 4 million individuals, directly affected nearly 1 billion people, and resulted in over US$600 billion in response and reconstruction costs.[1-3] A majority of these events occurred in the world's poorest nations. During this same period, the global population doubled, an estimated 90% of that growth stemming from the developing world.[4]

Widening wealth inequalities and shifting population demographics are redefining and expanding global disaster vulnerability. The effect of natural and manmade disasters on global development is so critical that the United Nations declared the 1990s the "International Decade for Natural Disaster Reduction."[5] The goal of the United Nations International Strategy for Disaster Reduction (UNISDR) was to develop "disaster resilient communities by promoting increased awareness of the importance of disaster reduction as an integral component of sustainable development."

The UN initiative drove efforts to professionalize disaster management education and training. Emergency physicians quickly emerged as leaders in the area of disaster operations management and medicine for a variety of reasons. First, the emergency department (ED) is the natural entry point into the healthcare system for most victims of disasters. Whether the scenario is a terrorist bombing, an earthquake, or a pandemic outbreak, patients will always enter the ED en route to definitive care. Second, emergency physicians oversee prehospital providers. This engagement with prehospital providers is critical during all phases of disaster management: mitigation, preparedness, response, and recovery. Third, the nature of emergency medicine is to triage, treat, and quickly discharge or admit patients. This operational model accounts for daily surges in patient volume. In disaster settings, this experience and mindset is critical. Finally, most emergency physicians have specialized training in mass casualty incidents (MCI), management of hazardous material (HAZMAT) exposures, toxicology, and trauma care. In addition, they have daily interaction with nearly every service in the hospital, from trauma surgery to infectious disease. The cross-disciplinary education of emergency medicine providers and their broad hospital-based network makes the specialty uniquely suited to lead disaster operations.

The successful management of local and regional disasters is directly related to the functional capacity of hospitals.[6] Damage to infrastructure, limited supplies, loss of staff, or inadequate surge capacity can all limit the hospital's ability to respond to immediate life threats as well as cope with subsequent public health outcomes. The role of a community hospital transforms from routine daily patient care to community support, assistance, and communication.[6] Accordingly, hospital personnel and emergency

*Emergency Department Leadership and Management*, ed. Stephanie Kayden, *et al.* Published by Cambridge University Press.
© Cambridge University Press 2015.

physicians in particular are critical for any effective disaster response. The American College of Emergency Physicians (ACEP) policy on disaster medical services states that "emergency physicians should assume a primary role in the medical aspects of disaster planning, management, and patient care." So critical is the role of hospitals in disaster operations that groups from the United Nations, the World Health Organization (WHO), the Pan American Health Organization (PAHO), and the World Bank have spearheaded a decade of international efforts to develop "safe and resilient hospitals."[6] Fundamentally, effective disaster operations management requires strong advocacy, administration, and execution. Emergency medicine providers are uniquely qualified to fill these roles.

## Key concepts in disaster operations management: the disaster cycle, hazards, risk, vulnerability, and resilience

The old axiom "disasters are chaotic" seems intuitive but deserves discussion. *Chaos* is a state of utter confusion and inherent unpredictability in behavior of complex natural systems. *Chaos theory* broadly addresses events or processes that cannot be modeled with conventional mathematics and focuses on how small local perturbations in one part of a complex system can have widespread and unpredictable consequences throughout.[7] Disaster operations management is an organizational framework on which disaster "chaos" is organized.

*Disaster operations management* (DOM) is the management of "activities that are performed before, during, and after the occurrence of a disaster with the goal of preventing loss of human life, reducing its impact on the economy, and returning to a state of normalcy."[8,9] A complete disaster plan accounts for the complex systems in which disasters evolve and creates a flexible structure upon which to transpose longitudinal management strategies. The goal of disaster operations management is to create strategy and techniques to reduce disorganization and strengthen community resilience, protect individuals, limit destruction of infrastructure, and protect local economies.

Key concepts that guide the practice of disaster operations management include hazard, risk, and vulnerability.

In the context of disaster operations, *hazards* are broadly defined as the source of potential harm to a community.[10] The first step in any effective DOM plan is to meticulously identify, categorize and rate hazards.

*Risk* is the threat that a particular hazard presents in terms of human, property, and economic impact. Risk can be generally quantified by the following equation:[11]

Risk = Likelihood × Consequence

*Likelihood* is the probability or frequency of an event and is based upon historical analysis and prospective modeling. Likelihood can be quantified and rated on a numerical scale. *Consequence* is the quantifiable outcome of a hazard (such as death, injuries, or damages). The product of *likelihood* and *consequence* is used to create a system of risk stratification: insignificant, minor, moderate, major, or catastrophic. This calculation is important, because communities and organizations will have different risk tolerances. Using this calculation allows DOM professionals to standardize risk assessments, determine priorities, and optimize investments in disaster-related activities.

*Vulnerability* refers to the "propensity of a group to incur [suffer] the *consequences* of a hazard."[10] There are four types of vulnerability: physical (infrastructure), social (social or cultural factors), economic (financial means of the community), and environmental (ecological health of the region).

Disasters are by nature local events. Therefore, the most successful emergency management systems have local operational control with mechanisms for integrating outside resources (regional, national, or international) as needed. The primary challenges in developing comprehensive DOM plans are money, time, and personnel.

Conventional thought holds that mitigation and preparedness efforts are generally at odds with organizational productivity. In addition, stakeholders frequently have competing priorities and interests. Overcoming these challenges is important. One strategy is to implement the principles of high-reliability organizations (HROs) into daily operations. The five parts of the HRO framework – preoccupation with failure, sensitivity to operations, resistance to simplification, commitment to resilience, and deference to expertise – allow institutions to create daily operating procedures that promote flexible response to changing disaster scenarios.[12]

These concepts will be discussed in further detail in the *Preparedness* section, below.

## Disaster operations management and the disaster cycle

The disaster cycle is a continuum of pre-impact, impact, and post-impact activities. It is divided into four phases: mitigation, preparedness, response, and recovery (Fig. 27.1). Advanced DOM programs include measures that build community and system resilience during all four phases of the disaster cycle.

New DOM programs often begin with the response phase to a major disaster. The urgent call to action unites response agencies (prehospital services, police, hospitals, clinics, the military, aid organizations, and government ministries) behind a common cause: preserving the community. Ideally, the response generates community awareness of the need to improve response systems. The development of a comprehensive DOM plan is circular and requires the identification of short-term, medium-term, and long-term goals. Short-term goals include the development of an elementary response mechanism that draws on local concerns and promotes civic engagement in community preparedness. As the plan develops, planners should conduct gap analysis and call upon the regional or national government to compensate for gaps in the comprehensive risk reduction plan. With proper foresight, local planners can gradually acquire and allocate resources to build capacity and proactively strengthen community resiliency.

This chapter will use the disaster cycle to discuss the theoretical foundations of DOM and provide functional guidance for effective operational implementation.

## Mitigation

Identification of the issues associated with a problem is the critical first step in the development of a decision-making strategy for addressing the problem.[13] *Disaster mitigation* is the process of designing and implementing procedures for reducing the risk associated with the occurrence of a disaster.[14] As discussed previously, reduction of risk can occur by decreasing either the likelihood or the consequence of a potential hazard.

Healthcare facilities face two broad categories of disasters: internal and external. *Internal disasters* include threats to daily operations such as power loss, disruptions in water supply, or security threats. Preparedness for these disasters begins within the facility and relies heavily on institutional support. *External disasters* include natural disasters such as hurricanes or floods, technological disasters such as failure of a power grid, and public health disasters such as pandemic influenza. External disasters are more complex and illustrate the critical role that healthcare facilities play in community DOM. The general process for disaster mitigation is similar in both situations. Emergency medicine providers play pivotal leadership roles throughout.

The first step in community-based disaster mitigation is to create a *local emergency planning committee* (LEPC). The LEPC is generally composed of representatives from hospitals, emergency services (fire, police, or ambulance services), local businesses, schools, elected officials, and community leaders. The LEPC helps to set community priorities and serves as an important resource to the DOM team.

The cornerstone of DOM is the *hazard vulnerability assessment* (HVA). The HVA is a comprehensive matrix used by disaster managers to identify threats, allocate scarce resources, create preparedness strategies, and craft a common language for responsible agencies. Developing an HVA is a team effort. The *HVA team* should be diverse, representing the major stakeholders while remaining small enough to act

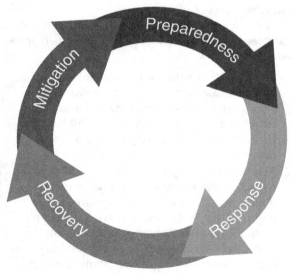

**Figure 27.1** The disaster cycle. Source: Federal Emergency Management Agency (FEMA).

efficiently. When building the HVA team, important members include the LEPC, emergency management, emergency medical services, healthcare facilities, public works, and local business or community leaders. Emergency physicians, given their unique position at the crossroads of prehospital and hospital medicine, are frequently critical team builders in this process.

A variety of online HVA toolkits exists. However, all HVAs consist of three basic steps:

(1) **Hazard identification**. The first step in creating an effective HVA is to conduct an exhaustive identification of *all* potential hazards (hurricanes, earthquakes, flooding, civil unrest, even computer failures). Each hazard is then described in detail, with emphasis on severity, expected direct effects of hazard, and projected impact on the community. This process allows for the generation of a risk statement that incorporates all relevant information, including political, geographical, economic, and medical impacts. Checklists are a simple yet effective tool for organizing hazard identification data.

(2) **Hazard profile creation**. During the hazard profiling phase, planners analyze organizational capacity, identify organizational resources and strengths, review past responses, and perform a gap analysis in order to determine a qualitative preparedness score. Potential hazards are then graded based upon risk (probability and consequence) and institutional preparedness.

(3) **Prioritized target list development**. From the hazard identification and profiling process, the HVA team creates a standardized metric to measure vulnerability and optimize allocation of resources for planning, preparedness, and response efforts.

In the USA, the Joint Commission on Accreditation of Healthcare Organizations (JCAHO) emergency management standards mandate that healthcare facilities have procedures in place to identify and respond to a variety of potential disasters based upon the HVA. The organization also requires that healthcare facilities participate in at least one annual community-wide training drill.[15] In many regions of the world, no such regulatory agency exists. It is therefore incumbent upon emergency medicine providers to advocate for disaster mitigation.

## Preparedness

Disaster preparedness measures are aimed at improving the expected capabilities of response and recovery efforts in advance of an actual disaster event.[16] Preparedness can reduce vulnerability and increase resilience. Emergency physicians are instrumental participants in the preparedness process, serving as subject matter experts in the hospital and, frequently, ensuring integration with local emergency response plans (LERPs).

In 2005, the United Nations Yokohama Strategy reaffirmed that "[the world] will develop and strengthen national capacities and capabilities and, where appropriate, national legislation for natural and other disaster prevention, mitigation and preparedness."[17] Most communities view healthcare facilities as the cornerstone of disaster preparedness. However, some organizations view dedicating resources to disaster preparedness as being at odds with productivity. Hospital funding often does not include allocations for the planning process, as it is seen as not adding to the institution's core function of direct patient care.

Effective organizations, be they local governments, hospitals, or corporations, operate differently. Instigating HRO principles can align disaster management priorities with daily operations in order to improve cost-effectiveness of the preparedness process. Viewed within the HRO context, preparedness creates a climate of safety that improves daily operations, avoids catastrophic failures, and enhances mission effectiveness.

The five pillars of the HRO framework, and examples of their application in disaster preparedness are detailed below:

(1) **Preoccupation with failure**. Imagine the unimaginable, then brainstorm mechanisms to prepare and respond. In practice, this means examining each component of the "all-hazards" HVA and mentally gaming various potential outcomes.

(2) **Reluctance to simplify**. Disasters are complex, but so are daily operations. Focus on process improvement and continuous quality improvement in daily operations. For example, if an institution utilizes just-in-time logistics to provide pharmaceuticals or equipment, recognize that this system will likely fail in disasters. Therefore, it is important to identify this operational gap, build redundancy in critical

supplies (intravenous catheters or sterile equipment), and incorporate this knowledge into training evolutions.

(3) **Sensitivity to operations**. Whenever possible, efforts should be made to create routine standard operating procedures (SOPs) that can expand or evolve to handle disasters. The focus on continuously improving daily systems allows for sustainable training, objective improvement in daily operations, and enhanced preparedness. Important, but often overlooked, components include developing staffing profiles, recognizing vital ancillary functions such as patient transport and maintenance, and planning to transition certain areas to continuous operations. Operations-sensitive training is critical in preparedness. Successful training cannot interfere with the daily mission. For example, large-scale MCI drills that interfere with daily ED operations cannot be routinely conducted at the expense of patient care. Partial task drills that test components of the system, such as patient registration or communications, are effective strategies to test systems, create staff awareness, and identify critical gaps.

(4) **Commitment to resilience**. Protect the staff and your constituents so that they can perform their duties and protect the community. This is both proactive (ensuring safe working conditions) and reactive (developing work–rest cycles and critical-incident stress debriefing plans). Examples of additional efforts include stockpiling critical supplies (pharmaceuticals), planning redundancy in communications, or negotiating contracts with multiple vendors to provide overlapping services.

(5) **Deference to expertise**. Effective disaster preparedness focuses on improving operational systems. An effective disaster operations manager creates a framework to engage component experts and effectively assimilate their knowledge into a broader plan.

## The disaster preparedness process

The disaster preparedness process generally is composed of four basic components: policy development, planning, training, and monitoring and evaluation. No one person or group can conduct all of these activities. However, emergency medicine personnel can serve as important advocates, subject-matter experts, and leaders within each arena.

(1) **Policy development** defines an organization's overarching strategy and establishes the legal and operational framework for disaster operations. The goal is to develop policies that clearly delineate responsibilities, ensure the pursuit of common goals, and protect victims, responders, and organizations. Effective policy is required prior to developing the written plan. Lawyers, hospital administrators, and physicians are important stakeholders in this process.

(2) **Planning** is a critical component of the preparedness phase. The written plan generally includes institutional policies, concept of operations, contingency operations, job-action sheets, and hazard-specific appendices.[18] The plan must be comprehensive, user-friendly, flexible, and able to be operationalized. Optimal plans focus on systems to identify which routine processes can be expanded, contracted, discontinued, or modified in response to disasters. The written document also defines the training priorities and strategies.

(3) The objective of **training** is to educate the community, the responders and the organizational leaders. Healthcare workers, and emergency physicians in particular, are at the vanguard of disaster management. Various efforts have been made to identify and codify core competencies for healthcare workers in disaster medicine.[19] The increased financial and medical burden of disasters is driving an evolution toward evidence-based disaster management practices. At the core of this movement is a desire to develop and validate core competencies and standardize global disaster management training.

Preparedness training varies in depth, substance, and style based upon the target audience. Various self-directed and professional educational programs exist for healthcare workers. These often provide adequate disaster operations familiarization training. Effective training builds upon this foundation with organization-specific training and drills. When developing a new program or evolving an existing system, it is important to review existing international standards and understand the individual student's knowledge base, preconceptions, and routine tasks.[19,20] Programs should be cross-sectoral, and at minimum should contain a didactic, tabletop exercise and an operational drill component.

There is also evidence that improved community education and preparedness builds resilience and decreases disaster vulnerability. One model advocates using the "village university" to train community members in basic life support in order to build local "chains of survival."[21] Likewise, in Cuba, the government trains school children in basic disaster preparedness and first aid. During hurricane season, these children, armed with local knowledge and basic first aid skills, are able to serve as force multipliers for first responders. As frontline providers in daily operations, emergency physicians are again uniquely situated to serve as leaders in community education.

The required frequency of training is unclear. However, a comprehensive hospital-based program should at minimum conduct annual community-wide drills, biannual interagency exercises, and monthly targeted system training. This can be augmented by formal expert lectures and awareness events. Ultimately, the program must address the multidisciplinary components of disaster management education, incorporating groups such as first responders, safety personnel, administrators, and business and community leaders.

(4) **Monitoring and evaluation** is essential to ensure that training is performed and is effective, new operational gaps are identified, and stakeholders have a mechanism for feedback. Generally, it is most effective to designate one person with strong administrative skills who can maintain the training matrix, assimilate feedback, and effectively communicate with the DOM team.

The 2006 earthquake in Bam, Iran, illustrates the importance of a comprehensive preparedness strategy. The earthquake destroyed nearly all of the schools and healthcare facilities and crippled 80% of the city. An estimated 30 000 people died. Despite the 2003 establishment of a disaster management framework, no integrated plan had been implemented.[2] A review of the response, published five years later, concluded that a "comprehensive disaster management plan must not be limited to the relief phase, but rather must include preparedness, recovery with optimal legislation and budgeting, improvement in healthcare facilities, and provision of organized communication channels."[22]

Implementation and sustainment of preparedness efforts can be challenging. All parties tacitly know that being prepared for a disaster is a good thing. However, the complexity of the task can be daunting and organizational leaders may be wary to commit the required resources (money, time, and services).[23] The first step is to bring together the key stakeholders and tailor the preparedness argument accordingly.

Flexible communication strategies are essential. Topic maps can be an effective tool in identifying stakeholder priorities and convincing leaders to invest in mitigation and preparedness.[24] For example, key issues for hospital administrators include cost-effectiveness, patient safety, and effects on the daily mission, patient care. Therefore preparedness plans must emphasize how the investment of resources can improve daily operations and strengthen the institution's role in the community. If meeting with local politicians, important components of the preparedness argument can include the ability to access national funds for local projects, serve as local or regional models of success, or create links to international funding opportunities consistent with UNISDR. Likewise, with local businesses, one can emphasize that investing in preparedness can promote continuity of operations, protect laborers and local markets, and provide financial benefit.

## Response

This section will outline the basic organizational principles of disaster response and key operational strategies. The response phase is the most complex component of DOM, marked by high stress, tight time constraints, and cognitive challenges. These operations seek to contain the event and reduce property loss, and to minimize loss of life and injuries.[16] Some authors divide the disaster response into *pre-hazard* (e.g., the day prior to a hurricane making landfall), *ongoing emergency hazard* (e.g., search and rescue response to an earthquake with ongoing aftershocks and infrastructure instability), and *post-emergency hazard* (e.g., medical efforts in Aceh after the 2004 tsunami).[10]

Coordination is the greatest challenge in disaster response. Disasters by definition overwhelm local resources and invariably require the integration of outside agencies into the response plan. Generally, the response is most effective when local leaders assume positions of authority and help to guide regional, national, and international support. Too often in developing nations, a lack of funding, awareness, and training limits the capabilities of locals to become effective response leaders. As a result, myriad outside groups descend upon the scene, inject their own priorities, and may not act in alignment with local goals. Frequently, these agencies do not proactively coordinate with each other or, at best, rely on the UN Office for the Coordination of Humanitarian Affairs (UNOCHA) or the UN Disaster Assessment and Coordination (UNDAC) teams to provide operational guidance. The emergency physician will universally be called upon to lead efforts in disaster response. This call to action may be as a medical provider, an administrator, an operational leader, or a combination of all three. It is imperative that local providers are equipped to meet this call and lead response efforts.

## Incident command structure (ICS)

Experience from Hurricane Katrina, the 9/11 attacks, and the Indonesian tsunami indicates that the successful development of hastily formed networks and implementation of an incident command system (ICS) can mark the difference between a successful and a failed response.[25,26] The incident command system (ICS) was developed by firefighters in the US during the 1970s to address the complex communication and coordination challenges that arise with multi-agency response to disasters. The ICS structure empowers local leaders while creating a common language and operational framework for integrating outside agencies. The ICS is a clear and relatively intuitive structure that has proven effective in hospital-based response, large-scale natural disasters, and complex humanitarian emergencies. The ICS is predicated on the concept of span of control, which ensures that each component remains focused and does not suffer "mission creep."

The ICS is built upon a five-component model that includes sections for command, planning, operations, logistics, and finance and administration.[27] The basic framework of the ICS includes the following (Fig. 27.2):

- **Command.** The incident commander (IC) is responsible for directing response efforts

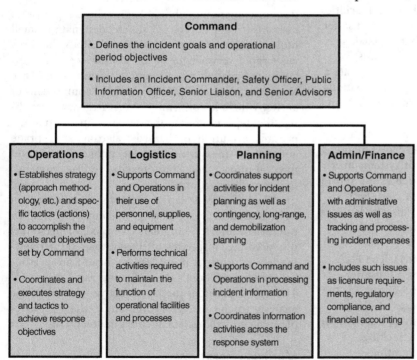

**Figure 27.2** Incident command system. Source: US Department of Health & Human Services. Public Health Emergency. Emergency Management and the Incident Command System. http://www.phe.gov/Preparedness/planning/mscc/handbook/chapter1/Pages/emergencymanagement.aspx.

throughout the event. The IC provides an initial incident briefing to responders and is responsible for maintaining lines of communication with outside agencies. There is generally only one IC at a time, though many systems will designate 2–3 ICs and create 8- or 12-hour IC shifts.

- **Planning**. The planning section collects information on the disaster, performs gap analysis, and creates the incident action plan (IAP). It is responsible for working in concert with the other sections to disseminate information and develop immediate response plans, long-term contingency plans, and demobilization plans.

- **Operations**. The operations section is responsible for executing the IAP and integrating responding agencies into the unified response plan. It conducts the tactical fieldwork, assigns resources, and provides the incident commander with "ground truth." The provision of medical care falls under the operation chief's span of control.

- **Logistics**. The logistics section is responsible for managing the critical supplies necessary for effective disaster response, including, but not limited to, vehicles, food, water, medications, volunteer and patient transportation, and facilities management. Logistics is the lifeblood of disaster response and the most frequently neglected component of a response. The system must be able to quickly inventory existing stocks, create a tracking system for incoming supplies, donations, and volunteers, and operate with transparency and accountability. Technology is becoming an increasingly important component of disaster logistics, and the evolution of web-based mapping systems and logistics management systems may revolutionize the field. Groups such as the World Food Program (WFP), UNOCHA, and the US military are leaders in the field of disaster logistics and provide a good starting point for further systematic study.

- **Finance and administration (F&A)**. The F&A section is responsible for tracking all disaster response-related expenses and accounting for the significant administrative challenges of disaster operations. This section must provide a system for respondent accreditation, patient tracking, incident record keeping, and accounting.

The Hospital Emergency Incident Command System (HEICS) is a specific ICS system that offers a general, flexible response structure for healthcare facilities.[28] The emergency physician plays a critical role in both multi-agency ICS (coordinating the medical branch or EMS operations) and HEICS (as a provider, section chief, or subject-matter expert). At times, the emergency medicine provider may be the only person who understands the ICS structure. It becomes imperative that he or she both understands the structure and is capable of filling multiple leadership positions.

During the response phase, the number of apparent stakeholders rapidly expands to include victims, local community leaders, elected officials, response agencies, and outside organizations (both private and public). Power abhors a vacuum. The ability to rapidly deploy an ICS improves an organization's capacity to acknowledge these stakeholders, optimize manpower integration, and reduce scene confusion. Functionally, success requires aggressive communication strategies (both internal and external), proactive on-scene education efforts, and clear operational protocols.

## Response operations

Response operations should begin with a *rapid needs assessment* (RNA). The IC should designate a small multidisciplinary team to conduct an RNA that provides rapid surveillance of the disaster scene, assimilation and analysis of data, and provision of guidance to responding agencies. In general, the components of an RNA include confirming the emergency, describing the type of event, the initial impact, and the possible evolution of hazards, alerting appropriate authorities, measuring current public health and medical impact, assessing capacity, and recommending immediate actions.

The basic four-step process for conducting an RNA includes (1) reviewing existing data (known number of injuries, buildings damaged, or personnel displaced), (2) inspecting affected areas, (3) interviewing key informants (local leaders, healthcare personnel, or victims), and (4) conducting rapid surveys.[29] The RNA provides both subjective and objective analysis to the incident commander that improves planning and allows for targeted interventions.

## Medical operations

For physicians, provision of medical care should generally be limited to triage and the hospital unless they are specifically trained in austere medicine. It is important that the overwhelming desire to help does not interfere with organized disaster response activities. Emergency physicians are frequently able to bridge this divide, working clinically across the entire spectrum of the disaster response. Further, the emergency physician is frequently called upon to fill critical administrative and leadership roles such as coordinating medical volunteers, deploying patient tracking systems, identifying operational gaps, and providing ongoing quality assurance.

## Recovery

Disaster recovery is the process of minimizing the long-term effects of a disaster situation and facilitating the efforts of individuals, families, communities, and countries to repair, reconstruct, or return to conditions that are as good, or better, than those in place before the disaster occurred.[16] Recovery efforts include both the physical rebuilding (provision of temporary or long-term housing, demolition of damaged structures, debris removal, inspection and repair of damaged structures) as well as the psychological healing of a community (addressing stress from loss of loved ones, jobs, cultural heritage, housing, or religious facilities).

During the response and recovery phases, there is great pressure for leaders to act, often sacrificing proper analysis and planning. Though ad-hoc recovery efforts can succeed, too often communities act reflexively and without proper analysis in an effort to quickly return to normal life. This behavior frequently leads to haphazard activities that may provide temporary solutions, but do not build community resilience.

The physical process of recovery proceeds through four basic phases: emergency, restoration, replacement, and development. In successful recovery efforts, these phases overlap and are mutually reinforcing. This process requires planning, organization, and execution. Pre-event planning for post-event recovery (PEP-PER) is an important process that dramatically increases the likelihood of effective, goal-directed recovery. Ideally the PEP-PER process begins during the mitigation and preparedness phase and articulates organizational priorities, action plans, and development goals. PEP-PER acknowledges community vulnerabilities and prospectively defines actions that can be undertaken during the recovery phase to build community resilience and limit future disaster consequences.[10] In healthcare facilities, recovery efforts frequently focus on similar infrastructure issues (restoring electricity, waste management, and water), return to daily operations including routine patient care, and completion of post-event assessments.

The Haiti earthquake illustrates a scenario in which PEP-PER could strengthen community resilience. Structural collapse was the major contributor to mortality after the 2010 earthquake in Haiti. This devastation is largely attributed to the well-known lack of building codes in Port-au-Prince. Though the hazard was identified, the systematic retrofitting of buildings or construction of new structures "to code" was not financially, politically, or logistically feasible. The result was that about 105 000 homes were totally destroyed, more than 208 000 were damaged, and nearly 1.3 million Haitians had to move into temporary shelters.[30]

Recovery is the most costly portion of disaster management. It is time-consuming, emotionally taxing, and economically burdensome. However, it can also present unique opportunities for strengthening community resilience. Rather than rebuilding to a pre-disaster state, implementing a PEP-PER plan that outlines a detailed plan for improving zoning, construction, and land use could significantly reduce future vulnerability. It is very important to incorporate mitigation practices into recovery and rebuilding efforts in order to avoid incurring the same losses in future disasters.

Many of the most visible stakeholders during the response phase are absent in the recovery phase. Partnerships in disaster response and recovery are often ad hoc and dynamic, but longer-term relationships are needed to incorporate mitigation and preparedness strategies into the long-term recovery effort. Especially in resource-poor regions, reliance on partnerships with non-governmental organizations and international aid groups becomes more prominent. Disaster managers with well-defined disaster plans, organized response efforts, and clearly articulated institutional goals are able to leverage these relationships more effectively.

Obtaining funding and managing donations in DOM programs is always challenging. Distinct strategies are required during each phase of the disaster cycle. Analogous to public health, investment during the mitigation and preparedness phases is essential and cost-effective. In reality, short-term economic constraints often pose significant hurdles. Accordingly, physicians and disaster managers must know their audience and often learn to speak a different language. In general, detailed plans that emphasize concepts such as return on investment improve success rates when soliciting funds. For example, when approaching organizational leaders, funding requests should articulate plans that both improve daily operations and strengthen response capabilities. A plan that identifies dual-use areas at a facility and outlines a process for rapid conversion to clinical space is more likely to get funded than one to build an additional care site. Likewise, when soliciting government funds, it can be helpful to emphasize the investment's social and political benefits. For example, a government-funded program to vaccinate children can demonstrate to the community a commitment to public health while simultaneously limiting the potential for a measles outbreak during a disaster.

In the aftermath of a disaster, there is frequently a large influx of economic assistance from private donors, international aid organizations, government agencies, and multinational groups such as the United Nations. Proper planning and ensuring the administrative capacity to integrate this funding allows for rapid implementation of predefined response and recovery efforts. The lack of these systems results in corruption, inefficiency, and loss of local control of recovery efforts.

## Conclusion

Emergency physicians are a critical component of effective disaster operations management. When disaster strikes, their roles may range from providers, to counselors, to incident commanders, to logisticians. A clear understanding of the disaster cycle, highly reliable organization principles, and the ICS structure, coupled with a flexible, mission-oriented mindset, is vital for success.

## References

1. Bacerra O, Cavallo EA, Powell A. *Estimating the Direct Economic Damage of Earthquake in Haiti.* IDB working paper series 163. Washington, DC: Inter-American Development Bank, 2010.

2. Djalali A, Hosseinijenab V, Hasani A, *et al.* A fundamental, national, medical disaster management plan: an education-based model. *Prehospital and Disaster Medicine* 2009; **24**: 565–9.

3. National Research Council. *Confronting Natural Disasters: an International Decade for Natural Hazard Reduction.* Washington, DC: National Academy Press, 1987.

4. Leaning J. Disasters and humanitarian crises: a joint future for responders? *Prehospital and Disaster Medicine* 2008; **23**: 291–4.

5. United Nations General Assembly. International Decade for Natural Disaster Reduction. 85th plenary meeting. December 22, 1989

6. Albanese J, Birnbaum M, Cannon C, *et al.* Fostering disaster resilient communities across the globe through the incorporation of safe and resilient hospitals for community: integrated disaster responses. *Prehospital and Disaster Medicine* 2008; **23**: 385–90.

7. Kiel LD, Elliot E, eds. *Chaos Theory in the Social Sciences: Foundations and Applications.* Ann Arbor, MI: University of Michigan Press, 1996.

8. Zobel CW, Wang GA. Topic maps for improving services in disaster operations management. *Journal of Service Science* 2008; **1**: 83–92.

9. Altay N, Green WG. OR/MS research in disaster operations management. *European Journal of Operational Research* 2006; **175**: 475–93.

10. Coppola DP. *Introduction to International Disaster Management*, 2nd edn. Oxford: Butterworth-Heinemann, 2007.

11. Ansell J, Wharton, F, eds. Risk Analysis, Assessment and Management. Chichester: Wiley, 1992.

12. Bigley GA, Roberts KH. The incident command system: high reliability organizing for complex and volatile task environments. *Academy of Management Journal* 2001; **44**: 1281–99.

13. Birnbaum ML. A model for all. *Prehospital and Disaster Medicine* 2004; **19**: 186–7.

14. Ridge TJ, United States Department of Homeland Security. *National Incident Management System.* Washington, DC: DHS, 2004.

15. Joint Commission on Accreditation of Healthcare Organizations. Revision to the Emergency Management Standards. http://www. trainforemergencymanagement. com/JCAHO.html (accessed November 16, 2010).

16. Rao RR, Eisenberg J, Schmitt T, eds. *Improving Disaster Management: the Role of IT in Mitigation, Preparedness, Response, and Recovery.* Washington, DC: National Academies Press, 2007.

17. UNISDR. *Yokohama Strategy and Plan of Action for a Safer World: Guidelines for Natural Disaster Prevention, Preparedness and Mitigation.* World Conference on

Natural Disaster Reduction, Yokohama, Japan, 23–27 May 1994.

18. Keim MA, Giannone P. Disaster preparedness. In GR Ciottone, ed., *Disaster Medicine*. Philadelphia, PA: Mosby, 2006; 164–73.

19. Hsu EB, Thomas TL, Bass EB, *et al*. Healthcare worker competencies for disaster training. *BMC Medical Educatio*. 2006; **6**: 19.

20. Hsu EB, Jenckes MW, Catlett CL, *et al*. Effectiveness of hospital staff mass-casualty incident training methods: a systemic literature review. *Prehospital and Disaster Medicine* 2004; **19**: 191–9.

21. Gilbert M. Bridging the gap: building local resilience and competencies in remote communities. *Prehosp and Disaster Medicine* 2008; **23**: 297–300.

22. Motamedi MH, Saghafinia M, Bararani AH, Panahi F. A reassessment and review of the Bam earthquake five years onward: what was done wrong? *Prehospital and Disaster Medicine* 2009; **24**: 453–60.

23. Petinaux B. Financial burden of emergency preparedness on an urban, academic hospital. *Prehospital and Disaster Medicine* 2009 Oct; **24**: 372–5.

24. Chesbrough H, Spohrer J. A research manifesto for services science. *Communications of the ACM* 2006; **49** (7), 35–40.

25. The Hastily Formed Network Research Group. http://www.hfncenter.org/node/117 (accessed November 20, 2010).

26. Natsios AS. U.S. Strategies for Relief and Reconstruction Assistance in Response to the Tsunami. Testimony before the Committee on Foreign Relations. Washington, DC: United States Senate. February 10, 2005.

27. Federal Emergency Management Agency Emergency Management Institute. *Basic Incident Command System (ICS) Independent Study*. Washington, DC: US Government Printing Office, 2000.

28. Zane RD, Prestipino AL. Implementing the hospital emergency incident command system: an integrated delivery system's experience *Prehospital and Disaster Medicine* 2004; **19**: 311–17.

29. Liu SW. Needs assessment. In GR Ciottone, ed., *Disaster Medicine*. Philadelphia, PA: Mosby, 2006; 224–8.

30. Crane K, Dobbins J, Miller LE, *et al*. *Building a More Resilient Haitian State*. Santa Monica, CA: Rand, 2010.

Chapter

# 28

# Working with the media

Peter R. Brown

## Key learning points

- Interacting with the media can be intimidating but it is necessary for an ED leader who is responding to a crisis or wishes to share a story with the public.
- Your institution's public affairs and communications (PAC) team can help you write effective press releases and prepare for interactions with the media.
- By understanding how the media works, you will better understand their role and their thinking when they are telling your story.

## Introduction

You may think you never will connect with the media, but in this fast-spinning age of the 24-hour news cycle, you never know. So why not be prepared? You could easily find yourself in a position to interact with members of the Fourth Estate, because your work – emergencies and trauma – naturally attracts media attention.

As you learned in your medical training, if you practice in advance, you will be in a much better position when the time comes to talk to a reporter. Do not dread the conversation. You are the expert. You are in charge. The goal of this chapter is to share some of the tools you can use if you interact with the media.

(Author's note: I believe it is important to state up front that I worked as a journalist in television news for more than 25 years. I am partial to talking with the media, because I see more benefit in doing so, and I have written this chapter through that lens.)

Before we provide the details, let us begin with a quick game that you might know as "word association."

What is the first thought that comes to your mind when you hear the word *media?* (Be nice, now.)

Did you think of any of these words?

- important
- investigative
- controversial

What about this word?

- *necessary*

The media can be useful, helpful, and yes, even necessary if you know how and when to engage them. However, there are some key steps to follow before you jump into any conversation with a reporter.

The first and most important: *No one should interact with the media alone.* Not that it is going to be a bad experience – in fact, odds are it will be a positive one – but you never want to make contact until you have an idea about what questions you are being asked to answer.

Chances are your organization has an office of public affairs and communications (PAC); count on this team to assist you in any and all conversations with the media, especially if this is the first time someone from a news outlet is calling you. The PAC group should have an experienced member who has the background to guide you through the process. If not, there are outside consultants who can help. Perhaps the most important assistance your communications team can offer is finding out from the reporter the story angle and the proposed questions.

One reason you do not want to engage the media alone is this simple rule: *Everyone needs an editor.* When you wrote papers for school, chances are you asked someone to look them over before you submitted them for grading. The principle is the same here.

*Emergency Department Leadership and Management*, ed. Stephanie Kayden, *et al.* Published by Cambridge University Press. © Cambridge University Press 2015.

You want someone to help you think through every one of your media interactions, no matter how many times you have spoken to a reporter before.

## The good/the bad

Let us stay optimistic and start with a positive media interaction. You or your organization has a story to tell and you are the chosen spokesperson. There are several ways to prepare and questions to ask:

- What is your "news nugget," or particular focus or angle to the story that the media will find interesting? The fact that you may think it is interesting or "news" does not mean that anyone else will. Rely on your PAC team to help shape your idea, or "pitch."
- Your pitch to the media needs to be compelling and relevant. Put yourself in the reporter's shoes; ask yourself if the story is interesting for a broad audience and state the reasons why.
- You need to identify a news organization or reporter to whom to make your pitch. Your PAC team should have an updated media list or an idea of which outlet or reporter would be open to the idea.
- Before you make any contact, you need to be certain you are ready. Once you make your pitch, if a reporter finds it interesting, be ready to speak immediately. Reporters are trained to think in a world where the news changes at least every 12–24 hours.
- Remember: Do not engage with the media until you are ready – PRACTICE, PRACTICE, PRACTICE!

This preparation is important if you are talking to a national news correspondent, a writer for a trade journal, or a web blogger. So what is the best way to prepare? First, think like a reporter. Ask yourself the basic questions and know how to answer them:

- who?
- what?
- when?
- where?
- why?
- how?

These last two, why and how, can create a trap for you. They can force you to speculate and to offer details before they are confirmed. Speak only to what

you know at that moment in time. You could write a news release and share it with the reporter. Doing this in advance of your interview will help you think through your message, which you want to keep to three or four key and compelling points.

When you write a news release, keep these tips in mind:

- The most important information must be first, defining your "news nugget" clearly and early.
- Less important information goes at the bottom.
- Write in simple sentences, using the names of the institutions or persons involved, but never referring in the press release to *I, me,* or *we.* Write in the third person.
- Keep the paragraphs short.
- Limit your release to one page.
- Add supporting facts with a quote from the newsmaker.
- NO jargon or acronyms.
- Include web links that support your story or provide further information.

Your news release, or "press release," most likely will wind up in the hands of an assignment editor. This is one of the key roles in the newsroom; this person helps decide what gets covered by the staff of reporters. Find out who the assignment editors are at your media outlets so you can address the news release to them. Better yet, find out their email addresses. An assignment editor has only a few minutes, often only seconds, to process a news release on any given day. You must get his or her attention in the first paragraph. Do not oversell your story, but do not understate it either.

If you have a relationship with a reporter, you can send the news release to that person instead. A reporter can be recognized by his or her boss for bringing a good story idea to an editor.

When you make your pitch, keep in mind whom you are addressing. Good editors and reporters are educated about many subjects, but they do not have the depth of understanding that you do on the topic, so do not talk above them. *Practicing your pitch with your PAC team is crucial.*

In all cases, you will want to think about your overall story, which will include a visual or audio element. Whether it is a reporter from television, newspaper, web, or trade magazine, all will want a picture. If it is a radio reporter, the need could be for the sounds of your story, if available. For example, if your story involved a patient's arrival in the emergency room, the radio reporter might want to get the sounds of an ambulance arriving. Finding the appropriate visuals for the story is always a little tricky. Rely on your PAC team to work directly with the reporter to find out what is desired and what is possible. One other point to remember is that many newspaper reporters today are asked to record video for their websites.

Reporters want every little detail of the story shared with them, but that does not mean you are obligated to give them everything. You are in control, to a degree. The point at which the reporter takes over is during the writing of the story. That is why it is so important to repeat your three or four key messages during your interview. You want to answer the reporter's questions, but you also want to make sure you get across your points.

## The interview

First, let us address the question of whether to do an interview in the first place. The potential benefits should be clear: an interview allows you to share a story that promotes your work, research, or institution. As you consider the benefits, you also need to think about the potential problems. There may be none, but be certain you have thought about it. It might be as simple as your colleagues' perception that you are taking credit for a story that includes their work, too.

After you have cleared these hurdles, think about the interview. The first rule of the media interaction is to remember that it begins at "Hello." Anything you say after that is considered "on the record," and the reporter can use anything you say in the story. If you do not want to talk "on the record" with the reporter, you must have clear ground rules before you begin your conversation. The best advice is to keep everything "on the record" unless you have a skilled PAC member with you, in person, helping coordinate the interview.

There are many definitions for the ground rules of what can be reported. Below are two examples. Each reporter you encounter will have his or her own definition; that is why you need to be cautious.

- "Off the record." This is supposed to mean that anything you share with the reporter cannot be used and you will not be quoted. This technique can be used to share a piece of information that might help shape a reporter's thinking about the story.

- "On background." This is information that the reporter can use in the story, but you will not be quoted. Often, you will see a reporter quote a source, but respected media outlets and editors are cracking down on unnamed sources in stories. There are other terms that fall into this category, such as "deep background." Unless you have training, it is best to avoid using this rule.

If you do find yourself in a conversation using these terms, be very careful to identify when you are "on background" and "off the record." If you do decide to use these phrases, only do so with a reporter you know and trust, and have a trained PAC member with you.

When you begin your interview, you may want to have an opening statement. This is not a long statement; it should be short (no more than one or two minutes) and compelling enough to help pull the reporter into your story. After your opening remarks, give the reporter an opportunity to ask you questions. Your PAC team should have prepared the reporter with background information that you approved in advance of the interview. This opening statement is designed to let you outline your three or four key points.

The interview will be conducted either with the reporter joining you in person, on the phone, or via the internet. If the reporter cannot see you, you should have a piece of paper in front of you that includes at least the bullet points for your opening statement and some possible questions the reporter might ask, along with your answers. You will be glad you did this. No one thinks they need this, but it is an important tool. If the interview is expected to involve some challenging and difficult questions, you should consider having a member of your PAC team on the phone. Your PAC person should not interrupt the conversation unless absolutely necessary, and the two of you should agree about the criteria for any interruption. If the interruption does not go well, it could harm the story and the reporter may write about it.

If you are meeting the reporter in person, there is much more to think about. First, you will need to know your topic very well. You do not want to have notes in front of you, because they could become a distraction for you. First impressions can make a difference. Be aware of your environment. If you are doing a television interview, your appearance matters. And I do mean down to what you are wearing as well as your hair; avoid anything that could take the attention away from what you are saying. Take a few minutes to prepare and remember to acknowledge the team that is working with the reporter. A cameraperson can make you look good – or not. If the interview is being held in your office, clear your desk of any confidential material, secure your computer with a screen saver image, silence your beeper and phone (mobile and office) and remove any pictures that you might not want in the background. No one ever looks over their shoulder before a TV interview is conducted or a photograph is taken; it is a good idea to be sure there is nothing behind you that you do not want seen in the picture.

## Effective messages

When you begin to create your three or four key messages, consider these points. You want your themes to be:

- concise
- credible
- persuasive
- repetitive

The message should be layered with facts and consistent with other available information that is known by the public. Be clear if you are sharing your opinion.

## Endorsements and challenges

Consider the role of "third-party endorsements." They are your friends or supporters who can bring an additional point of view or evidence to reinforce what you are saying. You need to speak to them in advance of the interview, and you should encourage the reporter to speak to them too. If your story has more than one point of view, expect the reporter to find the person who disagrees with you. If you know who that person might be and what he might say or has said in the past, you want to work with your PAC team to help shape your messages to address the counter issues that might arise during the interview. A reporter who has time to prepare may have spoken to your critics in advance, so you should not be surprised. A smart idea is to conduct a web search of your topic and even your name to see what has been said about you and the subject material. The bottom line is to know your weaknesses; the media will.

## Keys to success

You will do a good job in your interview if you consider the following criteria:

- Confidence – be decisive.
- Clarity – speak in terms that most people would understand; consider a conversation with a neighbor, not a colleague.
- Control – say only what you want and only what you know.
- Conviction – you should be interested and enthusiastic when talking to the reporter; if you do not care, no one else will.
- Repetition – underscore your important points.

There are points to avoid:

- **Don't** give too much detail. Let the reporter ask you questions. This is not a monologue.
- **Don't** use jargon or acronyms. The reporter could continue to interrupt you for clarification.
- **Don't** speak for anyone else.
- **Don't** speculate, or allow the reporter to lure you into speculation. Your comments could be taken out of context later.
- **Don't** debate the reporter or be defensive if the reporter challenges you; answer with your key messages. This reporter technique can be used to throw you off your message and get you to speak in greater detail than you wish to do.
- **Don't** accept misinformation, and correct misconceptions or mistakes during the interview.

The chance of you falling into any of these traps is small if you prepare. Remember that most interviews go very smoothly without any of these issues surfacing. If you practice you will be ready.

## Lures and traps

The next several paragraphs of this chapter are for those who may have to go beyond the typical, straightforward interview. The suggestions that are raised here should be discussed and coordinated with your PAC team.

You need to know that the reporter interviewing you is really not your friend, but that does not mean that he or she is your enemy either. Reporters have a job to do, and they all have their own unique styles of asking questions. Be cautious of the reporter who is extra-friendly, tries to get you to talk about yourself and your story, and nods in apparent belief at everything you say. The person could be just that, very polite, but the good ones use this technique to get you to open up to say more than you want to share.

Some reporters will want to paraphrase what you have said to them. If the phrasing is not accurate, speak up and say so. Do not let the reporter put words in your mouth. If the reporter does, make it very clear you are not saying that and continue to repeat the point you intended to make.

Reporters like to ask questions in different ways, just as you might when you want to understand a topic. A couple of the techniques used are multiple questions and yes-or-no options. These can be tricky if you try to follow their format. You do not have to; you control the conversation.

If the reporter asks several questions at a quick pace, pick one of them. If the reporter comes back with others, again, pick the one you wish to answer. If the reporter decides to go with the yes-or-no technique, do not get fooled. Consider this example:

- **Question:** "Yes or no: is the father of the murder victim guilty of the crime?"

You can see how you could get lured into a *yes* or *no* response, but consider this answer:

- **Answer:** "The investigation is ongoing, and we have reached no conclusion."

Control the situation and offer the response that fits your message and states the truth. A good rule to follow: Reporters talk to plenty of people; misinformation has as a way of coming back to bite you. If you do not have an answer for a reporter's question, it is fine to say so. "I don't know" or "let me check" are better than guessing.

## Other reporting techniques

The good reporters know how to work "the pause," that moment of silence that makes you feel awkward and might force you to say more than you want to reveal. If you are finished making your point, stop. No need to fill the silence. You can ask the reporter if he or she understood your point, but do not add any more information unless you want to do so.

If the reporter continues to use the pause, feel free to ask if you are speaking too quickly. You can also

use the opportunity to repeat key messages through a technique called "bridging." This is a technique that you can use to change the conversation to a topic that you are more comfortable talking about. For example, if you are given a challenging question and are not certain of the answer at that moment, you can "bridge" to one of your key messages using one of these examples:

- "Let's go back for a moment and focus on a point I made earlier . . ."

or:

- "Your question speaks to another point I want to make . . ."

This "bridge" carries you from a position of uncertainty to one of safety among your key messages.

Uncertainty also arises when you get a question that you were not expecting or one you did not prepare for and frankly do not want to answer. Your response could be:

- "That's a good question; I would like to think about it and get back to you . . ."

You should not use this more than once or twice in an interview, and only use it if absolutely necessary.

You might want to use it during an "ambush interview"; these often are the worst and, in most situations, are unfair to those who are being questioned. The "ambush" is rarely used by reputable reporters and news organizations anymore. They are saved primarily for those people who are ducking questions for an extended period.

There are several points to remember if you find yourself in an ambush. First, always be polite, even if a camera is pointed at you. A good response is, "Unfortunately, this is not a convenient time to answer your questions; let's arrange a time later that works for both of us." The "ambush" reporter will not take "no" for an answer. You, however, must continue to be polite. Do not put your hand up to try to block the camera; the reporter is hoping you will do this. It only will add to the drama. You should continue to repeat your message, "This is not a good time to speak, but perhaps there is a time later that would work best for the both of us." I know what you are thinking – "easier said than done" – and you are right. The key is not to lose your cool. The best advice is to avoid putting yourself in a situation where a reporter feels the need to ambush you.

This may not be an ambush technique, but it certainly can throw you off balance. Reporters have been known to call unannounced, especially if the story they are writing is not favorable to you or your organization. Until you are ready to speak to the reporter, here are some suggested responses:

- "Sorry, I was expecting someone else, let me call you back."
- "What is the best number to reach you?" The reporter will try to engage you right away, but you will want to get to your next question.
- "May I ask what your inquiry is about? My apologies, but I will need to call you back."

If you can get those answers without talking, you are in good shape. Do not be abrupt; be polite. Your next phone call is to your PAC team. Let them take it at this point to find out what the reporter wants to talk about and how it involves you or the organization.

Whatever you do, when you speak to a reporter – whether you are prepared or not – the words "no comment" are not acceptable for one simple reason: they make you look like you have something to hide. You and your PAC team must come up with a response that addresses the reporter's query even if it is not specific to the question. You should offer the reporter a statement that includes key points you wish to address.

At the conclusion of your initial interview with the reporter, take the opportunity to repeat your messages one more time. Remember to follow up if you promised you would do so and, more importantly, thank the reporter and the team for their time and attention to your story.

Your assignment once the story is complete, including any follow-up interviews, is to watch, read, or listen to the final product. Critique your performance. If the story met your goals, it is alright to send the reporter a note. Avoid abundant praise. The best choice is to say thank you for their time and their focus on the topic. Reporters do like to know they did a good job.

## Breaking news

What do you do when the news is not planned?

"Breaking news" is the most difficult to manage because it is unpredictable. Breaking news is defined broadly as an unscheduled news event, such as a fire or an accident. First, let us take a moment to offer a little history of the term "breaking news," which was coined by television newsrooms in the USA in the 1990s. Local TV news, in particular, has been known to take advantage of the drama of good visual stories since the emergence of electronic news gathering (ENG) in the 1970s. The brilliant engineers in television have gone on to master this technology so reporters can go live from anywhere in the world via small, portable satellite systems.

Some in the industry believe this has been a step in the right direction, taking viewers to stories as they happen. The critics in and out of the industry think this has been hurtful, saying that more attention is paid to the visual aspects of a story while there is less emphasis on the reporting and the written word. It is clear, however, that no one is talking about going backwards; the technology is only moving forward.

The media focus on "live" is crucial when considering your plans for how to handle breaking news and interacting with TV, newspapers, or any media outlet that is putting resources into their websites.

So what happens if you find yourself and your organization in the center of a "breaking news" storm? You will need to know how to react. Here is what news organizations want and need:

- **A rapid response from you**. You do not need to give them everything they want, but you need to give them some details (think minutes, not hours, as a guideline). Otherwise, they will turn to other sources of information. That could include the witness on the street who may know nothing but has seen something out of context. Think about the news release format. Can you answer the following questions safely and not jeopardize any crucial or private information?
  - What happened? Give only the basic information; if not answered, there will be media speculation. For example, if fire is involved, and reporters on the scene see trucks outside your building, they will count the number of them to decide how large the fire might be – the key words being "might be."
  - When did it happen?
  - Who was involved? Protect the innocent and children.
  - Where did it happen? Be sure to offer all contexts you can. For example, if a fire broke out in a patient's room make sure you can address the status of the patient, and of other

patients and rooms on that floor, in that wing, and in the building.

o How did it happen? Be very careful here. The phrase to use is "The investigation will determine what happened; it is too early to speculate."

o Why did it happen? Again, be careful, especially if there could be legal issues involved at a later time.

o Repeat the important details at the beginning and end of any release of information to the media.

- **Updated information**. It is not enough to say something once and then wait to report back to the media for hours. In a breaking news situation, your PAC team (some organizations in a crisis choose to designate a single person as the public information officer, or PIO, to coordinate communications) should stay in touch with reporters to let them know when briefings are expected.

- **Easy access to interviews**. The media wants to hear from the newsmakers who are directly involved in the story. Your local authorities, if they are involved in the story, can help guide you in this. You may decide that the people directly involved should not talk to the media right away. To the media, the newsmaker can be anyone who has direct knowledge of the situation. Your PAC spokesperson or PIO can play this role in the beginning, but at some point, someone making decisions will need to speak. The reason for this is to avoid a sense that your leadership has something to hide. A warning: This person needs to be a media-trained spokesperson. Do not put someone without training in this position; chances are it will not go well.

- **Meeting deadlines**. This is an intense pressure point for all reporters and all editors. The goal for the media is to be first and to be accurate. If they are not first, the intensity of that pressure increases, and your organization can be pressured by the reporters to offer information you are not ready to share. Do not favor one media organization over another during a time of breaking news. This will only lead to confusion if one organization has new or different information than the others covering the story. No reporter is looking to get it wrong, but the pressure to be live and first with any information is intense in the early minutes and hours of a breaking news story. Competition among the outlets drives this pressure. Do not underestimate it, because if it is not controlled, it could factor into how reporters cover the story.

Meeting a deadline has taken on a whole new meaning in the era of "live" and web reporting. Every media outlet has a new deadline: *right now*. Your best way to help ease that pressure is to answer the basic questions to the best of your ability. The media will appreciate it. That may sound like you are being asked to favor the media, but that is not the intent of this statement. If reporters are satisfied you are giving them the most current information, chances are they will stay satisfied until their editors call them looking for more information.

## To speak or not to speak

Let us take a break from the breaking news and focus on the topics that every organization struggles with during an interaction with the media. Should I speak to the reporter? What is the correct format – a written statement or a news conference? The answers are "yes" or "no" and maybe "both."

There is no right answer, as you probably know already. It really depends on each situation. Again, it is best to have your PAC team guide you through the process of determining the correct steps for you and your organization. So much depends on what the questions are, who is asking them, and why the questions are being asked in the first place.

If you have nothing to gain from talking to media, you should not ignore their inquiry, but do limit your response. You should always have something to say to help frame a story, even if it is a negative one.

## Should I speak to the reporter?

Sorry to say this again, but it all depends. If there is a clear benefit, then the answer is certainly "yes." If there are concerns that the focus on you or your organization could be negative, you want your PAC team involved immediately. Your PAC team can engage the reporter to find out the line of questioning. If the team is prepared with enough background information, it can use, with caution, the tools of "off the record" or "on background" to share information that can inject your point of view into the reporter's thinking about the story. As I stated at the opening of this chapter, as a former journalist, I have a bias. I believe you always want to say something, even if it is delivered to the reporter as a written statement. If you say nothing, then the reporter will write that or worse by noting that you offered the dreaded phrase "no comment." No matter what you do, think it through with your PAC team, and if you do talk, no matter how easy you think it may be, review your thoughts and practice with your PAC team.

## News conferences versus one-on-one interviews versus written statements

The news conference is an important and useful venue, but if not managed it can be a dangerous one. The news conference allows you to talk to the media, so all outlets are hearing the same story at the same time. In times of breaking news that can be helpful, but at other times it can be a challenge. Each situation must be judged on its own merits.

If the story is a negative one, you can lose control of your message at a news conference. With any negative story, you want to have a trained professional giving the answers. That trained professional needs to be a key member of your organization, not an outsider, and someone who has direct knowledge of the situation and is in a leadership role. The public wants to see their leaders take responsibility and not hide behind a public relations consultant or lower-level spokesperson from the organization.

If you commit to a news conference to explain a negative story, practice sessions with members of your PAC and leadership teams are critical. Ask members of your organization to play the roles of the reporters so the person speaking to the media can be ready. This approach is not intended to give the spokesperson a pass in practice. Your team needs to think like reporters and ask tough questions. A news conference that does not provide reporters with enough information could lead to more questions, and if the spokesperson appears evasive, you can count on a negative tone filling the paragraphs of the reporters' stories.

The other danger with news conferences is something called "piling on." Piling on happens when reporters compete with one another at a news conference. There is always a small minority of reporters who want to sound smarter than their media colleagues. If one reporter asks a good question, that could actually spark an idea for a more difficult question from another reporter. This could turn into an extremely difficult news conference for your spokesperson.

The best way to try to take control of the news conference, whether it is a good or bad topic, is at the beginning. Start with an opening statement. Do not make it too long. A couple of minutes – no more than three or four – should be plenty of time, but make sure it has enough detail to answer most of the reporters' basic questions. Set boundaries for reporters. For example, the spokesperson could initiate this phrase in the opening statement:

- "We understand you want to know more details about this particular aspect of the story, but we are not ready to talk about that yet. We are still investigating."

The spokesperson should feel free to refer back to that statement if a question along that theme or any similar theme is raised.

The goal is to build gradually on your public statement. The reason to move slowly is that you never want to back away from or alter your original statements; this can create mistrust with all your audiences, especially the media. This is why you start by answering the basic questions of what, when, who, and where, if you can. Reporters and editors love inconsistency; it propels them to ask more questions and keep a story alive. You certainly have seen the examples in the media. One day a person is telling the media this happened and then, two days later, the person is confessing to something else. Not a good way for your story, if a negative one, to go away. Be truthful and accurate from the start.

In this initial process of building your statement, be careful not to bring any other party into the story. In other words, do not blame anyone else along the way. If someone else, outside your organization, might hold some responsibility for what happened, keep them out of it until you have all of the facts and the proper legal advice.

The one-on-one interview is a good tool to use when appropriate. It takes a lot of time and energy, especially with your designated spokesperson, but in the right environment it gives you better control over your story. The one-on-one is simply what it says: a one-on-one interview with a reporter. This cuts down on the potential for the spokesperson to lose control. This does not mean it could not happen in a one-on-one, but the ability to look someone directly in the eye can be a powerful controlling agent.

The written statement is another technique to share your side of the story. Organizations tend to use this method if they never talk to the media, or if the reporter's questions have a negative focus. The written statement is one way to avoid saying "no comment," but it at least gives you the opportunity to have a point of view. One danger is that it can result in the reporter asking more questions if there is not enough substance in the message. Again, you want to consult your PAC and leadership teams when preparing any written statement.

With all these methods, you want to make sure that what you are saying is consistent with what you and your organization have said in the past. Reporters are very good at research and finding past public statements. To catch you in a contradictory message adds more substance to the reporter's story. A web search is a necessary step to protect you and your organization.

## The event may be over, but …

The event may be over, but the media coverage is not. You have spoken; the story is complete from your perspective. But for the media outlets the story may not be. For websites, newspapers, TV newsrooms, and radio news outlets, there is plenty of space and time to fill, from early morning, through the day, to late at night. If your story is big enough to warrant national coverage, remember the 24-hour cable news networks. The bottom line is to make sure the story is wrapped up from the media's point of view before you decide it is over.

## Don't forget your internal audience

However you decide to interact with the media, do not forget about your own community of employees. They certainly have a right to know, especially if the story has warranted a fair amount of media attention. The balancing act is critical, though. If you give your

internal community more than the media received, chances are a reporter will hear from someone in your organization. The person might simply be a next-door neighbor with no malicious intent. The employee might communicate on any of the social media websites; you know how quickly news can spread via those outlets. *A good rule to follow is that anything internal is also external.*

## Sharing with outside agencies

If you have interacted with a government or public safety agency during the development of your story, it is important that you coordinate all public statements. The worst scenario would be conflicting messages. Best for your team to coordinate all statements with the agency's PIO.

## Conclusion

This chapter has outlined the depth of material needed to process when you connect with the media. Each point is as important as the next. It is almost impossible to remember every detail, so count on your common sense to be your guide during your interactions.

As noted at the beginning, the media, intimidating at times, can be helpful and, yes, necessary during times of crisis. They can be your outlet for sharing information with a broad range of audiences. They can deliver vital answers to key questions the public may have as they work directly with you and your organization in providing the information. The goal of the media is to inform the public and capture their attention; it is a business, after all. If you have a story to tell, let them hear it from you.

If you do not have a relationship with your PAC team, develop one. If for some reason your organization does not have a PAC member or team, I encourage you to find a public-relations consultant who can be called on at a moment's notice. This consultant should have background about your organization so that if any tricky media interaction develops, the person can move in quickly to help. Time is your enemy when a reporter is calling looking for answers. As you know so well in your role as a healthcare provider, the better prepared you are in advance, the better the outcome will be for everyone involved

# Special teams in the emergency department

David Smith and Nadeem Qureshi

## Introduction

Historically, the emergency department (ED) has been the first stop for patients with undifferentiated medical problems. However, the first decade of the new millennium witnessed the growth of specialized teams within, and associated with, the ED. This chapter will consider specialization in the ED as demonstrated by the development of three special teams covering trauma, stroke, and sepsis.

Typically, these teams are formed to deal with unique types of patients that require a special skill set of treatment modalities, the interaction of multiple departments, and quick response times. Once the need for special teams is recognized, a multidisciplinary committee or planning team is formed to study the process and make protocol recommendations. Based on the committee's recommendations, a response or treatment team is created and an activation plan developed. Then, the team's planning committee meets to monitor the process, identify problem trends, and recommend corrective action.

## Trauma team

One of the earliest specialized teams to be employed in the ED is the trauma team. Multiple trauma patients, most commonly from motor vehicle accidents, present without warning, have multiple organ-system involvement, and are frequently the sickest patients in the hospital at that moment.

Trauma teams have been described in the literature as far back as 1990.[1] The rationale for a trauma team is easily understood when considering a patient who is unconscious, hypotensive, and tachycardic with respiratory distress secondary to a pneumothorax, frank hematuria due to a pelvic fracture, and a thigh deformity secondary to a broken femur. The usual model of an ED physician doing an initial exam, ordering tests, and calling an appropriate consultant when results are back simply does not apply. The following problems are encountered in dealing with this type of patient:

(1) multiple labor-intensive injuries
(2) prioritization of intervention
(3) immediate access to pan CT scans
(4) immediate access to the operating room (OR)
(5) immediate access to multi-specialty care

The experience of one tertiary-care hospital in dealing with trauma patients is illustrative: an ED physician needed about 50 minutes on the phone to get the OR open, the OR staff in place, and all the necessary consultants present to take care of a typical trauma patient. This, of course, was in addition to being at the bedside taking care of the patient.

---

*Emergency Department Leadership and Management*, ed. Stephanie Kayden, *et al.* Published by Cambridge University Press.
© Cambridge University Press 2015.

Establishing a trauma-code system to activate a trauma team involves the following components:

(1) formulating criteria for initiating a trauma code

(2) a "burst" paging system, enabling multiple preselected people to be called to the ED simultaneously

(3) expedited lab and basic plain-film radiography immediately available

(4) pan CT scan immediately available

(5) after-hours OR activation system in place

(6) command expectations pre-established – when does the ED physician turn over the care of this patient, and to whom?

While these system requirements can be listed in a simple paragraph, there is a great deal of planning that must take place before the first trauma patient arrives. The process starts by establishing a multidisciplinary committee to address all of the above issues.

## Criteria for calling a trauma code

While there are many variations of trauma-code criteria, they generally involve the following elements: multiple organ-system involvement, hemodynamic instability, an altered level of consciousness, and compromised airway/respiratory system. Some trauma activation protocols contain mechanism-of-injury criteria, but this has not been shown to be effective apart from consideration of the patient's clinical condition. Naturally, it is important for all of the stakeholders to agree on these criteria in advance.

Two other factors are important. First, the ED physician should be allowed to call a trauma code even when the patient in question does not exactly fit trauma-code criteria. Second, the ED physician must be able to call a trauma code after the patient's arrival in the ED when deterioration is noted or injuries are discovered to be more severe than initially suspected.

## Burst paging system

As in a military operation, communication with all of the involved parties is critical. There is a finite group of people whose presence in this situation is crucial, or likely to be so, with any given trauma patient. These people are as follows:

(1) Enhanced ED staff. Depends on the size of the ED, but typically 3–4 ED nurses are diverted from other patients for the initial stabilization process in addition to another ED physician, if there is more than one in the department.

(2) Respiratory therapist. Airway involvement requiring immediate intubation is common.

(3) X-ray technologist. The standard three-view x-ray series required to provide immediate basic information are lateral C-spine, chest, and pelvis x-rays.

(4) Nursing supervisor. A dedicated person must coordinate extra-departmental needs and open the OR after hours.

(5) General surgeon. A surgeon can help make an immediate decision on whether to go to the OR or conduct more diagnostic testing in the ED.

(6) Anesthesiologist. In some EDs, an anesthesiologist may be needed to assist with airway management, or should be available if the surgeon decides on an immediate trip to the OR.

(7) Neurosurgeon and orthopedic surgeon. Depending on typical patient presentations, some hospitals add these physicians to the trauma team.

## Expedited laboratory and radiology

A trauma lab panel and basic x-rays are required immediately. These are preselected and performed without waiting for the physician to place the orders. Lab and x-ray protocols do save significant time in critically ill patients, but have the disadvantage that some patients may undergo unnecessary tests and x-rays unless the trauma team is vigilant and conservative in their management.

## Immediate availability of pan CT scanning

The radiology department must agree to several essential concepts. The first is the concept of "pan CT scanning," in which head, neck, chest, abdomen, and pelvis CT scans are performed as a unit to save time. Second, the radiologist must understand the need to give intravenous contrast without first obtaining BUN and creatinine levels, and that oral contrast is not required for the abdominal and pelvic portions of the CT scan. Obtaining a pan CT scan in a severely injured patient is not a new concept, but there are still radiologists who are not accustomed to trauma patients and may need to be convinced of its necessity. Also, as with expedited lab and x-ray protocols, it soon becomes easy to pan CT scan any patient from a motor vehicle accident by ambulance, including those who do not warrant this level of radiation exposure. Establishing a protocol for pan CT scanning requires discretion on the part of the ED physician or trauma team.

## After-hours OR activation system in place

Hospitals vary in their after-hours capabilities. If the OR is closed after hours, there must be a plan to open it quickly when required by a trauma patient. When there is an in-house nursing supervisor, this is an ideal task for that person. The nursing supervisor is usually a senior person who knows the staff well, and should be included in the initial burst paging list. He or she should be involved in the initial deliberations by the general surgeon and the anesthesiologist about surgical plans. Typically a hospital will have after-hours contingency plans, so it is essential to have the person who can execute these plans in the ED as soon as possible.

## Command expectations pre-established

Most ED physicians are very familiar with the difficulties of getting an admitting physician to accept a patient from the ED. Trauma patients are no different. In addition, trauma patients are more likely to be uninsured, or at least to have incomplete insurance and medical information, and are likely to have an extended stay in the hospital. Traditionally, newly arrived, undifferentiated trauma patients have been the responsibility of the general surgeon. However, at hospitals that do not typically receive trauma patients, the ED physician may be expected to call the general surgeon if there is an abdominal injury, the thoracic surgeon if the chest is the primary organ injured, the neurosurgeon if a nervous system injury seems to predominate, and so on. This practice is outdated. The result is that urgently needed patient care is delayed, and the ED physician may be left with a critically ill patient with a low Glasgow Coma Score, borderline vital signs, and serious abdominal injuries that require serial exams. For this reason, it is now common policy for the general surgeon on call to be responsible for admitting new trauma patients for the first 24 hours. If it becomes clear in the ED that the patient in question has an isolated organ-system injury, such as a subdural hematoma or pelvic fracture and is hemodynamically stable, an appropriate specialist can assume care of the patient. The ED physician is expected to stabilize and resuscitate the patient until the arrival of the general surgeon. At that point, the general surgeon assumes care of the patient, and the ED physician takes on the secondary role of assisting with procedures and team organization as required. The trauma protocol must be very clear on this point, or the results are chaos. The nursing staff will be uncertain as to whose orders should be followed, and the general surgeon may leave too early if it appears that there is no intra-abdominal injury.

## Stroke team

Other rapid-response teams are modeled on the trauma-team concept. Each has a list of patient criteria, designated team members, and an activation process. Multidisciplinary teams caring for stroke patients, or "stroke teams," were first described in 1998.[2] Originally designated primarily for inpatients, stroke teams in the ED have become popular, particularly since the advent of thrombolytic therapy. As with trauma, the treatment of stroke is time-sensitive. Stroke teams have been shown to decrease the time to examination and CT (required before the initiation of thrombolytic therapy). Stroke teams also decrease hospital length of stay, complications, and mortality.[3,4] Finally, a hospital that is designated a "stroke center" typically experiences a decrease in time from presentation to physician contact, an increase in patients treated with thrombolytics, and no significant increase in complications.[5]

Typically, a stroke team is composed of three or more staff members led by a neurologist or neurosurgeon. Team members may include other physicians, physician trainees, and nurses. Most of these teams respond to hospital-wide calls and are available 24 hours a day.[2]

In 2005, the American Stroke Association Task Force on the Development of Stroke Systems noted that stroke teams are a critical element in providing systematic care for these patients.[6]

Areas of concern for stroke teams include the following:

(1) public education
(2) early patient identification
(3) immediate CT scan on arrival to the hospital or discovery of symptoms in inpatients
(4) prompt study review and transmission of results
(5) availability of thrombolytic medication for qualified patients

## Public education

The work of the stroke team begins – even before the event occurs – with educating the public. Only a small fraction of patients who are potential candidates for thrombolytic therapy arrive at a healthcare facility within the treatment time window of three hours (recent evidence suggests that this may be extended to 4.5 hours). If this therapy is to be made available to the maximum number of patients, the public must be educated about the signs and symptoms of stroke.

## Early patient identification

There are many similarities between the treatment of acute myocardial infarction (AMI) patients and stroke patients. Both of these treatable diseases involve a recognizable event pattern. Training health-care providers in the field or at the bedside to recognize the pattern is essential for early treatment. Just as it has become emergency medical services (EMS) policy to obtain a 12-lead ECG in the field to enable system preparation for the arrival of an AMI, trained EMS providers can give the ED advance warning of arriving stroke patients.[7] Appropriate patient identi-fication extends beyond EMS and nursing. Physicians must be reminded that there are stroke mimics, or disease processes that appear to be cerebrovascular in origin but which are actually seizures, hypoglycemia, psychiatric symptoms, or other conditions. In the well-intentioned rush to treat within the therapeutic window, physicians must avoid exposing patients who do not have a stroke to the potential side effects of thrombolytic therapy. Finally, stroke teams must be notified early of a stroke patient's identification and arrival at the hospital. Early involvement of a neurolo-gist, if he or she is not a member of the stroke team, is essential in patient selection for treatment.

## Immediate CT scanning

The third area of focus for the stroke team is imme-diate CT scanning on arrival to the hospital or iden-tification on the ward. Since the early 1990s, the primary treatment for stroke has been thrombo-lytic therapy. Obtaining a CT scan to rule out hemor-rhage or signs of tissue edema is an absolute prerequisite. Without a stroke team, the ability to obtain an urgent CT scan often is mired in slow test-ordering processes. Finding creative ways to move stroke patients to the front of the queue and expeditiously transport them to the CT scanner quickly requires a multidisciplinary approach.

## Prompt study review and transmission of results

Once the study is obtained, the diagnostic process is not finished. Radiology departments must be edu-cated regarding the need to immediately read and transmit the results to the ED. All of the preparatory work in early identification and CT performance is for naught if it takes the radiologist an hour to read the study or the results sit ignored on an ED fax machine. A direct call from the radiologist to the treating physician after the CT scan is performed and read is essential.

## Availability of thrombolytic medication

The final link in the chain of treating an acute cere-brovascular accident is administration of the throm-bolytic agent to the patient. The stroke team needs to evaluate pharmacy and nursing processes to enable rapid and safe administration. A "stroke packet" is useful. When a patient presents to the ED with stroke symptoms, the stroke packet is automatically placed on the patient's chart. The packet includes everything from CT scan orders to thrombolytic medication dosing information. For the physician, who may not order this medication often, the packet provides a list of perquisites and contraindications to thrombolytic therapy and a reminder of stroke mimics to consider.

## Sepsis team

In 2000, the Institute of Medicine published its land-mark paper on the state of healthcare in the USA.[8] This study suggested that every year 100 000 lives were lost because of provider error. The appropriate management of sepsis was one of the foci of this study. In 2002, the European Society of Critical Care Medicine, the International Sepsis Forum, and the Society of Critical Care Medicine joined together to form the Surviving Sepsis Campaign (SSC). SSC is devoted to educating medical, nursing, and support staff on optimal recognition and treatment of sepsis. An essential part of this effort is the formation of sepsis teams to provide an additional level of technical expertise in the management of septic patients. As in the case of the trauma and stroke teams, the sepsis planning team must be multidisciplinary, involving all of the primary stakeholders in the planning process. Effective teams include a hospital administrator, to remove barriers and overcome obstacles that inevitably arise and to provide necessary time and resources.[9] Sepsis teams typically include an ED physician, several nurses, and a lab technician. One large institution found that having a pharmacist as a member of the team facilitated drug selection and dosing issues.[10] The essential elements of a successful sepsis program include:

(1) early patient recognition
(2) streamlined diagnostic and treatment processes
(3) continual monitoring of processes and outcomes

## Early patient recognition

The goal of the team is the identification and treatment of septic patients within two hours of arrival in the ED. On arrival to the ED, patients with systemic inflammatory response syndrome (SIRS) often look very similar to patients with a viral syndrome, so accurate and early patient recognition is crucial. In 1991, a consensus panel of the American College of Chest Physicians/Society of Critical Care Medicine established criteria for a diagnostic continuum from early sepsis (SIRS) through septic shock.[11] Their criteria provided EDs with a framework for patient identification.

## Streamlined treatment processes

The next step for the sepsis team is the establishment of a protocol or clinical pathway to use for identified patients. The MUST (multiple urgent sepsis therapies) protocol is one such protocol. The MUST protocol has at its core the idea that a properly designed protocol allows the nurse at the bedside the freedom to identify and treat the patient within designated limits. When an appropriate patient is identified, the nurse pages the members of the sepsis team, including ED and ICU physicians. Once the central venous pressure (CVP) line is inserted, the ED nurse administers fluids as necessary to attain a CVP pressure of 8–12 mmHg. If the mean arterial pressure is still low after adequate fluid administration, the nurse begins pressor administration as directed by the protocol. The obvious advantage, in a busy ED, is that early detection and early goal-directed therapy are in the hands of the nurse at the bedside, who is operating within the confines of a protocol.[12]

One large institution experienced a 50% reduction in mortality after the establishment of a detailed sepsis protocol. This protocol focused on three major areas: recognition of the septic patient, resuscitation priorities, and ICU management. The hospital then prepared a packet, to be pulled when a patient met pre-established criteria, which included a care management guideline, a treatment algorithm, an ED order set, and multiple adjuncts to streamline patient identification and management.[13]

A common theme in hospitals that have improved sepsis care is the careful search for, and removal of, obstacles to expeditious care – from ease of order entry by ward clerks to ease of determining and obtaining antibiotics. This illustrates the absolute need for widespread representation of all involved parties on the sepsis team.

## Process and outcome monitoring

Every institution is unique, and every process, while having common features, requires local modification. The sepsis team committee must continue to meet on a regular basis to monitor and adjust the process. Performance review data will guide the continuing education efforts of nurses and physicians. Deficiencies that are identified must be corrected, and staff informed and educated. One institution documented a drop-off in algorithm compliance as the interval between educational updates increased.[13] Frequent review and a rigorous approach to maintaining and improving quality are essential if the sepsis team is to make a lasting difference to the outcomes of these critical patients.

## Summary

As in any other system or modality in medicine, there are pros and cons. On the plus side, especially in the case of the trauma patient, the use of a specialized team provides nearly simultaneous multi-specialty care at the bedside. Stroke and sepsis teams apply their unique combination of skill sets to augment ED operation and can bring additional assets to bear on a sick patient in an often overwhelmed ED. As noted above, however, trauma patients may receive unnecessary lab studies and CT scans. In addition, there is the potential for loss of control for ED physicians when physicians from other departments are involved.

Special teams in the ED are here to stay. Trauma, stroke, and septic patients present with multifaceted clinical problems that require the time-sensitive, comprehensive efforts of multiple departments. ED managers must be able to direct the efforts of multidisciplinary committees. Organizing and orchestrating these efforts is a dynamic, labor-intensive, frustrating, but immensely rewarding component of the medical director's job. This chapter provides the framework for ED managers to begin the task of setting up special teams to deal with these challenging subsets of critically ill patients.

# References

1. Deane SA, Gaudry PL, Pearson I, *et al.* The hospital trauma team: a model for trauma management. *Journal of Trauma* 1990; **30**: 806–12.

2. Alberts MJ, Chaturvedi S, Graham G, *et al.* Acute stroke teams: results of a national survey. *Stroke* 1998; **29**: 2318–20.

3. Schouten LM, Hulscher ME, Akkermans R, *et al.* Factors that influence the stroke care teams's effectiveness in reducing the length of hospital stay. *Stroke* 2008; **39**: 2515–21.

4. Birbeck GL, Zingmond DS, Cui X, Vickrey BG. Multispeciality stroke services in California hospitals are associated with reduced mortality. *Neurology* 2006; **66**: 1527–32.

5. Gropen TI, Gagliano PJ, Blake CA, *et al.* Quality improvement in acute stroke: the New York State Stroke Center Designation Project, *Neurology* 2006; **67**: 88–93.

6. Schwamm LH, Pancioli A, Acker JE, *et al.* Recommendations for the establishment of stroke systems of care. *Stroke* 2005; **36**: 690–703.

7. Kidwell CS, Starkman S, Eckstein M, Weems K, Saver JL. Identifying stroke in the field: prospective validation of the Los Angelos Prehospital Stroke Screen (LAPSS), *Stroke* 2000; **31**: 71–6.

8. Institute of Medicine. *To Err is Human: Building a Safer Health System.* Washington, DC, National Academies Press, 2000.

9. Surviving Sepsis Campaign. http://www.survivingsepsis.org (accessed January 2014).

10. Lowry F. Dedicated team helps to improve outcomes in severe sepsis patient. *Pharmacy Practice News* 2010: **37** (03).

11. Bone BC, Balk RA, Cerra FB, *et al.* Definitions for sepsis and organ failure and guidelines for the use of innovative therapies in sepsis. The ACCP/SCCM Consensus Conference Committee. American College of Chest Physicians/Society of Critical Care Medicine. *Chest* 1992; **101**: 1644–55.

12. Picard KM, O'Donoghue SC, Young-Kershaw DA, Russell KJ. Development and implementation of a multidisciplinary sepsis protocol. *Critical Care Nurse* 2006; **26**: 43–54.

13. Zubrow MT, Sweeney TA, Fulda GJ, *et al.* Improving care of the sepsis patient. Joint Commission on Accreditation of Health Care Organizations. *Joint Commission Journal on Quality and Patient Safety* 2008; **34**: 187–91.

# Interacting with prehospital systems

Scott B. Murray

## Key learning points

- Understand the major responsibilities of the prehospital medical director.
- Describe the essential components of a prehospital system.
- Discuss examples of organizing, funding, staffing, and assuring quality in a prehospital system.

## Introduction

If you are currently working in a hospital emergency department (ED), then you realize the essential need for an undifferentiated patient to receive prompt assessment and treatment. The same rationale applies to patients who are so ill or injured that they cannot reach a hospital under their own power, especially trauma patients who are otherwise healthy people who could have a complete recovery if provided with timely care. The World Health Organization estimates that 5 million people per year die from traumatic injuries. In 2002, among the 15 leading causes of death in ages 5–44 were road traffic injuries, self-inflicted injuries, violence, burns, and drowning.[1]

If you are considering getting involved as a prehospital (PH) medical director, there are many reasons to do so. It allows you to begin and control the care of your patients before they arrive. You can train a prehospital provider (PHP) to recognize emergent conditions, start treatment, and stabilize the patient before arrival in the ED. You can prevent inappropriate delays in care when time is of the essence and prevent inappropriate treatment that complicates the care of the patient. You can avoid unnecessary "lights and sirens" responses by ambulances that could jeopardize the health of bystanders,

patients, and PHPs. All of this will make your job in the hospital's ED easier and improve patient care.

There are reasons not to get involved, also. It will require much of your time. It may take a lot of political capital to start a PH system or cause significant political upset when you begin instructing PHPs on how to perform their job when they were previously operating without any oversight. Financial resources may not be sufficient to initiate a PH system or improve an existing PH system. The quality of the ED and the people working there may need to be improved before developing or advocating for a PH system that brings the sickest of patients to the hospital.

## Variation in prehospital systems

PH systems encompass any planned out-of-hospital response that is designed to care for patients and transport them to a hospital or other center for further treatment. It is important to note that there is no single "perfect" PH system that should be used as a model for the rest of the world; in some countries physicians are PHPs, while in others bus drivers are PHPs. There is usually an ambulance involved to transport a patient who is so ill that he or she needs to be moved in the supine position. However, any convenient transportation modality can suffice, such as the undertaker's hearse, buses, taxis, police cars, water ferries, and private boats or cars. A PH system could include fire, police, military, dedicated ambulance services, and the dispatch center that receives the call that a patient is in need. The general community is also part of a PH system that needs to be taught how to recognize a medical emergency, how to perform CPR, and how to activate the rest of the PH system.

PHPs are specifically trained to be out-of-hospital caregivers. They may have differing levels of training,

*Emergency Department Leadership and Management*, ed. Stephanie Kayden, *et al.* Published by Cambridge University Press. © Cambridge University Press 2015.

but can usually be classified into several general categories. There are many potential "first responders" who are geographically spread out, so they are very close to any emergency when it occurs. Outside of the USA, first responders are not often used. In those areas that use a formal system of first response, these personnel will usually arrive prior to an ambulance or other higher level of PHP, and have very basic medical training consisting of simple first aid, bleeding control, and CPR. First responders usually have another primary function (firefighter, police, military, other civil servants) where they are already present in a geographically dispersed fashion, are cross-trained for medical emergencies that arise intermittently, and are inexpensive to train. The goal of the first responder is to get to an emergency very quickly and start caring for a patient before PHPs with higher training arrive, who will then accompany the patient to the hospital in an ambulance and provide a higher level of care.

These higher-level PHPs can be roughly divided into "basic PHPs" and "advanced PHPs," recognizing that in-between categories do exist, and that a basic PHP in one country may be able to perform skills that an advanced PHP is not allowed to do in another country. Depending on the country, basic PHPs may perform basic fracture and spinal immobilization, oxygen administration, bag-mask ventilation and oral-pharyngeal airway insertion, hemorrhage control, scene management, and extrication techniques to remove patient from buildings or damaged vehicles. In addition to basic PHP skills, advanced PHPs are usually taught advanced airway techniques (laryngeal mask airway, double-lumen tracheal-esophageal airway, or intubation), IV line placement, IV fluid and medication administration, cardiac arrhythmia interpretation and defibrillation, emergent childbirth/delivery techniques, and so on. In some countries the advanced PHP role is filled by physicians, while in others it is filled by nurses or specially trained technicians. Some PH systems will routinely partner a basic PHP and an advanced PHP together and send this team to care for every patient. Other systems will have a tiered response in which an advanced PHP will be sent only when those skills are needed, and basic PHPs will be sent to all other patients. This triage process requires the person receiving a call for help (call-taker or dispatcher) to have medical knowledge or to follow specific scripted questions to elicit information from the patient,

bystanders, or first responders in order to determine the correct level of tiered response to send to the patient. Basic and advanced PHPs need not be tethered to the ambulance; they may come as part of the fire department or in a separate vehicle from the hospital. In Hong Kong, it can take an ambulance 30–40 minutes to reach a patient because of traffic congestion. In order to reach cardiac patients within minutes, PHPs respond to patients on motorcycles that are equipped with defibrillators.[2]

## Setting up a prehospital system

Which system and level of PHP training you choose will ultimately depend on your budget and on what existing systems have already evolved to fill the need locally. Incorporating existing systems and personnel into an integrated PH system allows you to learn the lessons that these groups have already discovered; should result in less political resistance from these groups when they are assimilated, rather than being left out; and allows one to take advantage of existing infrastructure, training programs, ambulances, knowledgeable personnel, and possibly an existing funding stream. The system you choose should reflect the type of illnesses and injuries that patients suffer locally, the treatment that is available at local hospitals, how fast treatment is needed, and the length of time to transport the patient to the hospital. For example, in a city where opiate overdoses with respiratory arrest are frequent, allowing basic PHPs (who do not start IVs) to administer intranasal naloxone makes sense even if there are many hospitals nearby. Training this same urban basic PHP to give intranasal fentanyl for acute pain would not make much sense, but it might if this same basic PHP was working in a rural area that is far away from a hospital or an advanced PHP.

Your PH system should strive to bring the greatest good to the most people with the limited resources that are available (see Case study 30.1). A PH system may compete for finite funds with other public health priorities such as vaccination, safe drinking water, or sewer sanitation that would save far more lives than employing and training advanced PHPs. Implementing an advanced PHP program is expensive and should not be implemented if that means not having basic PHPs available to the majority of patients in a timely fashion (see Case study 30.2). Choosing where to station first responders, basic and advanced PHPs, and ambulances should be made with the goal of reducing response time to the scene of an emergency. This requires historical data of the geographic and temporal frequency of emergencies in the area. Be prepared for political influences (the country's leadership wants most of the advanced PHPs stationed visibly in certain political and financial areas of the country, despite most of the need coming from an industrial district) or financial influences (ambulances are over-represented in affluent neighborhoods, at the expense of poor neighborhoods where the ambulance bill is less likely to be paid) to compete with this goal. Ambulance transport is sometimes a free public service rendered by volunteers or government employees. In other cases it is provided by private companies and "cash-up-front" payment may be required prior to transporting the patient.

---

**Case study 30.1. Imitating external PH models**

A Malaysian city was studying the creation of a PH system that would result in 85% of cardiac arrests having defibrillation capability arrive on scene within six minutes. It was determined that staffing and outfitting a system like this would cost US$2.5 million per year. The models predicted the new system would save only seven additional lives, three of them with severe neurologic injury.[3] This illustrates the importance of obtaining a cost–benefit analysis prior to developing what would seem to be a prudent system change. Because of different illness and injury patterns and patient populations, what works in one PH system does not necessarily translate to another PH system.

---

**Case study 30.2. Technology hunger**

A consultant, assisting an international municipal EMS service, recommended first purchasing basic and advanced airway management equipment, and that a defibrillator should be purchased when more funds became available. When the consultant returned later, all of the money allocated for airway management and defibrillators was instead spent on a single portable ventilator, and even simple basic airway equipment was still unavailable. VanRooyen has labeled this phenomenon "technology hunger": there always seems to be enough money in the budget for the most cutting-edge piece of equipment, but never enough for the more necessary mundane items.[2] Certainly it is impressive to pose in a photograph next to a shiny new ambulance, but appropriating money for improved

---

training is more important, if less glamorous. In certain parts of the US, basic PHPs can administer an epinephrine auto-injector for life-threatening anaphylaxis, but rarely use them, given the infrequency of the condition. One particular basic PHP ambulance service lobbied to get rid of the auto-injector, citing the expense of frequent replacement of expired unused medication. The same ambulance service seemed to have sufficient funds to request PH medical director approval to purchase a fingerstick blood glucose detector, even though the basic PHPs were unable to treat hypoglycemia beyond giving oral glucose, and hospital transport times were short.

When choosing what type of PH system you want, it is only natural to look at existing systems around the world. Most societies have developed some way of bringing ill patients to get medical care, even if it is not well organized (a private vehicle or a pushcart). It is important to realize that no PH system is perfect, even the more developed ones with helicopter systems, advanced PHPs, and physicians who respond to out-of-hospital emergencies. Nor is it necessary or desirable to implement everything that these other systems have done, all at once. It is better to phase in portions of a PH system, starting with the least expensive, most beneficial portions first. Some have criticized the advanced PHP role as unnecessary and expensive, as data suggest there is no improvement in patient outcomes for many clinical conditions when compared to a basic PHP who can use an automatic external defibrillator.[4,5] This is controversial, and in fairness there is a paucity of literature to evaluate the efficacy of the prehospital care given by advanced PHPs. Even without significant resources it is still possible to have a PH system as seen in Ghana (see Case study 30.3).

---

**Case study 30.3. First aid training for commercial drivers**

During the 1990s patients who were injured in Ghana were taken to the hospital by bus or taxi, for cash or for free. The drivers were sometimes providing care but did not have any medical training, and care was sometimes harmful to the patient. Between 1998 and 2000, 335 drivers participated in an education program that used demonstrations and hands-on activities to teach first aid principles. Of those drivers surveyed after the class, 61% said that they had used

---

their training when transporting patients. Thirty-five percent of the trained drivers reported having performed automobile crash scene management (up from 7% before the class); external bleeding control was provided by 41% of drivers (up from 4% pre-training); and 16% had splinted extremity injuries (1% before training). Two years after the class, hospital nurses who received the injured patients were asked to rate the care provided by the trained drivers on a scale of zero (potentially harmful care) to ten (perfect care). Drivers who had been trained two years ago were given a median rating of 7, while untrained drivers were given a rating of 3. It cost only US$4 to train each of the drivers. Even with little existing PH infrastructure and funding, PH care quality can be improved.[2]

## Advanced PHPs

There are several options when determining who should fill the role of the advanced PHP. Having a physician be the advanced PHP obviously supplies a caregiver with a higher level of training and better diagnostic skills, who could provide superior treatment. Physicians directly responding to out-of-hospital emergencies may require less oversight of their skills and medical knowledge. However, if the advanced PHP-cum-physician was not specifically trained in emergency care or does not have wide enough experience with the variety of emergencies that can arise, then care would be suboptimal. For example, a cardiologist may provide excellent arrhythmia management but manage trauma poorly; the anesthesiologist may excel at managing airways but be unable to deliver a baby. Physicians may have longer on-scene times as they try to fully determine and treat the exact cause of the patient's condition, when the best treatment would be immediate transport to the hospital. Physicians may deviate from protocols of care, since they are accustomed to being decision makers. Trying to remediate another physician's behavior or skill set could be politically awkward or impossible, since in this case the advanced PHP physician and the PH medical director could be viewed as equals. There may not be enough physicians for this model to exist, or it may be cost-prohibitive. One hybrid solution is to have the advanced PHP role filled by a general practice physician at the local clinic (who has been given some additional specialized training), and a basic PHP-staffed ambulance that would bring a patient

to the clinic for brief stabilization by the advanced PHP before continuing to a more distant hospital.

Nurses are usually abundant and can be cross-trained in the additional advanced PHP skills needed to care for a patient out of hospital when a physician is not present. Nursing is an existing profession with its own education and training infrastructure that may make the advanced PHP-cum-nurse model politically easier to implement than creating a new "technician" or "paramedic." The usual nursing training would need to be adapted to include more skills, assessments, and treatments that are not currently taught. However, nurses operating in the advanced PHP role would not use much of the education and skills that they are currently taught in order to function as a traditional nurse. Simply adding the new advanced PHP skills on top of the regular nursing training may make the training process too long or too expensive, and may be inefficient.

A new class of trained technicians could be created to specifically fill the advanced PHP role. Retraining or cross-training existing government personnel (medical corpsmen seeking to transition out of the military, firefighters, and so on) looking for the next step in their career can provide a useful pool of experience. Given that the education of these technicians would be specifically tailored to emergent PH situations, the training interval could be shorter and less expensive than in training nurses, thus providing an adequate workforce more quickly and more cheaply. Creating a new category of healthcare provider risks creating rivalry with other providers with overlapping skill sets, especially when a technician (with fewer total years of education than a nurse) is allowed to perform actions such as intubation that nurses might not perform. There may be political challenge in creating a new healthcare provider role and creating an educational infrastructure. With fewer total years of education, technicians may have less overall medical diagnostic acumen than other providers, but may have better, more relevant medical knowledge as it relates to medical emergencies. One problem with creating the technician role is career advancement. Where do skilled technicians go, and what will they do when they are emotionally "burned out," have a physical injury that prevents lifting patients, are intellectually ready for something bigger than their current role, or need a break from PH care? Nurses and physicians can cycle back into the traditional world of health care, but these paths are limited for technicians, and may cause technicians to become stuck in a job that they grow to resent.

## Protocols and procedures

Regardless of who the PHP is, your PH system may employ the use of protocols, previously agreed-upon plans of action or treatment for certain conditions. These protocols may be "standing orders" or "off-line," where the PHP follows a plan if the patient fits certain criteria. Some parts of a protocol may be "online" or require "direct medical control," requiring live orders from a supervising medical person (who may or may not be the PH medical director) who is consulted by the PHP via radio or phone. For example, a cardiac chest pain protocol might require an advanced PHP to obtain an ECG, place an IV line, start oxygen, and give aspirin on standing orders, but require permission from a medically more senior person (usually a physician at the hospital ED if the PHP is a non-physician) after consultation over the radio to give nitroglycerin or morphine. The benefit of standing orders is that care can start quickly, without waiting for the PHP to reach someone by phone or radio. Studies looking at online direction for advanced PHPs have shown that they can lead to delays in care, often do not result in the PHP receiving any orders that were not already part of the standing order protocol, and require a lot of time on the part of the person providing the online medical control consultation.[6] Using online medical control does have benefits, as it allows closer supervision of more complicated patients requiring nuanced treatment, or consultation if the diagnosis is in question and the PHP is uncertain which protocol to follow. Some PH medical directors use minimal standing-order protocols, and require PHPs to contact online medical control on all patients, so that the supervising medical person can assign a protocol for the PHP to follow. Online and standing-order protocols can be created locally by the PH medical director, may be specific to a certain hospital, or may be the same for an entire region of the country. Confusion can occur, and errors can be made, when PHPs are expected to follow different protocols for the same diagnosis based purely on the hospital to which the patient is being transported. This author advocates for a robust, clearly defined set of offline standing-order protocols, with defined circumstances as to when online consultation should be obtained, and the option to obtain an online medical control consultation at any time if requested by the PHP.

## Dispatch, coordination, and cooperation

There are several activities that the PH medical director will need to become involved in, which are not immediately recognizable as supervising patient care, but which are very important to the quality of the overall PH system. The dispatch center is critical in gathering the correct information from the site of the emergency and making sure that the closest PHPs and ambulance are sent. Dispatch needs to determine when to send advanced PHPs, firefighting units to assist in extrication of patients, and police to maintain safety. Dispatchers should be able to provide pre-arrival medical advice to those calling for help until the first responders arrive. Under-triaging and over-triaging of conditions by dispatchers should be monitored, and consideration should be given to using pre-scripted questions (emergency medical dispatching) to prevent ambiguous or redundant questions and answers. There are commercial products available that use templates both for pre-arrival instructions and to assist dispatchers in determining the correct level of response. Maturing PH systems realize the advantage of having a universal access number (a single, easily remembered short sequence of digits dialed on the phone that, regardless of geographical location, will always reach a dispatch center). Communications is sometimes lumped into dispatch, but it is also important for PHPs to be able to reach hospitals, their fellow ambulances, firefighters, and police in order to coordinate emergencies. Communications solutions range from very expensive redundant networks to less expensive transmitting radios or cell phones. Cellular phones are easily used, but airwaves may be swamped and unavailable to PHPs in major disasters when they are needed most.

The PH medical director may need to advocate for mutual aid, system status management, and regionalization strategies in order to maintain PH system quality. Mutual aid assumes that at some point all efficient PH systems will be overwhelmed due to an unusual surge in emergencies or a local disaster, and that this is best managed by having pre-arranged plans with other neighboring PH systems to send additional resources in this time of need. Each PH system mutually agrees to send a certain number of ambulances and PHPs to each other when the other's resources are unavailable. This may involve redeployment of resources by several nearby regions so that each of the assisting regions is adequately covered for their emergencies, even if only one region is in need of assistance. System status management means moving waiting ambulances and PHPs to different locations in order to minimize the response time to any one emergency. Each time an ambulance is committed to an emergency, potential response times are reassessed, and available resources may shift position (they are not fixed at any one single ambulance station) based on the historical likelihood of an emergency call occurring in a certain location on a certain day at a certain time. Computer modeling programs are commercially available to assist with this, but it may be as simple as realizing that extra PHPs and ambulances will be required during the week of a large soccer match or during commuting time. Using system status management allows more efficient use of available resources compared to hiring more PHPs based at static locations when trying to meet response-time goals.

If multiple PH systems have evolved in parallel fashion, there may be unnecessary duplication or redundancy, and regionalization should be considered. Consider two adjacent towns, each hiring its own PHPs and running its own PH system, but with neither town having a high volume of PH emergencies. For half the day an advanced PHP in each of these towns may sit idle or perform non-medical tasks, when a single advanced PHP would be busy, but could adequately cover both towns. In this example, and in a system that must hire more PHPs to compensate for a lack of system status management, the medically idle PHP's skills deteriorate due to inadequate patient care contacts, IV lines placed, airways managed, and ECGs interpreted. Local town pride, budgetary disagreement in how to share costs between towns, and even the PHP union or collective bargaining agency may prevent enacting system status management and regionalization methods.

The question of to where an ambulance should transport a patient is not as straightforward as one might imagine. It is the PH medical director's responsibility to make sure that the patient is being taken to the closest medically appropriate hospital so that the ambulance and PHP are rapidly available again for the next PH emergency. In some cases the closest hospital should be bypassed in favor of a hospital where specialized care is available (a burn, trauma,

or pediatric center), or if the patient's usual hospital is just a little further from the closest hospital. The problem with allowing ambulances to routinely bypass the closest hospital is that the patient may benefit by being brought to any physician and hospital, even if it is not the best one for the patient. For example, a trauma patient would benefit from a thoracostomy (chest tube) that was emergently placed to relieve a tension pneumothorax at a small nearby hospital, even though the patient would benefit from the care at the larger trauma center hospital that is further away. There may be financial or political incentives for ambulances to transport patients to one hospital but not another, such as bringing poor patients to government hospitals and not to private hospitals. The ambulance or PHPs, if employed by a hospital, may have a financial incentive to bring the patient to "their" hospital. It is even possible that ambulances cannot find a hospital to which to bring their patients, as has happened in the United States during diversion periods, when EDs send out a radio announcement to PH systems that they are closed to new patients due to overcrowding – which is usually due to patient boarding (admitted patients being kept in the ED for longer than normal). Some areas in the US have banned the use of diversion (forcing hospitals to resolve their boarding problems), placed limits on the number of hospitals that can be on diversion at once, or started a triage team that directs ambulances to the most appropriate hospital when hospitals are on diversion (see Case study 30.4) The PH medical director will find that large system issues like this are best worked out with other PH medical directors from different hospitals who advocate at the national and regional government level. Gaining such representation blends into public health efforts in that the PH system has unique first-hand knowledge and data that are useful in identifying injuries and illness patterns that occur in the home, workplace, and transportation sectors that could be prevented with improved safety regulation.

### Case study 30.4. Diversion

In one country, a patient must be accepted by a physician in the hospital's ED before PHPs transport the patient to that hospital. Local law states that "physicians are required to examine patients unless an appropriate reason is present," but prior to 2009 there were no specific rules governing ambulance patient acceptance.[7] It is at the discretion of the physician whether or not to accept the patient. The physician is not legally liable if he or she refuses to accept the patient, but once a physician accepts transfer and starts caring for a patient, that physician may be subject to legal penalties if the patient is not cared for correctly. The "appropriate reason" standard is vague – it may be that the ED is too busy, does not have enough staff, or does not anticipate having the appropriate consultants available, or that the ED physician feels uncomfortable in caring for the patient.[8] EDs in this country are varied in the scope of care that they can provide, and some physicians may not feel capable in procedures such as childbirth. In the past, even the larger, tertiary hospitals (a hybrid of intensive care and trauma units) would sometimes refuse to accept neurosurgical emergencies if the ED physician was uncertain whether a neurosurgeon was available or on call. The malpractice system dissuades physicians from accepting and caring for some patients who need immediate medical care, even if it is not rendered by the most trained person. Hence, a practice has evolved in which ambulances make multiple requests for acceptance to several different hospitals and sometimes drive great distances with unstable patients, bypassing many hospitals that have refused to accept the patient. After several examples of patients having bad outcomes due to delays from this practice, hospital EDs have addressed the problem by agreeing to accept the patient if the ambulance has already been refused by two other hospitals. Patient acceptance now occurs more smoothly. Hospital ED issues, such as consultant availability and malpractice or legal concerns, frequently trickle down and affect PH systems.

# Finance

One of the largest barriers to running an effective PH system is its financing. When explaining the need for a PH system to policy makers, it is useful to point out the lost economic productivity that comes from patients who have needlessly died or become severely disabled simply for lack of good and timely emergency care. Besides the immediate loss of a family member who earns income, the remaining family members may now be prevented from working and contributing to the economy because they are consumed with caring for a permanently disabled patient. Governmental and charitable welfare programs could end up paying to assist these families. However, there is a greater societal question: who should pay for PH systems? Is it the responsibility of the government, similar to police and fire services, or a personal privilege?

Internationally, PH systems are funded and provided by a mix of national, regional, and local government; non-profit groups; for-profit private companies; and volunteers who do not charge for their services. Different branches of the same government may even claim overlapping authority or provide funds: transportation, public health, disaster agencies, public safety/law enforcement, and so on (see Case study 30.5). This author believes it is appropriate to allow PH systems to attempt to collect reasonable fees from patients after care is rendered, but unethical to demand payment prior to transporting the patient to hospital, or to refuse to provide care if it is suspected that the patient cannot pay. Such "cash-up-front" policies were not uncommon in the very early days of US ambulance operations. Some allowance or public funds should be made available so that people are not dissuaded from seeking lifesaving care because of a self-perceived inability to pay for PH care. Some sort of liability protection should be provided to protect PHPs who are acting in the best interest of the patient.

The importance of political capital cannot be overemphasized when seeking funding for a PH system. It is important for the PH medical director to be integrated into the local and regional governmental leadership so that the PH medical director is consulted as an expert resource on PH systems. Serving on committees and task forces, making time for small pleasantries or dinner, and writing friendly but informative letters to policymakers are all crucial to building relationships to help advocate for the PH system. It is important to make sure that someone is touting the PH system's successes to the public. The paramedic movement in the US did not really grow until the government allocated funds to start up paramedic programs in response to public demand from a nation that enjoyed a new a television show, *Emergency!*, which was based on a then-rare paramedic PH system.

> **Case study 30.5. Successfully funding a private PH system**
>
> Each state in India has its own method of providing PH systems, including government, charitable, and private "cash-up-front" ambulances. Confusion can occur when a patient or bystander does not know

which of many possible numbers to dial when needing help or is unable (or unsure if they will be able) to pay for the ambulance when it arrives. In the early 2000s the level and quality of care provided by the different services was highly variable, and in many places ambulance transport was still being delivered in hearses. In 2005, Ziqitza Health Care's "Dial 1298 for Ambulance" program started providing advanced and basic PHP ambulance services in one city with 10 ambulances. Their development and rapid expansion is a success story of innovative PH system funding.

The 1298 model provides ambulance service for anyone regardless of his or her ability to pay. It works because of a differential pricing model: the affluent are charged full rates, while the charge is reduced by a sliding scale for others. Hospital destination is used as a proxy for the ability to pay. Patients going to expensive private hospitals are felt to be able to pay the full rate, while patients going to government hospitals with an emergency are deemed to be less affluent. Regardless of one's ability to pay, the ambulance will transport any accident or disaster victim to the government hospital for free, leading to rapid recall of the number 1298 by the public.

When starting the business, the owners were unable to secure traditional bank financing and were forced to put most of their own savings into the business. They rented out the space on the sides of the ambulances for brightly colored advertisements (which were often featured during television news coverage of emergencies), and this practice currently accounts for 40% of the company's revenue. The Acumen Fund, a non-profit venture capital organization that invests in financially self-sustainable companies that are trying to solve the problems of global poverty, provided a large capital infusion for Ziqitza Health Care to improve marketing and expand operations. Ziqitza has since expanded to several other Indian states in public–private partnership with "Dial 108 in Emergency," where the ambulance company is paid by the government to provide care for free for a fee set by the government. In 2010, Ziqitza, with over 300 ambulances, set out to obtain additional capital funding for expansion from another large foreign ambulance company.[9]

## Other roles for the prehospital system

Though we have focused on the emergent PH system (unscheduled care and transport of the acutely ill or injured from the scene to a hospital), there are other times when ambulances and PHPs are used. PHPs are uniquely trained and equipped to transport invalid people even if they are not acutely medically decompensated but instead simply cannot sit up, need oxygen, or require suctioning. Patients may need to be routinely transported from their home to their routine medical appointments. Occasionally a patient is too ill to stay at one hospital and will require transport to another hospital. This patient may have been only partially stabilized, may have medical devices inserted, or medications infusing, all of which are unfamiliar to the PHP. In order to prevent errors during transport, the PHP operating in this role should be trained in these medications and devices, and liberal consultation with a knowledgeable physician should occur. PHPs may be used in other capacities, such as providing first aid at mass gatherings, working in hospitals as assistants, or providing medical coverage at sporting events.

## The role of the director

You should always be aware of how strong the PH medical director role actually is; how much influence you may or may not have with certain people; who your allies are; who does not understand the PH system but should be informed about it; and who has the political power in your hospital, government, or ambulance service to accomplish things. Your hospital or department leadership needs to understand the role of the PH medical director so that they will financially support your time. It may be necessary to explain the nuances and details of your PH system to educate them on why everything cannot change all at once. Ambulance services and PHPs may or may not want your input, even if your ideas are needed and correct. You should, but may not be allowed to, determine which PHPs are allowed to work in the PH system and have input into the training of PHPs. You should, but may not, have control over which medical devices are purchased and used by the PH system (ventilators, NIPPV, glucometers, cardiac monitors, cricothyroidotomy kits). You should, but may not, have significant input into the creation of care protocols and deciding the medications that will be carried by PHPs and when they should be administered. If you are responsible for a PH system, you should have access to medical records and response-time data, even if the ambulance transported the patient to a hospital at which you do not work. You should have representation at governmental or regional meetings where your PH system is being modified or discussions are had about credentialing or licensing PHPs operating under your oversight.

## Quality assurance and improvement

Even though there are many different ways to design a PH system, the underlying approach in setting up a program to ensure quality is the same. Prospective education can take the form of education on protocols, reviewing the differential diagnoses to consider for a given chief complaint, focusing on the care of a specific illness or injury, or reviewing challenging non-medical scenarios such as extrication techniques or dealing with an intoxicated patient. Medical education speakers should make the medical knowledge relevant to the PHP, but avoid "speaking down" to the PHP. For example, a vascular surgeon who is a gifted speaker could speak about the latest surgical techniques in treating a rupturing abdominal aortic aneurysm, but this may not be relevant or helpful. When an expert who is less familiar with PH systems assists with education, it is helpful for the PH medical director to create learning objectives for the expert in order to make the education relevant and to make sure that PHPs are not being instructed to perform procedures or give medications that they are not permitted to do. "Skill labs" are the backbone of honing procedural skills before a PHP is required to perform them. PHPs may practice placing IV lines in the hospital or be taught intubating and bag-masking techniques in the operating room. Extremity splinting, spinal immobilization, and ECG or rhythm-strip interpretation can easily be done in small groups. Simulation, with mannequins, can be used to review critical steps in severely ill patients without the need of expensive high-fidelity equipment. Anyone operating an emergency vehicle needs to be trained in the safe operation of these vehicles, especially if operating in "lights and sirens" mode. To identify PHPs who need extra help, or determine future education needs, it may be helpful to routinely test PHPs in these topics as part of an ongoing credentialing program.

Retrospectively, quality assurance is usually performed by chart review. There should always be some record of the patient's encounter with the PH system that at a minimum includes basic demographic information, location of the emergency, nature of injury or illness, any exam findings including vital signs,

care that was rendered by the PHP, and where the patient was taken. If possible, certain key times should be recorded: the time the call for help arrived at the initial call-taking point/dispatch center, the time the ambulance and/or PHPs each were dispatched, the time the ambulance and/or PHPs each arrived to the scene of the emergency, the time the ambulance left the scene, the time the ambulance arrived at the hospital, and the time the ambulance and/or PHPs were available to respond to another call. Calculating these intervals (especially dispatch-center time, ambulance and PHP response time, on-scene time, transport-to-hospital time) allows one to look broadly at system efficiency and determine appropriate PHP staffing levels. Response and transport-to-hospital times should be separated by emergent (light/sirens) and routine (regular driving patterns) if the dispatch center and PHPs are trained in dual dispatch/ response modes. There is good discussion elsewhere of these intervals, and what data points should be captured on the PHP's chart.[2],[10]

One can review a random general sampling of charts for overall quality, or a rotating clinical topic might be chosen (for example, this month: for all patients with cardiac chest pain, what percentage of patients had an ECG, received aspirin, were given oxygen; next month: in motor vehicle accident patients what percentage had cervical spine immobilization and complete vitals taken). One can also target high-risk or low-frequency conditions, since something that is rarely done or is being performed under high stress has an increased probability of being performed incorrectly. Procedures such as needle decompression of suspected pneumothorax, external pacing, airway management, childbirth, and care of young children might routinely be reviewed. Reviewing the appropriate use of skills includes calculating the percentage of patients who had an IV line placed when it was indicated, or who had an ECG performed when indicated and whether it was interpreted correctly.

Two special cases of retrospective review involve deaths and refusals. Your PH system may or may not allow a PHP to declare a patient to be dead and thus stop resuscitation efforts. Besides wasting resources, PHPs and bystanders would be placed at unnecessary risk by ambulances rapidly transporting an unsalvageable patient to the hospital. However, nothing is more politically damaging and demoralizing to the PH system than erroneously declaring a patient dead, only to discover later that the patient is alive but critically ill. There are well-publicized cases in the US of patients with hypothermia, toxic ingestions, and hypoglycemia who had a delay in care after mistakenly being presumed dead by PHPs. Severe bruising can present as lividity, and arthritis masquerades as rigor mortis. If your system does allow PHPs to declare death, this author recommends that a structured checklist protocol be followed via phone or radio consultation with a supervising physician.

Depending on the resources available to the PH system, local medicolegal risk climate, and local culture, you may decide to review cases in which the patient refuses transport to the hospital, or the PHPs determine the patient does not require ambulance transport to the hospital. There are many activations of the PH system in response to which the patient may decline transport to hospital after PHP intervention: hypoglycemic diabetics who improve after IV dextrose, dyspneic asthma patients who feel better after nebulized albuterol, an elderly patient who fell and only needs assistance standing up, a person in a car accident who is uninjured but a concerned bystander has activated the PH system. As appropriate as this may seem, there is some risk when patients who appear ill enough to generate a PH system activation are not transported to the hospital. The diabetic may have hypoglycemia because he or she takes a sulfonylurea medication, and may become hypoglycemic again; perhaps the elderly patient fell because of an underlying urine infection and may fall again and fracture a hip; the asthmatic may need a course of systemic steroids; the uninjured motorist may be intoxicated on alcohol and not perceive his spinal fracture. In the US (where the PHP is a non-physician technician), one study examined the outcome of patients who refused PHP medical assistance and found that about half of the refusing patients required some other medical attention for the same complaint within a seven-day period, with 7% of them actually admitted to the hospital, and 0.5% died within a week.[11] Realizing that there is medical need in the refusing population, researchers sought to discover how patients could be convinced to be transported to the hospital for further evaluation. Having a physician who is knowledgeable in PH systems check the PHP's assessment of the patient (over the phone or radio) increases the transport rate of high-risk patients tenfold.[12] About a third of patients who initially refuse care will change their minds and be transported to the hospital after they speak directly over the phone to a physician knowledgeable in PH systems.[13] A doctor who is assertive and asks questions when providing radio guidance to PHPs results in a much higher transport rate (81%) than a doctor who is more passive (19%).[14]

Having a senior medical provider knowledgeable in PH systems provide online medical control allows the PH medical director (or whoever is providing the online medical control) to influence care in real time and to give feedback to the PHPs in the moment. It need not be a physician providing online medical control, provided the person is well trained. Some oversight and review of the person providing the online medical control should be performed, the most useful way being to listen to recorded conversations with the PHPs. Other ways of providing concurrent guidance are ambulance ride-alongs with PHPs or having other supervisors observe and teach while providing PH care.

Inevitably a situation will occur in which a PHP will have made an error, and the PH medical director will be charged with either remediating or disciplining the PHP. Remediation assumes that the PHP wants to do a better job next time and that most error is due to lack of knowledge, or that a latent error in the PH system design is to blame (for example, two different medications have similar packaging). Remediation requires the PH medical director to create an atmosphere where the PHPs want to continually improve themselves. Creating peer review committees at the PHP level is useful for this, but it is critical to reinforce that everyone errs and that it is important that everyone learn from mistakes. This requires one to judge a decision prospectively (based upon the information that was known to the PHP at the time), not retrospectively by details or diagnoses that were learned later. Remediation requires, but also creates, openness and honesty about errors. Intentionally malicious acts to harm the patient or egregious neglect are not remediable. Deciding that someone is not remediable usually has financial or disciplinary consequences, and should not be undertaken lightly. If someone commits the same error repetitively or does not acknowledge the error, despite re-education, then that person may not be remediable. It is then the PH medical director's duty to protect future patients from harm by preventing the PHP from being put in a situation where he or we would make the same error.

Using discipline at the time of the error (loss of pay, change in job status, demotion in clinical operating level) assumes that the PHP will be less likely to cause the same error again. This may be useful for obvious willful performance issues that are due to attitude or are obviously incorrect (being late, purposefully damaging equipment, lying, stealing), as it can send a strong message to the PHP's peers that such behavior is not tolerated. However, using discipline as a primary deterrent for medical error will result in PHPs hiding their future errors or being afraid to ask if they have potentially made an error. A blend of both remediation and discipline is needed. This author favors the PH medical director primarily being a remediator in medical error in order to foster a culture of openness in medical decision making and quality assurance, while having other administrators handle discipline of non-medically related errors or behavioral issues. However, this author believes that the PH medical director needs to have the authority to determine whether a PHP can continue to care for patients or whether a PHP is irremediable, which would result in discipline.

## Summary

PH systems are needed to convey non-mobile patients to the hospital, and to initiate care for patients who cannot wait for treatment. Every PH system is different and needs to be tailored to the needs of the patient community, local geography, proximity and skill level of surrounding hospitals, PHP skill level and abundance, political climate, and financial resources. Involvement of in-hospital emergency physicians as PH medical directors is critical in guiding PH systems and PHPs. At times, you may find yourself in conflict while simultaneously trying to represent the hospital you work at, the ambulance services, governmental bodies, and PHPs. When conflicted, the PH medical director should always ask, "What is best for the patient?" The answer will guide you true.

## References

1. World Health Organization. *Prehospital Trauma Care Systems.* Geneva: WHO, 2005.

2. VanRooyen M. Development of prehospital emergency medical services: strategies for system assessment and planning. *Pacific Health Dialog* 2002; **9**: 86–92.

3. Hauswald M, Yeoh E. Designing a prehospital system for a developing country: estimated costs and benefits. *American Journal of Emergency Medicine* 1997; **15**: 600–3.

4. Isenberg DL, Bissell R. Does advanced life support provide benefits to patients? *Prehospital and Disaster Medicine* 2005; **20**: 265–70.

5. Stiell IG, Nesbitt LP, Pickett W, *et al.* The OPALS major trauma study: impact of advanced life support on survival and morbidity. *CMAJ* 2008; **178**: 1141–52.

6. Wuerz RC, Swope GE, Holliman CJ, Vazquez-de Miguel G. On-line medical direction: a prospective study. *Prehospital and Disaster Medicine* 1995; **10**: 174–7.

7. O'Malley RN, O'Malley GF, Ochi G. Emergency medicine in Japan. *Annals of Emergency Medicine* 2001; **38**: 441–6.

8. Interview with Dr. Takashi Nagata, Director, Department of Emergency Medicine, Himeno Hospital, Fukuoka, Japan.

9. Interviews with Sweta Mangal, CEO, and Ruchika Beri, Assistant Manager of Ziqitza Health Care, India.

10. Brennan J, Krohmer J, *et al.* Principles of EMS Systems 3$^{rd}$ ed. Massachusetts. 2006

11. Burstein JL, Henry MC, Alicandro J, *et al.* Outcome of patients who refused out-of-hospital medical assistance. *American Journal of Emergency Medicine* 1996; **14**: 23–6.

12. Alicandro J, Hollander JE, Henry MC, *et al.* Impact of interventions for patients refusing emergency medical services transport. *Academic Emergency Medicine* 1995; **2**: 480–5.

13. Stark G, Hedges J. Patients who initially refuse prehospital evaluation and/or therapy. *American Journal of Emergency Medicine* 1990; **8**: 509–11.

14. Burstein JL, Hollander JE, Delagi R, Gold M, Henry MC, Alicandro JM. Refusal of out-of-hospital medical care: effect of medical-control physician assertiveness on transport rate. *Academic Emergency Medicine* 1998; **5**: 4–8.

Chapter

# 31

# Emergency medicine in basic medical education

Julie Welch and Cherri Hobgood

## Key learning points

- Knowledge of emergency medicine is critical to modern medical practice, and there are many ways to integrate emergency medicine into every stage of basic medical education.
- Emergency medicine's broad practice base makes emergency physicians ideal teachers for today's medical students.
- Early and consistent exposure to emergency medicine benefits both medical students and the specialty.

## Introduction

Emergency medicine is an essential component of modern medical practice and must be incorporated into basic medical education. Because there is a critical demand for emergency physicians and training worldwide, developing a universally accepted curriculum covering the delivery of high-quality lifesaving interventions in a timely manner is a necessity.[1,2] Of all specialties, emergency medicine encompasses the broadest spectrum of medical care and patient experience. It serves as the hospital's primary diagnostic unit for the undifferentiated patient. The door to emergency care is literally open to everyone, and does not discriminate based on age, race, disease process, socioeconomic status, or patient condition. Whether acutely or chronicly ill, critically injured, mentally unstable, or in need of basic medical care, the patient defines the emergency. In response, an emergency physician is trained to approach every patient in the same way and to serve not only as the safety net for many patients without other access to care, but also as the front line for diagnosis, stabilization, and treatment of acute emergent conditions. This creates the perfect environment and faculty for integrating the specialty of emergency medicine into all stages of basic medical education.

## Integration of emergency medicine into basic medical education

Basic medical education varies the world over but essentially two major models exist, the US and the British. In the US model, the traditional medical school training program matriculates students who have completed a preliminary four-year university degree (bachelor's degree) into a four-year course of study at medical school. The first two years of medical school are centered in classroom courses covering the basic sciences as a foundation for studying medicine and the correlation to the human body. Additionally, students are introduced to clinical medicine and the fundamentals of the history and physical exam. Years three and four of medical school typically consist of 4- to 8-week-long clinical rotations, or "clerkships," through a variety of core and specialized practice environments with graduated responsibilities in patient care. In the British model, students are matriculated at age 18 or 19 without a preliminary bachelor's degree. The medical education itself takes five years, and consists of an aggregate of two years of preclinical training in an academic environment and three years of clinical training in a teaching-hospital environment. Other course work may be completed during the first two years, extending the length of study. The Canadian system adheres most closely to the US training model and typically matriculates students after acquisition of a full bachelor's degree, but may also allow students to enter after as few as two years of university study. The basic medical education framework parallels that of the USA, in

---

*Emergency Department Leadership and Management*, ed. Stephanie Kayden, *et al.* Published by Cambridge University Press.
© Cambridge University Press 2015.

**Table 31.1** Educational experiences and essential skills offered by exposure to emergency medicine[4,5]

1. Approach to undifferentiated patient
2. Highly varied clinical experience and pathology
3. Acute care resuscitation
4. End-of-life care
5. Intergenerational care
6. Basic and Advanced Life Support
7. Procedural skills
8. Unique educational content (such as toxicology)
9. Prehospital care
10. Disaster preparedness and medical readiness
11. Healthcare system understanding and management
12. Leadership, management, diplomacy
13. Communication skills
14. Cultural competency
15. Research and scholarly activities
16. Multidisciplinary collaboration
17. Fostering independent study and learning
18. Acquiring skills of critical judgment (evidence-based medicine)
19. Advising and mentoring
20. Training of effective teachers

**Table 31.2** Examples of opportunities to integrate emergency medicine into basic medical education

1. Integration into basic science curricula
2. Integration into intro to clinical medicine course
3. Addressing the core competencies to be effective physicians
4. Emergency medicine clinical rotations
5. Clinical elective rotations affiliated with emergency medicine
6. Job shadowing or physician extender opportunities
7. Emergency medicine student interest groups
8. Student advising and mentoring
9. Research opportunities

which the first two years are spent in classroom study and the final two years in clinical clerkships. The Australian system is much more closely aligned with the British model. Understanding these medical education frameworks and the maturity level of the student is essential to designing a strategy to integrate emergency medicine into the course of study.

The importance of integrating emergency medicine into medical school is not only to enhance the student's medical education, but also to shape the student's perception of the specialty and give them an appreciation and understanding of its principles.[3] The experiences gained by students through exposure to emergency medicine have been described in detail.[4,5] Essential skills range from communication skills and cultural competency to acute-care resuscitation and the approach to the undifferentiated patient (Table 31.1).

Engaging students in a variety of learning environments during medical school will broaden the possibility of exposure to emergency medicine. Students move through the classroom, laboratories, simulated medicine arenas, inpatient hospital medicine, outpatient clinics, the emergency department (ED), and out-of-hospital or prehospital medicine environments. Emergency medicine faculty must

consider using both traditional and creative methods of teaching students in a variety of these learning venues. Exposing medical students to the experiences and core concepts of emergency medicine during every phase of medical education can include, but is not limited to, integration into the basic science curriculum, teaching introductory clinical medicine courses, addressing the core competencies, offering emergency medicine clinical rotations, creating clinical elective rotations affiliated with emergency medicine, forming an emergency medicine student interest group, student advising/mentoring, and research opportunities (Table 31.2).

## Basic science curricular integration

Emergency medicine faculty are well positioned to take on central roles in course leadership, development, and formal teaching during years one and two of medical school. The format of the didactic teaching often includes a variety of approaches, not only traditional lecture halls but also small-group formats using case-based or problem-based learning, and high-fidelity simulation sessions.[3] Curricula for basic science, introduction to clinical medicine, and additional courses can be enhanced by using clinical emergency medicine examples within these learning formats.

Many basic science courses now integrate an organ-system approach to teach core topics, such as gastrointestinal, cardiovascular, pulmonary diseases. The corresponding physiology, pathology, and pharmacology are taught in the context of that organ system. Because this approach mirrors the practice of emergency medicine in many ways, faculty can bring clinical cases into the classroom to integrate these topics. Demonstrating the clinical application of basic science can lead to improved retention and understanding.

To enhance the gross anatomy course, emergency medicine faculty can teach a procedure-based anatomy experience. Teaching surface anatomy can include thoracotomy tube placement, approach to a lateral canthotomy, obtaining central venous access, performing an arthocentesis on various joints, and defining landmarks for a lumbar puncture. As the anatomy dissection advances, pertinent emergency medicine cases can reinforce learning. Examples include relating the most common organs injured in blunt trauma, performing an open thoracotomy, and teaching the steps of a crichothyrotomy.

During the physiology course, emergency physicians can teach pathophysiology as it pertains to many common clinical presentations. The science of resuscitation explores shock in all of its forms (cardiogenic, hypovolemic, neurogenic, septic), oxygen transport, and oxygen delivery. The concept of acid–base balance can be taught using cases of diabetic ketoacidosis, advanced chronic obstructive pulmonary disease, and aspirin overdose.

Making the basic pharmacology course relevant can be achieved using emergency medicine case presentations. The simulation lab is a key resource for emergency medicine cases because of its unique ability to create the timeline of clinical events, including changes in the vital signs, physical findings, and electrocardiogram. Toxicology cases explore many common medications, their physiologic presentation or toxidromes in overdose, and specific antidotes or treatments. Teaching neuropharmacology can include the role of GABA neuroreceptors in alcohol withdrawal and the use of benzodiazepines. The pharmacologic management of cardiac arrhythmia, including atrial fibrillation with rapid ventricular response or supraventricular tachycardia, can enhance the cardiology section.

Additional didactic courses for first- and second-year students to interface with emergency medicine might include radiology, electrocardiogram interpretation, basic life support, advanced cardiac life support, and biostatistics with an evidenced-based medicine approach to common clinical scenarios.[3] Emergency medicine uniquely offers the breadth and depth of cases necessary to reinforce pertinent educational experiences during the first and second foundation years of training.

## Problem-based learning integration

Many medical schools use problem-based learning (PBL) formats to cover key content areas and more closely align the preclinical learning styles with those of a practicing physician. PBL is a group learning style developed at McMaster University.[6] The focus of PBL is to stimulate students to develop more flexible effective problem-solving skills in a team setting. One of the major benefits of this pedagogy is that early in their medical education students learn skills such as effective collaboration, how to parse knowledge into known and unknown, and how to acquire new information. This educational format mandates that students use intrinsic motivation to expand their understanding and gain mastery of the problem, a key professionalism skill required for successful medical practice. Emergency medicine faculty are outstanding mentors for this teaching format, as it closely aligns with our daily practice. The actual practice of emergency medicine, where information is limited and often not known, mandates that successful emergency physicians seek additional knowledge to resolve problems. When core content is taught in this manner, emergency physician tutors bring significant credibility to both the format and the usefulness of many of the tacit learning objectives such as teamwork.

## Introduction to clinical medicine integration

Hands-on instruction during introduction to clinical medicine is a perfect fit for an emergency physician. As the student is learning to approach history taking and the physical exam for the undifferentiated patient of any age, there is no better instructor than one who practices this daily. The emergency physician is an ideal tutor for a variety of chief complaints in a diverse population of patients. Practicing and reinforcing the key elements of the history and physical exam are essential, whether on active patients, on standardized patients, or in a simulation session. In addition, students should be offered opportunities for bedside modeling of real patient interactions with emergency medicine faculty.

## Integration of emergency medicine into the clinical rotations of medical school

The second half of medical school represents the clinical years of training. Typically, students spend 4–8 weeks in clinical rotations, experiencing a variety

**Table 31.3** Common goals and objectives of an emergency medicine clinical rotation

1. Understand the management acute emergency conditions (specific dx)
2. Take a history and physical exam
3. Diagnosis
4. Create an evaluation plan
5. Create a management/treatment plan
6. Manage multiple patients
7. Understand the flow of ED and triage system
8. Participate as a member of team in patient care
9. Develop key attributes of professionalism
10. Develop effective communication skills
11. Engage in systems based learning
12. Seek and accept feedback
13. Develop basic emergency medicine procedural skills
14. Demonstrate cultural awareness and sensitivity to unique patient situations

**Table 31.4** Didactic lecture/module topics for emergency medicine clinical rotation

- Approach to resuscitation
- Approach to chest pain
- Approach to abdominal pain
- Approach to the trauma patient
- Approach to the febrile/crying child
- Approach to outpatient infections
- Approach to dyspnea
- Approach to pain management
- Approach to the violent patient
- Approach to toxicology
- OB/GYN emergencies
- Neurologic emergencies
- Orthopedic emergencies
- Approach to wound care/management
- Approach to headache
- Approach to the septic patient
- Approach to anaphylaxsis
- Approach to syncope
- Approach to testicular pain
- Approach to gi bleed
- Substance abuse
- Domestic violence/child abuse
- Environmental emergencies
- Mass-gathering medicine
- Rashes/dermatology
- Arrhythmia management

of core and specialized practice environments with graduated responsibilities in patient care. Each rotation immerses the student into a specific medical discipline with clinical duties, patient care, and required reading and study.

A clinical rotation in emergency medicine is charged with the task of introducing and training the medical student in the basics of emergency medical care. It is offered as either a core or an elective rotation. For many reasons, emergency medicine should be a required core rotation for every medical student. Emergency medicine arguably sees the greatest variety and diversity of patients, disease states, and social conditions. What better way to prepare medical students for nearly every specialty of medicine than exposure to the ED? Additionally, emergency physicians interact with nearly every other field of medicine, and therefore offer a good perspective of integrated medical care for students new to the healthcare system.

An emergency medicine rotation should contain several key features in order to be effective and efficient in training students during a 4- to 8-week block of time. Students are often assigned 14–16 shifts per month on a circadian cycle. Common goals and objectives of the rotation are outlined in Table 31.3. Didactic lectures should address acute-care medicine topics, focusing on problem-oriented case management, often based on chief complaint (Table 31.4). Study resources typically include a notebook of articles or lectures, a study guide, or

online lecture modules and references pertinent to emergency medicine topics. To enhance the rotation, students should be invited to participate in journal clubs or other evidence-based medicine modules. Additional teaching venues might include high-fidelity simulation sessions, mock codes, procedure labs (Table 31.5), radiology, and prehospital care experience with emergency medical services (EMS) ride-alongs.

The clinical component of the emergency medicine rotation should involve direct patient care and clinical teaching in the ED, overseen by an emergency medicine-trained faculty physician. Senior residents who have been trained to teach can assist with trainees' instruction. Students must be engaged in direct patient contact as an essential component to guide and evaluate their history and physical skills, medical knowledge, and ability to integrate findings with a differential diagnosis and management plan. Additional bedside modeling of patient interactions by faculty, residents, or nurses can enhance and reinforce learning. Students should be required

**Table 31.5** Procedural skills lab for an emergency medicine clinical rotation

1. Airway management
   - Endotracheal intubation
   - Rapid sequence intubation
   - Rescue airway devices
2. Vascular access
   - Peripheral IV access
   - Central venous line placement
   - Arterial line placement
3. Lumbar puncture
4. Splinting
5. Joint reduction
6. Arthrocentesis
7. Suturing
8. Incision and drainage
9. Ultrasound (FAST exam)
10. Foley Catheter
11. NG/OG placement
12. Nasal packing
13. Slit lamp exam

to keep a log of patients, chart their history and physical exams, and do patient follow-up reports for complete learning.

## Addressing core-competency-based frameworks

Medical students, during each phase of their medical school career, are required to attain KSA (knowledge, skills, abilities) in several core competencies. These competencies address the qualities required to be a successful, effective physician with improved patient outcomes. They provide students with clinical, scientific, and relational abilities to transition into the next stage of their career. There are two major competency-based frameworks which are used internationally: the CanMEDS Framework and the Accreditation Council for Graduate Medical Education (ACGME) Core Competencies (Table 31.6).[7,8] CanMEDS is used primarily in Commonwealth nations. While these were developed primarily for graduate medical education, many medical schools have adopted these frameworks and use them to structure the curriculum or assess the knowledge, skills, and aptitudes of medical students prior to their graduation.

Faculty in the ED can easily fulfill content that falls along any of the framework nodes. They are poised to guide the development of the curriculum for these core competencies while engaging as instructors and evaluators. For instance, emergency medicine faculty have a unique capacity to design and measure KSA in the systems-based practice and manager domains. As emergency medicine is a hospital-based specialty caring for patients in an acute-care environment, it requires that physicians be able to deploy the resources of the system to advance the care of both individual patients and populations. In addition, the ED exposes students to the social and community contexts of health care, as these are central themes in the mission of emergency medicine as it interfaces with society. Furthermore, demonstrating and teaching effective communication is achievable because of the numerous opportunities to interact with patients, consultants, nurses, staff, chaplains, social workers, families, and the media. Emergency medicine faculty can become masters in training and analyzing these critical skills and core competencies.

Although many specialties have the opportunity to introduce the benefits of seeking, comprehending, and maintaining a breadth of medical mastery, addressing the core competencies is arguably a perfect meld with the practice of emergency medicine. Emergency medicine faculty might have to take the initiative to approach institutional leaders in order to demonstrate the usefulness of the specialty in medical education at each stage. Whether teaching the basics of effective communication, clinical skills, and problem solving or demonstrating hands-on complex medical cases integrated with moral reasoning and ethical judgment, emergency medicine covers it all.

## Additional emergency medicine engagement for all medical students
### Research electives and special electives

Engaging students in academic activity within the department is often very appealing to students who seek careers in emergency medicine. To achieve this goal many faculties create special electives in research or in fields related to emergency medicine. These elective rotations can include: EMS rotations, mass-gathering medicine experiences, international medicine elective/global medicine, toxicology, ultrasound and emergency radiology, critical care, administration,

**Table 31.6** CanMEDS and ACGME core competency frameworks[7,8]

| CanMEDS Educational Framework[a] | |
| --- | --- |
| Medical expert | As medical experts, specialist emergency physicians integrate all of the CanMEDS Roles, applying medical knowledge, clinical skills, and professional attitudes in their provision of patient-centered care |
| Communicator | As communicators, specialist emergency physicians effectively facilitate the doctor-patient relationship and the dynamic exchanges that occur before, during, and after the medical encounter |
| Collaborator | As collaborators, specialist emergency physicians effectively work within a healthcare team to achieve optimal patient care |
| Manager | As managers, specialist emergency physicians are integral participants in healthcare organizations, organizing sustainable practices, making decisions about allocating resources, and contributing to the effectiveness of the health care system |
| Health advocate | As health advocates, specialist emergency physicians responsibly use their expertise and influence to advance the health and well-being of individual patients, communities, and populations |
| Scholar | As scholars, specialist emergency physicians demonstrate a lifelong commitment to reflective learning, as well as the creation, dissemination, application, and translation of medical knowledge |
| Professional | As professionals, specialist emergency physicians are committed to the health and well-being of individuals and society through ethical practice, profession-led regulation, and high personal standards of behavior |
| ACGME Core Competency Educational Framework[b] | |
| Patient care | Residents must be able to provide patient care that is compassionate, appropriate, and effective for the treatment of health problems and the promotion of health |
| Medical knowledge | Residents must demonstrate knowledge of established and evolving biomedical, clinical, epidemiologic, and social-behavioral sciences, as well as the application of this knowledge to patient care |
| Practice-based learning and improvement | Residents must demonstrate the ability to investigate and evaluate their care of patients, to appraise and assimilate scientific evidence, and to continuously improve patient care based on constant self-evaluation and lifelong learning |
| Interpersonal and communication skills | Residents must demonstrate interpersonal and communication skills that result in the effective exchange of information and collaboration with patients, their families, and health professionals |
| Professionalism | Residents must demonstrate a commitment to carrying out professional responsibilities and an adherence to ethical principles |
| Systems-based practice | Residents must demonstrate an awareness of and responsiveness to the larger context and system of healthcare, as well as the ability to call effectively on other resources in the system to provide optimal health-care |

[a] The CanMeds educational framework is used by the majority of Commonwealth nations as the format for organizing the goals and objectives for graduate medical education training (used with permission from *CJEM*).
[b] The core competency educational framework is used in the United States as the format for organizing the goals and objectives for graduate medical education training.

medical ethics, pediatric emergency medicine, sports medicine, hyperbaric medicine, and emergency medicine research. These more focused offerings can be done between first and second year or designed as a regular portion of the clinical curriculum. Allowing students to take the lead on a portion of a project and following the project all the way to publication or presentation is a great way for students to gain a close working relationship with an emergency medicine faculty member while providing evidence of significant interest in the discipline for postgraduate recruitment purposes.

## Interest groups and emergency medicine clubs

Whether a medical student in her first or second year with limited exposure to clinical medicine, or a student in his later years seeking additional clinical experience, emergency medicine faculty have the opportunity to provide unique activities to engage these students early in their medical careers. Many faculty have found that informal settings are the best places to engage a student's imagination and begin the process of having them see emergency medicine as a career opportunity. Medical schools often have an emergency medicine student interest group (EMSIG), which engages students during all years of training. Emergency medicine faculty should be available to serve as group advisors for such clubs or groups. Ideas for activities include offering lunchtime talks on interesting emergency medicine topics, procedure labs, suture sessions, volunteering at homeless clinics, and physician extender programs.

## Mentorship

Emergency medicine faculty should be available to provide mentorship to medical students. Studies show that mentoring is not only crucial to career satisfaction and success, but a strong mentoring relationship can positively influence a student's ultimate career choice.[9,10] Emergency medicine faculty serving as advisors and mentors should be prepared to fulfill the roles of teacher, sponsor, guide, and role model. Students' needs vary from career counseling, guidance on CV and personal statement preparation, selection of rotation schedules, and tips for residency interviewing and selection, to writing letters of recommendation. Table 31.7 offers a more extensive list of mentoring topics that an emergency medicine advisor might encounter pertaining to the personal and professional development of his or her mentee. Having emergency medicine faculty involved and invested in students will enrich both the student's and the faculty member's career.

**Table 31.7** Mentoring topics for emergency medicine advisors[10]

1. Career choice, including fellowship training
2. Course work, clerkships, and electives (EM and non-EM)
3. Application process
4. Residency programs
5. Clinical issues (including interpersonal skills with physicians, nurses, and staff)
6. Medical errors, ethics, professionalism
7. Academic advancement (research and administration roles)
8. Career satisfaction
9. Financial advice
10. Wellness, balance, life skills
11. Time management skills

## Conclusion

Integrating the field of emergency medicine into basic medical education is practical and possible at every stage of medical student instruction. Although training students to manage the acutely ill and injured is essential, understanding the needs of the institution, the administration, and the students is paramount in advocating for teaching emergency medicine specific content. This chapter addresses several means by which emergency medicine faculty can create a rich learning environment for students while enhancing proficiency in basic science courses, evidence-based medicine, procedure labs, core competencies, and clinical rotations. Adapting a curriculum that includes emergency medicine prepares students with the necessary skills to care for every patient regardless of age, gender, status, or disease state. This constructs a winning situation for the trainee, the patient, the emergency medicine department, the community, and the institution. Engagement at every possible level will pay rich rewards for emergency medicine as a discipline and assist in the integration and recognition of emergency medicine as a full partner in the academic program.

## References

1. Hobgood C, Anantharaman V, Bandiera G, et al. International Federation for Emergency Medicine Model Curriculum for Emergency Medicine Specialists. *Emergency Medicine Australasia* 2011; **23**: 541–53.

2. Singer A, Hobgood C, Kilroy D, et al. International Federation for Emergency Medicine model curriculum for medical student education in emergency medicine. *CJEM* 2009; **11**: 349–54.

3. Tews MC, Hamilton GC. Integrating emergency medicine principles and experience throughout the medical school curriculum: why and how. *Academic Emergency Medicine* 2011; **18**: 1072–80.

4. Russi CS, Hamilton GC. A case for emergency medicine in the undergraduate medical school curriculum. *Academic Emergency Medicine* 2005; **12**: 994–8.

5. McLaughlin SA, Hobgood C, Binder L, Manthey DE. Impact of the Liaison Committee on Medical Education requirements for emergency medicine education at U.S. schools of medicine. *Academic Emergency Medicine* 2005; **12**: 1003–9.

6. Neville AJ. Problem-based learning and medical education forty years on. *Medical Principles and Practice* 2009; **18**: 1–9.

7. Frank JR, Danoff D. The CanMEDS initiative: implementing an outcomes-based framework of physician competencies. *Medical Teacher* 2007; **29**: 642–7.

8. Accreditation Council for Graduate Medical Education (ACGME). Core Competencies, 2011. http://www.acgme.org/acwebsite/RRC_280/280_corecomp.asp (accessed January 10, 2011).

9. Sambunjak D, Straus SE, Marusic A. Mentoring in academic medicine: a systematic review. *JAMA* 2006; **296**: 1103–15.

10. Garmel GM. Mentoring medical students in academic emergency medicine. *Academic Emergency Medicine* 2004; **11**: 1351–7.

Chapter

# 32

# Emergency department outreach

Meaghan Cussen

## Key learning points

- A strong emergency department outreach program is an important tool that can be used to engage the community and ensure the success and longevity of your emergency department.
- Before launching an outreach program, do your research and evaluate current resources and limitations within the emergency department staff, the hospital, and the community.
- Choose one or two large initiatives, or three or four small initiatives, to start during the first year of your outreach program. Plan them carefully and execute them well.

## Introduction

A strong emergency department (ED) outreach program is an important tool that can be used to engage the community and ensure the success and longevity of your ED.[1,2] Outreach is defined as the act of extending services or benefits to a selection of the population. ED outreach is defined as the process of engagement with individuals, community organizations, and healthcare providers by the ED with the primary purpose of serving as a resource, and the secondary purpose of creating a mutually beneficial relationship in which the targets engage or increase their engagement with the ED. While advertising campaigns are largely unidirectional, ED outreach is a marketing tool that seeks to create sustainable growth and patient loyalty through two-way engagement.

There are many types of outreach programs. Examples include providing an information booth at a local community event, working with schools on a

bicycle safety campaign, working with local women's groups on domestic violence prevention, and organizing first aid lessons for the community. Any activity that engages community members, puts them in dialogue with your ED, or allows them to recognize your ED as a generous and helpful resource is an activity that will have positive effects for your department.

The corporate world has long recognized the benefits of community outreach and involvement and their positive effect on profits.[3–6] It can thus be inferred that a well-organized ED outreach program that effectively engages the local community can have significant effects on the mix and volume of ED patients presenting to your department.[1]

In addition to community engagement and good public relations, which we will discuss later in the chapter, ED outreach programs have additional benefits for your department such as increased visibility within your hospital, improved interdepartmental communications, and improved relations with providers and with local government. Let us explore these benefits now.

## Benefits of an outreach program
### Increased visibility within your hospital

A successful ED outreach program increases the ED's visibility within the hospital, gaining your department respect among the hospital's leadership team, administration, and, if applicable, the fundraising or foundation management team. When the administration sees that the efforts you are making in the community positively represent the hospital's name and brand, goodwill will be created with them which you can use to your advantage later when looking to improve patient services and clinical excellence with the

*Emergency Department Leadership and Management*, ed. Stephanie Kayden, *et al.* Published by Cambridge University Press.
© Cambridge University Press 2015.

purchase of new equipment, the development of training programs, or the addition of staff. Depending on your organization, this may be a good political strategy.[2,6]

## Improved interdepartmental relations

Outreach programs help foster collaboration and goodwill between the ED and other hospital departments. Many physicians say that the most difficult part of their job is working with other departments and with physicians from different "competing" medical specialties. Using an outreach project as a way of reaching out to other departments will help create goodwill and therefore help build bridges that lead to a more productive and collaborative working environment. One hospital in Florence, Italy, began offering pediatric patient transport training to local ambulance workers and volunteers. In addition to courses on spinal immobilization and head trauma prehospital treatment protocols, the ED added a course on prehospital treatment of burns. They then invited the burn specialists from the pediatric surgery department to develop and teach the course, providing them with all of the administrative and organizational support necessary. In an ED which had only recently made the change from a surgeon-staffed department to a department staffed solely by emergency specialists with the call-in of surgeons as needed, this type of collaboration was important in strengthening the relationships between the ED and surgical departments in order to better deliver high-quality patient care.

## Improved healthcare provider collaboration

A well-functioning ED outreach program can be an effective way of solidifying and strengthening relationships between the ED and local healthcare providers such as ambulance workers, local primary care physicians, and transferring hospitals. ED staff members rely on these people to provide accurate patient data, including the patient's medical history, history of illness, treatments, and so on. When healthcare partners are recognized and treated as the respected colleagues and valued team members that they are, communication is facilitated and goodwill is fostered, both of which lead to more accurate patient information, better cooperation in protocol and treatment practices, and, ultimately, improved patient care.[1]

## Government support

A well-functioning ED outreach program will positively represent your hospital and ED in the eyes of the local government. In a government-run system, this might lead to additional funding, additional attention and consideration from public institutions, or additional cooperation in dealing with political issues or funding initiatives. In a private healthcare system, local government support can help you receive funding from local charities (when charities know that the government is backing your injury prevention program, they may be more likely to donate to your hospital's foundation). Support from local government can also serve private hospitals well when applying for grants or national funding, from which monies can be obtained to improve a hospital's physical and technological infrastructure, better train current staff, or recruit new specialists, all in the interest of improved patient care.

## Community engagement and good public relations

Finally, and most importantly, an ED outreach program will positively affect your target population's view of and attitudes toward your hospital and emergency service. Outreach programs increase visibility among the local population, help strengthen the hospital brand, and increase patient satisfaction. A well-executed outreach program can help bring about many desired outcomes:

(1) First, it will help solidify and strengthen your community message. Perhaps your hospital's slogan is "we care about the city of Charlestown." Outreach programs such as prevention programs, health initiatives, and layperson safety classes will show that your hospital does, in fact, care about the city.[7]

(2) It will increase visibility and positive associations with your hospital and therefore drive more traffic to your ED.[8] In private hospital systems, this is an obvious motivator: more patients mean more income. However, in a public system it can also be a good thing. Increased patient load can help bring attention to your ED from hospital administration and local government, which will hopefully drive more funds and resources your way and ultimately increase the quality of care and level of services you can offer your patients.

In public systems where the hospital is paid by the government per patient visit, increased traffic is another obvious incentive.

(3) When patients and their families know that their healthcare providers are interested in their long-term health and obviously care about the community in which they work, shown through your outreach efforts, they are more likely to become loyal to your ED.

## When should you, or should you not, initiate a community outreach program?

### When is it not a good idea?

First, let us begin by discussing when starting an outreach program is *not* a good idea. While there are obviously many positives associated with ED community outreach, ED leaders must first make sure their operation is stable before diving into any outreach initiatives. If your ED is not well organized, efficient, and secure, or if you have any major deficiencies in service delivery and infrastructure, or if your ED is going through major leadership, staffing, protocol, or infrastructure changes, this is not the time to begin outreach activities. Most efforts made without the backing of a stable infrastructure and staff will risk being poorly supported and will ultimately fail. In addition, adding stress to staff members during times of change – keeping in mind that staff members are usually the face of the outreach program – could potentially negatively affect patient care. Even if outreach efforts have a chance of succeeding during a major transition phase, they might only bring more traffic to your ED – and if the transition means that you are not prepared to handle the new patient load, service will be poor and patient satisfaction lower than before. In addition, if you have limited resources in your ED and cannot afford to pay for structural changes that would be needed to deal with more throughput, at least the public portion of your outreach should hold off until proper resources can be obtained.

### When is it a good idea?

(1) When you have strong, dedicated staff that are happy in their jobs and are not overworked, this is the best time to start. Staff are essential to outreach efforts. They are the people who will primarily be supporting the initiatives, so take care of them first! The program will not work without them. Consider incentivizing individuals who participate in prevention programs – monetarily (as budget permits), honorably (recognizing their efforts formally in front of the team and hospital leaders), or with perks such as choice of shift or funding for outside training or educational programs.

(2) Starting an outreach program is also a good idea if you desire or need to increase patient volume in your ED. As mentioned earlier in the chapter, outreach is an excellent way to market your ED.[1]

(3) You should strongly consider starting an outreach program if there is good potential to tie in to local government efforts or programs in order to take advantage of the benefits that come with shared goals. For example, if your local government is known to be making efforts on prevention in order to lower long-term healthcare costs among the population, make your programs known to the local healthcare system. Become a part of their efforts and share ideas with them and volunteer to collaborate in their programs as well. Funding will most likely come your way, which you can direct to further your ED's outreach efforts.

## How to build an effective outreach program

### Part 1. Do your research

First of all, do your research. Before deciding how many and which specific initiatives you would like to launch, research and evaluate your current resources and limitations within your staff, the hospital, and the community.

#### Step 1. Figure out who the stakeholders are in your ED and hospital

Think about who the stakeholders will be in your outreach program: city and regional government, your hospital administration, your hospital partners, and any hospital-associated foundations. Are any of them already working on outreach efforts? Will your outreach efforts appear to be in direct competition to theirs? What are their opinions on ED outreach initiatives? Do as much fact finding and informal information gathering here as possible. Share your initial thoughts and get their opinions on how to proceed. They may have a lot of experience to offer and, even if you think you do not need it, you can never go wrong by asking a "powerful person" to guide you or offer advice on a new project. It is essential for obtaining and maintaining support for your future programs. The author of this chapter ran into difficulty when skipping this step in one hospital. Stakeholders who had previously been involved in less-than-successful outreach efforts quickly viewed the new initiatives as an insult and threat and put up logistical barriers that took months to overcome. Do not make the same mistake by skipping this important step.

Remember, once you launch an initiative, you will want to make sure to always factor stakeholders into your planning, invite them to be featured in or participate in any planned events, and make sure not to compete with any of their existing initiatives. It is essential that you obtain their support from the start; you will certainly need it when negotiating with outside organizations, when pursuing potential partners or donors, and when dealing with any interdepartmental conflicts that might arise with your new programs. The goal should be to establish a collaborative working relationship with them rather than a competitive one.

### Step 2. Meet with hospital public relations and communications staff

If your hospital has a public relations or communications office, even if this is just one person, approach its staff at the beginning of your efforts. Find out if there are already marketing or outreach programs in place that you can add to or expand. Run your initial ideas by them. They most likely have advice to offer and experience you can learn from. If your hospital has a foundation or a separate fundraising office, meet with them as well. They will most likely be very happy to use you and your department to strengthen publicity and fundraising efforts. In these initial meetings, look for ways to run your own outreach program in collaboration with them and, possibly, other departments. Figure out what resources they already have that you can tap into. Do they have graphic designers in-house that you might use? Do they have discounts at local printing services, or memberships of organizations of national/international healthcare or prevention programs that might be a good resource for you in developing your outreach programs?

The communications office will also most likely provide you with helpful guidelines about using the hospital's logo and about any communication protocols to follow. Make sure that you are clear on the hospital's message and mission, how it wants to be represented in the public eye, and what its philosophy on community outreach is. Ask them to give you updated logos and slogans, with the understanding that you will run significant publications or usages by them beforehand. Remember, when you get to a point in your programs when you may consider advertising through distributing press releases, the communications office will be a valuable asset in these efforts.

### Step 3. Assess, and add to, the resources of the team

Your ED staff is made up of physicians, nurses, technicians, administrators, and others – all of whom, outside of work, have additional talents and interests. Who is a good public speaker? Who is a good instructor? Who works well with children? Who is a good writer? Who has computer skills or organizational skills? Is someone an artist in his or her free time? Perhaps this is the person whose talents could be used to develop advertisements and printed materials. Understanding which resources are potentially available to you through your staff will help you determine which outreach programs would be best to concentrate on.

Be prepared to offer training to interested staff members. Is there a nurse who is interested in launching a parenting course for prospective parents but lacks curriculum planning skills or public-speaking training? Is there a staff member who is interested in organizing an ED "open house" but lacks confidence in event planning? As the budget allows, offer necessary support and education to your staff members to encourage them to become more involved in outreach efforts and keep them motivated.

### Step 4. Develop a network of community advocates

An important part of forming a strong base of support for your programs is to take the time and energy to develop advocates for your ED within the community. Having a base of local people, organizations, businesses, and clubs who support your ED is essential to the success of your outreach initiatives. You will eventually use this network to help publicize your events or recruit volunteers to help organize or staff any outreach events or efforts you develop.

While the idea of advocate network development may seem overwhelming at first, remember to use the connections of your staff members, who most likely live in, and are therefore involved in, the local community. At a staff meeting, brainstorm a list of local businesses and organizations that your staff members have personal connections to and that might want to partner with your ED. Choose appropriate community organizations which might share in your mission, and begin to work on forming and cultivating relationships with them. Consider the organization's size, influence, and demographics, and pick ones that are best suited to your target population.[1] Community organizations you might think about contacting or collaborating with include scouts, schools, local colleges/universities, local community groups/social clubs, charitable organizations, local churches/synagogues, other organized religions, and businesses that might want to sponsor outreach efforts in exchange for the publicity of being associated with your hospital.

It is also a good idea to assign a network member to each staff member, having your staff member "adopt" a group or organization. Once your outreach program starts, he or she can be the main contact, the one to send announcements and news to the organization. A good idea is to track the success of these networking relationships at monthly meetings, and award staff members who create the best relationships and opportunities.[1,9]

# Part 2. Choose your initiatives and launch

Now that you have done your research, it is time to start choosing which outreach initiatives you are going to launch for the first year of your program.

### Step 5. Choose the outreach initiatives for the first year

Choose one or two large initiatives, or three or four small initiatives, to start with during the first year. Plan them carefully and execute them well. Assign a team member to oversee each initiative, based on time, resources, and talents. Distribute a calendar and information to all staff and administration at the beginning of the year and make sure you have everyone's full cooperation. In the next section, we will discuss a variety of outreach initiatives from which to choose. When choosing your programs for the year, you also must look at your audience and your target population, and choose initiatives that are appropriate for them. Remember, when developing communication materials and programs, to keep in mind the various literacy levels and languages you may find in your target population, and design materials and programs appropriate for them[10]. Also keep in mind the differing health awareness levels of different immigrant groups in your population (see Case study 32.1).

---

**Case study 32.1**

A pediatric hospital in Italy decided to start an outreach program to promote its new trauma center. Funding only provided for 10 hours per week of administrative support and some physician compensation for teaching hours. With this limited budget, the hospital chose four easy things to do in the first year to boost community recognition:

(1) **Injury prevention brochures**. Graphics and content were generously provided by several US prevention organizations. Translations and cultural edits were done in-house while, after some lobbying, printing was donated by a major hospital donor. Brochures were distributed in the ED, at local physician offices, and at other scheduled outreach events.

(2) **Injury prevention lessons for parents**. Once presentations and curriculum were written, physicians took turns teaching this monthly class.

(3) **Pediatric medical transport classes** for ambulance workers. Once presentations and curriculum were written, physicians took turns teaching this monthly class.

(4) **Network building**. Over the year, the center's director traveled with one or more physicians to each of the 35 hospitals in the regional trauma network to announce the new center. Protocols and contact information were discussed, and this in-person contact proved invaluable to ongoing network building and future collaboration.

Together with timely press releases, these simple activities generated word-of-mouth publicity that resulted in a significant increase in transfers and ED visits.

---

### Step 6. Communicating within your hospital

Meet with heads of other departments to let them know what your planned initiatives are. Find out if there is anything they might be doing in terms of outreach that your preparatory research did not already tell you, and if there is potential for collaboration. Perhaps you are planning on presenting at a local event on injury prevention or first aid. You might ask them to help develop some of the material, or to help staff the event in exchange for a co-sponsorship opportunity. If you are developing an injury prevention brochure, check with other surgical departments (such as the burn unit) and ask them to write the section or review the section of your brochure dealing with their area of expertise ("how to prevent/care for burns").

### Step 7. Make sure you have a strong administrative organization and support

While physicians and nurses will play an integral role in executing outreach efforts, they cannot be expected to coordinate the logistics of your planned events. Also, while interns and hospital volunteers can certainly assist and participate in efforts, you should still have one person who is assigned to be the "front line" for all outreach efforts. EDs with many resources might have a dedicated staff member for this role. Others might use a department secretary or nursing staff member to coordinate. Make the outreach portion of the job clear. Write a revised job description with clear and detailed responsibilities and expectations for the year. Make sure that the relevant person has a certain number of hours per week in the schedule to dedicate to outreach program coordination. If not, the efforts will most likely fail.

Choose one email address for public communication and have your dedicated administrator respond to it. If you have the capability, dedicate a page of your hospital website to the ED and outreach programs. Create a social media page for ED community outreach and another for ED–ambulance or ED–provider relations, if you choose to concentrate on this area (see ideas in next section). Post events, articles, and news there. Social media websites have become an easy way to share information with a large group, but events must be current and information must be updated regularly.

While your patient care always takes priority, do your best to provide good response times to any

public inquiries, especially those regarding your outreach programs. Make sure email is checked regularly and phone messages returned. Staff members often have to be instructed to do this and given tools to help them respond quickly. Post information about your activities all over your ED, and make sure staff members are informed so they are capable of offering informed responses. Make it easy for the public to get in touch with your organization. Make a rule that you will respond to emails and calls within 24 hours.

### Step 8. Publicize your initiatives

There are a variety of low-cost ways to publicize your initiatives.

(1) **Press releases.** Instructions on how to write a well-crafted press release can be found on the internet. If you are planning to organize an event or launch a lecture or course series, consider a press release. Your communications office will be able to help you distribute it to local papers, which very well may pick up the story; this provides you with free advertising. A small press release announcing child safety courses for parents at one hospital generated four published articles, one radio spot, one television spot, and hundreds of phone calls. It truly got the program off to a strong start.

(2) **Articles for community newsletters, local papers, and magazines.** Think about writing small articles to contribute to local publications. It might be a simple synopsis of research your physicians are doing, information about a new piece of equipment your ED has purchased, or an announcement about one of your outreach initiatives. Consider also writing a "health tips" or "prevention tips" section as part of your outreach. New York Weill Cornell Medical Center has used this technique hospital-wide with excellent publicity results.[11] Preparing a small article for a local newsletter (university newspaper, club journal, church bulletin) is generally well received by often busy and overworked editors looking for new content, and it is free publicity for you.[1,11]

(3) **Create an email or mail distribution list** of people within your community and with community organizations so that, when you do have an event to announce, you can send information flyers to the public or to local clubs, schools, public offices, or doctors' offices for help with distributing.

(4) **Communicate electronically**. Have a page on your hospital website dedicated to the ED. If it is not easy or convenient to make changes to the hospital website, have your ED page link to a free online calendar created by you, featuring your outreach initiatives, which you can update regularly. You can also link your ED page to a social media webpage open to the public and dedicated to publicizing your events. Do your best to have your brochures and flyers available in PDF form for people to download so they can easily be shared and distributed online. While the internet is a fantastic way of sharing information, it only works if events and information are current and updated regularly. Make sure one of your staff members is assigned to do this.

### Step 9. Critically evaluate your programs

Obviously, the last phase of any good marketing strategy is the evaluation phase. It is important to evaluate the success of each program you do, with a user survey or another evaluation method you find appropriate. This will help you decide which initiatives to repeat next year, which initiatives to improve upon, and which initiatives to set aside.[12]

## Outreach initiatives

It is important to choose one or two large initiatives, or three or four small initiatives, to start with during the first year. Below is a list of ideas of potential activities and initiatives to help you decide what to plan for your first year.

(1) **Health booths**. Undoubtedly, part of your hospital's mission is to improve general health and well-being in your local community. Meet with the local town hall and get a list of events that might be happening in your area for the year. Organize booths or exhibits at local events, targeting specific prevention topics such as violence prevention or the importance of wearing seatbelts or bike helmets.[13–18] Perhaps organize "blood pressure check" booths or an exhibit on how to be "heart healthy."[1]

(2) **Information tables**. Organize a health-related display at your local library, school, or community center once every few months on different health topics. Get local science or medical students to help you with the information gathering and display, in exchange for your physicians' guidance

and expertise on this project. Work in collaboration with the head librarian. They are an excellent resource and may be very interested in a co-sponsored information table or campaign.[19]

(3) **Health speakers**. Host speakers at your hospital. Invite local sports figures or medical experts to present on topics that might interest the community. Collaborate with local universities or schools if you need assistance contacting or paying for the speaker. Remember, many local groups will want to co-sponsor projects with a hospital. You do not have to do it all alone.

(4) **Physician education**. Encourage your own physicians to speak on health topics that are meaningful to your community and that are within their specialty area. Offer to organize these at local events, local colleges, community organizations, or the public library. If you are an academic hospital, with an obligation to provide residents and new physicians with teaching experience and practice, it is a good idea to form a partnership between your institution and a community organization. The community organization may take care of publicizing and organizing healthcare learning events, while your ED provides the content and physician lecturer. This is a win–win situation. ED publicity/outreach and teaching experience for you, and a meaningful learning event for a community organization focused on improving a local health issue.[20] Make sure to have your staff bring flyers to these events to publicize other future outreach efforts.

(5) **First aid**. Organize first aid lessons or cardiopulmonary resuscitation (CPR) lessons for lay people at your hospital. Even if you have to charge a small fee in order to pay for the instructor's time and equipment, the initiative will be much appreciated by the community. Teachers, childcare providers, and parents should all be encouraged to attend.

(6) **Open house**. Host an ED or hospital open house. Locals might be interested in learning more about the hospital that their tax dollars or donations support. Offer them tours of the ED and demonstrations of new equipment. While physician and ED leader time is certainly precious, an open house could be organized once a year for a few hours. Ask hospital communications staff to help you organize something like this. Perhaps an ED-initiated effort will become a major hospital-wide activity and you will be seen as a great collaborator.

Medical student volunteers or others could be recruited to assist with the logistics of the day.

(7) **Pediatric outreach**. If your hospital is a pediatric hospital, or has pediatric emergency services, it is a great opportunity to promote pediatric injury prevention and get the community behind you. Some ideas to get you started:

(a) Host a teddy bear clinic. The concept of "teddy bear clinics" has taken off in the United States. Many hospitals, both pediatric and adult, use these events to improve visibility within the community, spread their message of health and well-being, provide information and skills to children and families that can help lower their risk of illness or injury, and help familiarize children with the hospital environment. The desired result is that, in the unfortunate case that children have to return to the hospital or ED as a patient, it will not be viewed as such a scary place (see Case study 32.2).

(b) Bike safety campaign with sponsored helmet giveaway.

(c) Peer tutoring program (see Case study 32.3).

---

### Case study 32.2. Teddy bear clinic

Teddy bear clinics are an excellent outreach program that can be organized by the ED alone, or in collaboration with the entire hospital.[21] Teddy bear clinics are a great way to involve the entire community – children, parents, schools, and community organizations – and organizational costs can often be reduced through community donations. The benefits of teddy bear clinics are explained in a paper published in the *Journal of Emergency Nursing*: "In one study of children's depictions of hospitals, children drew dark, stark buildings. Teddy bear clinics can change that image . . . [In fact], the children's post-event pictures showed hospitals as light, sunny buildings with smiling people . . . [Teddy bear clinics] are successful 'play therapy' that provide young children with an opportunity to prepare for their inevitable contact with hospitals as a helping, normal life experience. [During a Teddy bear clinic], acting as surrogate parents, children ages 4 to 7 describe their teddy bear's or doll's 'symptoms' and get 'treatment' from healthcare providers."[22] Healthcare providers may explain the illness and treatment of the teddy bear to the child, take teddy's temperature, dress teddy's wound, or give prescriptions such as "3 hugs a day."[22]

---

Not only are these events a great hospital marketing tool and helpful to families, but researchers have also noted an important side benefit: children who have participated in these clinics are more cooperative when they subsequently visit the ED.[22] These events can also build staff morale; in fact, in one study, "participating nurses become very enthusiastic because of the children's responses."[22]

---

### Case study 32.3. Junior trauma educators

If you have relationships with local schools, your public health education agency, or with health-focused community organizations, and if you can obtain their partnership and assistance, you might think about organizing a "junior trauma educator" program. One hospital used its ED physicians to train a group of 16- to 22-year-olds to become junior trauma educators (JTEs). JTEs were trained on pediatric trauma and basic injury prevention techniques. Once trained and given the proper presentation, script, and materials, these JTEs educated 5- to 11-year-olds in local elementary schools on the importance of bike and road safety, focusing particularly on bike-helmet use, reinforcing the rule "under 12 years old in the back seat," and the proper use of car seats, booster seats, and seat belts.[14–18] The JTEs (supervised by an adult program leader) delivered 45-minute interactive presentations involving projected slides, skits, and games to a maximum of 30 participants per lesson. At the end of each lesson, bike helmets (donated by a local foundation) were distributed to participants, along with a prevention brochure targeted at parents. The hospital's ED and trauma center received excellent publicity for this outreach project, and the effort generated several news articles. Not only did 2300 students (and therefore almost 4600 parents) receive a valuable lesson on injury prevention, they also witnessed a generous effort coordinated by their local ED. It should be noted that the use of cross-age education has proven to be an effective methodology with benefits for both the younger students and the presenters.[23–25]

---

(d) Child safety lecture series or training taught by your ED physicians once a month. Develop a slide presentation on domestic and road injury prevention topics related to your community. Use your physicians' experience in the ED to determine areas on which to concentrate. If your ED collects data on the cause of injuries that present to the ED, use this as your guide. Potential topics include bike helmet safety, seatbelt/car-seat/booster-seat use, drowning, poisoning, suffocation, fire, and falls. Look at World Health Organization (WHO) statistics to get a better idea of what problems your nation is currently facing in terms of injury prevention.[26]

(e) Develop a series of pamphlets and brochures that state and expand your message of injury prevention. Remember, as ED staff members, you are the experts in what causes accidental injury. Share this knowledge with your community. If funding and resources are limited, and you do not have a communications or graphics team at your hospital that can help you, consider asking for help. Perhaps graphic design students from a local college would jump at the chance to add this to their portfolio. UNICEF, WHO, and injury-prevention non-profit organizations often have resources you can use for free (and edit and translate into your own language). Local organizations or businesses may want to work on a joint project with you in which your ED provides the expertise while they provide or fund the graphics and printing.

(f) Since car seats are frequently installed improperly, sponsor a "car-seat check day." Train a local garage on how to inspect for properly installed car seats and allow them to advertise this event in collaboration with your hospital. Or set up a car-seat check day with your physicians and trained volunteers at a toy store, shopping center, carnival, or other event. Again, doing this once or twice a year will be enough to create awareness of the need for car seats to be properly installed, and will put your ED at the forefront of this safety initiative.[27]

(8) **Design a quarterly newsletter**. If you have administrative workers, interns, students, or others who have writing or photography skills, involve them in this project. Be clear on the messages you want to convey to the community and suggest ways they might start to gather stories. Potential articles include:

- an update on your outreach programs
- a new piece of hospital equipment purchased
- interviews with new ED staff members
- an article highlighting one of the nursing staff
- an article highlighting another hospital department and an important collaboration

that occurred between that department and the ED for a particular case. Remember, you do not have to do the writing yourself; you can delegate. However, make sure to be clear about your message with the staff, offer to write an introduction or closing letter or statement, and have regular meetings to review drafts.

Another option is to approach a magazine or newspaper in your area. Have one of their staff take charge of writing the newsletter in exchange for publicity in your newsletter. Make them a part of the team to ensure you do not lose control of the message or content. Make sure to include other departments, hospital administration, and the hospital communications office to make sure your ED message is in line with hospital policy and messages. Distribute the newsletter to the public through your website, social media sites, and mailings. Make it available in various locations in the hospital or around the city. Send it to transferring hospitals, local physicians, and ambulance workers.

(9) **Donate to local raffles**. Approach organizations and schools in your advocate network about donating something to one of their raffles for one of their events. You can offer no-cost or low-cost gifts such as "follow an ED physician for the day" (for children or teens)[1] or a free health scan (for adults). This will create goodwill with your advocates and will encourage them to participate more in your efforts.[1]

(10) **First aid support**. Provide free first aid support at local events, perhaps using your trained medical students or residents. In exchange, have a small table to publicize your ED and its events and outreach efforts. Or provide first aid kits with your logo on them and distribute them at schools and local events. Ask a medical supplier to co-sponsor this initiative with you in order to cut or eliminate costs.[1]

(11) **Social media campaign**. If members of your target population are active users of social media, an obvious and successful way of engaging them is through this means. If your ED can create a compelling social media voice and presence, the two-way engagement results you are hoping for in your outreach campaign will be achieved. The

*Harvard Business Review* offers a guide for healthcare organizations to develop social media strategies that is applicable to your ED.[28]

(12) **Healthcare provider network outreach**. As mentioned, a well-functioning ED outreach program can be used as an effective way of solidifying and strengthening relationships between the ED and local healthcare providers such as ambulance workers, local physicians, and transferring hospitals. ED staff rely on these providers to provide accurate patient history and symptomology. Here are some ideas on how to outreach to this network:

(a) **Hospital networking.** If you are a referral hospital, go out and visit transferring hospitals. Take the time out of your schedule as a busy ED leader to do this – and actually *go* to them, showing a willingness to collaborate. Form relationships with them and even attempt to work on some research or quality improvement projects with them to improve the network and enhance collaboration (see Case study 32.4).

(b) **Primary care physician relationship building.** The local physicians in your area are an excellent referral source for your ED, and so maintaining a relationship with them is beneficial to you. Think about hosting educational sessions for them at the hospital. During the event, take the time to ask them how accessible your ED services are, and if they have any patient feedback to offer. Provide them with prevention brochures you may have developed and ask for their cooperation in distributing them to patients. These physicians are an important part of your network and an important ED referral source. Treat them as such and make them a part of your team.

(c) **Prehospital community outreach.** Form good relationships with ambulance workers. These professionals need to be respected and recognized for what they are: the first system contact a traumatized or ill patient has. Their actions in the first 10 minutes significantly affect the outcome of patients. The information they collect during the prehospital transport is essential to patient care. Treat them as professionals and with respect in order to foster the relationship. Make sure some of your staff members are assigned to cleaning and returning any equipment they might need to leave behind after transport (such as backboards).[1] Follow up with them after severely ill or injured patients have recovered. Thank them for the information and treatment they provided and give them feedback on ways to improve the collaboration. In short, your patient was their patient too – so let them know how the patient is doing after they left him or her at the hospital. Give them constructive feedback on their care. Based on their current skill level and need, offer to participate in their training sessions, and perhaps even host lectures or training on special topics at your hospital for them. Remember, they are an important part of your team and your ED and have a big influence on the type of care you provide, so reaching out to them is essential.

---

**Case study 32.4    Take your ED on the road**

Large referral or specialty EDs that rely on hospital transfers to increase admissions, or that are in need of improvements in hospital transfer procedure in order to improve process and flow, may consider in-person marketing and relationship building with their referring or potential referring hospitals. Have you recently expanded your ED, added new equipment, improved ED processes, or implemented new hospital transfer protocols? These are good excuses to launch a networking initiative to start to build and to better relationships with other EDs.

One regional hospital with a potential referral network of 38 hospital EDs, unfortunately, had a poor reputation for handling transfers and for emergency clinical care in general. However, the hospital and ED had recently undergone some major administrative, staffing, and procedural changes and was now ready to effectively, efficiently, and safely handle incoming transfers. They developed a brochure and poster that outlined their new capabilities, highlighted their growth and expansion, and provided a direct-access number, available at all hours, where a transferring physician could speak directly with a receiving ED physician. The hospital had solved the problem of transfer communication by staffing this number; however, it would take much effort to change a longstanding poor reputation. The department director organized in-person meetings with ED staff in each of the 38 hospitals. Some hospitals accepted invitations to visit the new facilities and take a tour. Others requested that the director visit them at their hospital. The willingness and openness of the director to discuss past problems, offer solutions, and request better working relationships clearly impressed ED colleagues. Transfers dramatically increased within the year, and a second round of meetings was scheduled the following year, with similar positive results.

## Conclusion

A strong ED outreach program is a key factor in ensuring the success and longevity of your ED. A well-functioning ED outreach program will allow you to increase visibility within your hospital, improve interdepartmental relations, improve healthcare provider collaboration, gain government support, and, most importantly, engage the community.

## References

1. Suter RE. Community relations and organizations. *Emergency Medicine Clinics of North America* 2004; **22**: 183–94.

2. Frabotta D. Community outreach. *Managed Healthcare Executive* 2003; **13** (4): 24.

3. Martin RL. The virtue matrix: calculating the return on corporate responsibility. *Harvard Business Review* 2002; **80** (3): 3–4.

4. Mescon TS, Tilson DJ. Corporate philanthropy: a strategic approach to the bottom-line. *California Management Review* 1987; **29** (2): 49–61.

5. Ullmann AA. Data in search of a theory: a critical examination of the relationships among social performance, social disclosure, and economic performance of US firms. *Academy of Management Review* 1985; **10**: 540–57.

6. Birchard B. Doing well by doing good. *Harvard Management Update* 1999; **5**: 5.

7. Pillow DJ. Public relations. In RF Salluzzo, TA Mayer, RM Strauss, PS Kidd, eds., *Emergency Department Management: Principles and Applications*. St, Louis, MO: Mosby, 1997.

8. Buschiazzo L. Marketing the emergency department. *Nursing Management* 1985; **16** (9): 30B–30D.

9. Holtan N. How partnering benefits health care workers, physicians, and patients. *Journal for Quality and Participation* 2003; **26** (1): 44.

10. Bodie GD, Dutta MJ. Understanding health literacy for strategic health marketing: eHealth literacy, health disparities, and the digital divide. *Health Marketing Quarterly* 2008; **25**: 175–203.

11. Botvin JD. In New York, the early bird gets the holiday "plum." News releases bear fruit for N.Y. Weill Cornell Medical Center. *Profiles in Healthcare Marketing* 2001; **17** (2): 27–34.

12. Aghababian RV, Volturo GA. Marketing and outreach. In RF Salluzzo, TA Mayer, RM Strauss, PS Kidd, eds., *Emergency Department Management: Principles and Applications*. St, Louis, MO: Mosby, 1997.

13. Holdsworth G, Criddle J, Mohiddin A, *et al.* Maximizing the role of emergency departments in the prevention of violence: developing an approach in South London. *Public Health* 2012; **126**: 394–6.

14. Gesten EL, Jason LA. Social and community interventions. *Annual Review of Psychology* 1987; **38**: 427–60.

15. Morris BP, Trimble NE. Promotion of bicycle helmet use among schoolchildren: A randomized clinical trial. *Canadian Journal of Public Health* 1991; **82**: 92–4.

16. Klassen TP, MacKay JM, Moher D, Walker A, Jones AL. Community-based injury prevention interventions. *The Future of Children* 2000. **10** (1): 83–110.

17. Liller KD, Smorynski A, McDermott RJ, Crane NB, Weibley RE. The MORE HEALTH bicycle safety project. *Journal of School Health* 1995; **65**: 87–90.

18. Britt J, Silver I, Rivara FP. Bicycle helmet promotion among low income preschool children. *Injury Prevention* 1998; **4**: 280–3.

19. Dutcher GA, Hamasu C. Community-based organizations' perspective on health information outreach: a panel discussion. *Journal of the Medical Library Association* 2005; **93** (4 suppl): S35–42.

20. Meyer D, Armstrong-Coben A, Batista M. How a community-based organization and an academic health center are creating an effective partnership for training and service. *Academic Medicine* 2005; **80**: 327–33.

21. Santen L, Feldman T. Teddy bear clinics: a huge community project. *American Journal of Maternal Child Nursing* 1994; **19**: 102–6.

22. Zimmerman PG. Teddy says "Hi!": teddy bear clinics revisited. *Journal of Emergency Nursing* 1997; **23** (1): 41–4.

23. Cohen J. Theoretical considerations of peer tutoring. *Psychology in the Schools* 1986; **23** (2): 175–86.

24. Gaustad J. Peer and cross-age tutoring. *ERIC Digest* **79** 1993.

25. Jostad CM, Miltenberger RG, Kelso P, Knudson P. Peer tutoring to prevent firearm play: acquisition, generalization, and long-term maintenance of safety skills. *Journal of Applied Behavior Analysis* 2008. **41**: 117–23.

26. Health Statistics and Health Information Systems. Child mortality. http://www.who.int/healthinfo/statistics/mortality_child/en (accessed May 28, 2012).

27. Edward CR, Gyulay JE. Parental compliance with car seat usage: a positive approach with long-term follow up. *Journal of Pediatric Psychology* 1981; **6** (3): 301–12.

28. Kane GC, Fichman RG, Gallaugher J, Glaser J. Community relations 2.0.

*Harvard Business Review* 2009; **87** (11): 45–50, 132.

## Further reading

Bloch YH, Toker A. Doctor, is my teddy bear okay? The "teddy bear hospital" as a method to reduce children's fear of hospitalization. *Israel Medical Association Journal* 2008; **10**: 597–9.

Botvin JD. Trick or treat and ho, ho, ho! Marketing campaign for Emory ER reflects the holiday spirit. *Profiles in Healthcare Marketing* 2001; **17** (2): 8–12.

Burke L, Logsdon JM. How corporate social responsibility pays off. *Long Range Planning* 1996; **29**: 495–502.

Graber TW. Structure and function of the emergency department: matching emergency department choices to the emergency department mission. *Emergency Medicine Clinics of North America* 2004; **22**: 47–72.

Mayer TA, Tilson W, Hemingway J. Marketing and public relations in the emergency department. *Emergency Medicine Clinics of North America* 1987; **5**: 83–102.

Paul DP, Honeycutt ED. An analysis of the hospital–patient marketing relationship in the health care industry. *Journal of Hospital Marketing* 1995; **10**(1): 35–49.

Porter ME, Kramer MR. The competitive advantage of corporate philanthropy. *Harvard Business Review* 2002; **80** (12): 56–68.

Proctor J, Hall P, Carr J. The business of emergency medicine: a model for success. *Emergency Medicine Clinics of North America* 2004; **22**: 19–45.

Zasa RJ. Marketing health services. *College Review* 1984; **1**(1): 23–53.

**Special topics**

# 33

# Planning for diversity

Tasnim Khan

## Key learning points

- Patient and staff cultural diversity is increasing in emergency departments worldwide, and informed management is needed to avoid dangerous or disruptive misunderstandings.
- Differences in values and beliefs are not always apparent but can have serious effects on patient care, family satisfaction, and workplace morale.
- Staff can use simple techniques to prevent stereotyping patients and ensure high-quality care.

## Introduction

The world is becoming a global melting pot of cultures and people or, arguably, a pot of soup – a mix of different discrete ingredients all contained in the same vessel. Increasingly, this blend of interactions is seen in healthcare work settings worldwide. Coincident to this evolution of the workplace is a notable increase in chronic diseases, rising healthcare costs, technological changes, and continued fragmentation of healthcare. Today, the scenario of an Indian doctor and an Irish nurse, both working in a South African hospital, stabilizing and caring for a 53-year-old Somali patient with a myocardial infarction, uncontrolled diabetes, and congestive heart failure is not an uncommon occurrence. This kaleidoscope of encounters is prone to significant mishaps arising from communication breakdown due to the barriers of culture, nationality and language.

The unifying goal of most healthcare systems around the world is to provide optimal, effective, and safe patient care. Many people erroneously believe that if they just treat everyone with respect they will avert most cultural problems. An essential requirement for fulfilling the aspiration of skilled culturally sensitive health care is that frontline healthcare providers, such as those in the emergency department (ED), strive to attain ongoing literacy in culturally competent health care. In turn, ED leaders also need to focus on multi-ethnocentric staff development to foster high-quality care. Diversity in patients and in the workforce has significant impacts on patient and system-wide outcomes. It is important for the ED leader to understand these meaningful nuances in order to effectively improve staff productivity, patient care outcomes, and retention of ED staff.

## An anthropologic perspective

The hegemony of the current medical education system has largely marginalized the concepts of social and cultural anthropology as critical aspects of health care.[1,2] The strategy of healthcare education has largely focused on the hard sciences as the core of medical education, with the soft sciences of cultural anthropology and ethnography largely relegated to public health.[3] However, the subject remains important when caring for many different kinds of people, and a basic framework of anthropological definitions is a reasonable vantage point from which to begin.

The first concept is one of generalizations and stereotyping people. These two concepts differ from each other based not on the *content* but on the *usage* of the knowledge.[4] For example, Majid Al Sayyid is a Kuwaiti gentleman, and his German emergency doctor's first thought is, "Mr. Majid is an Arab, so he must have many wives." The doctor is stereotyping. However, if instead he thinks, "Mr. Majid is an Arab, and they often have more than one wife," and then asks Mr. Majid if he has more than one wife currently, then the doctor is generalizing. Stereotypes

---

*Emergency Department Leadership and Management*, ed. Stephanie Kayden, *et al.* Published by Cambridge University Press. © Cambridge University Press 2015.

are fixed, commonly held notions or images of a person or group based on an oversimplification of some observed or imagined trait, behavior, or appearance. Stereotypes do not allow exceptions and reflect rigid counterproductive prejudices that are often derogatory. Stereotyping can be dangerous. A generalization is an idea or statement that places emphasis on general characteristics. Group generalizations are flexible and permeable to new, countervailing, knowledge – ideas, interpretations, and information that challenge or undermine current beliefs.[5]

The journey towards cultural competence involves lessons in appreciating, understanding, and respecting the values and beliefs of others, and then being able to apply the knowledge to provide better care for patients of diverse ethnic backgrounds. Health care delivered in this context can be extremely rewarding, and it adds a pleasurable dimension to the job of the ED healthcare professional. Patients exhibit greater adherence, visible satisfaction, and, ultimately, superior health. There are steps that are required to build the foundation of cultural competency. Each step leads to another, and competency should be sought at each level prior to moving on to the next. This type of incremental learning draws from basic tenets of the field of social anthropology. The first step calls for an exploration of one's own culture, its biases and value system. Second, using this enlightenment as a background, a healthcare provider can acquire knowledge of other cultures and their belief systems. Finally, these two areas of knowledge are reconciled and amalgamated to use in caring for ED patients in an effective manner. It is critically important to remember that cultural adeptness is an ongoing journey and not a final destination.

In today's climate of formalizing and expanding the concept of patient-centered care, it is important to begin with an approach of care that addresses what Slavin called the 4 C's.[4] This technique formalizes the dimensions of an illness from the patient's viewpoint and is especially useful when approaching patients of diversity. The four C's are:

(1) CALL: What do you call your problem? What do you think is wrong? This allows for a patient's interpretation of the problem.
(2) CAUSE: What do you think caused your problem? This allows the patient to review what he or she thinks caused the present state.

(3) COPE: How are you coping with this illness? What have you tried to make yourself feel better? Whom else have you visited for treatment?
(4) CONCERNS: What concerns do you have about this problem? How serious do you think it might be? Does it interfere with your current functioning?

## Patient diversity: looking beyond the vital signs

Language and cultural barriers become critical weak links in providing effective care and achieving positive outcomes in the ED. Patients need to have the right tools to be able to communicate with their providers, and providers, in turn, need the resources and skill sets to be able to deliver care and minimize disparities. EDs that embrace all aspects of diversity provide better care, as patients will be more apt to seek treatment in an environment where communication and trust are enhanced. Expanding the knowledge base for effectively caring for diverse patients in the ED is a continuous process. Using vignettes that arise in the course of patient care and then examining group generalizations within analytical dimensions can help develop culturally competent care.

Within the context of the Tower of Babel of intercultural medical care, it is not too uncommon for language and communication differences to arise and result in communication breakdown. Take for instance the example of a word that sounds the same in two different languages but has two different, sometimes contradictory, meanings.

---

**Case study 33.1**

During a routine discharge from the ED, Gabrielle asked Mr. and Mrs. Venkatesan and their son to reiterate her thorough instructions for aftercare of Mr. Venkatesan's diabetic foot ulcer. She was surprised when they could not repeat anything she had just discussed with them. After all, they smiled and nodded during her entire discourse, and she knew that they spoke English well. Gabrielle later learned from an Indian physician friend that in the South Asian culture dignity and self-esteem are considered extremely important. In such "face cultures,"[6] the preservation of dignity, especially as a group or family unit, is highly important. Thus, the Venkatesan family would rather avoid admitting their lack of understanding of the disease and discharge

---

instructions or, perhaps, Gabrielle's inability to explain things clearly. Gabrielle misunderstood their nodding, smiling and occasional laugh as a sign of understanding. These were just cultural buffers to avoid loss of face and dignity. Additionally, the family did not want Gabrielle to be embarassed because she had not explained the instructions in an understandable way. Gabrielle was perceptive and did the right thing by making them repeat her instructions for clarification. She also addressed and learned from the cultural communication barrier.

### Case study 33.2

Caleb was an eight-year-old boy of orthodox Jewish parents. He presented to the ED with his father complaining of an asthma attack. Shortly after his evaluation by the nurse, the father came out and requested a change in the nurse assignment. Linda, the initial nurse, was confused but respected his wishes and assigned another nurse to care for the little boy. The physician probed the father for the reason behind the nursing change, and the father reported that Linda kept asking Caleb where his "mommy" was, a question he thought was offensive. The physician later discovered that *mami* in Hebrew (which sounds like "mommy") means "sweetheart." Nurses from the Philippines will often call geriatric patients "mama" or "papa," which can be endearing to Middle Eastern patients, yet invasive or rude to patients of Dutch origin.

Patients of different cultural backgrounds can sometimes appear non-compliant with recommendations and appointment times because of cultural beliefs and traditions.

### Case study 33.3

Mr. Kwang, an elderly Chinese man, was seen in the ED and diagnosed with an excacerbation of heart failure. He refused admission, and given that he had responded to treatment in the ED an appointment was arranged for him by Dr. Pamela Jones, the emergency physician, with a reputable cardiologist the next day. However, three days later Mr. Kwang returned to the ED short of breath. It was discovered that he had not attended his appointment with the cardiologist. Further probing by another emergency physician revealed that Mr. Kwang had agreed to the appointment but never intended to go as he felt

better in the ED. However, he did not wish to let Dr. Jones know of his intentions as this would be considered dismissive and openly confronting an authority figure, especially a Caucasian woman. In many Asian cultures, people are taught to be highly accommodative and to avoid confrontational interactions. Being cognizant of this at the time of the appointment, and clearly stating that he would achieve better health and less cost if he kept the appointment, might have been a useful strategy towards compliance.

The communication style and body language of the healthcare provider has tremendous implications to patients of different backgrounds. A quiet, unhurried, but purposeful demeanor and pleasant facial expression is part of normal professional decorum that is particularly reassuring to Southeast Asians and Arabs because it symbolizes characteristics that are highly valued, such as wisdom, good judgment, and dignity. Such a demeanor commands respect, and to many of these people it is critical to the success of the treatment plan.

Correctly addressing the decision maker, who may not be the patient, is also critical. The situation described in Case study 33.4 illustrates the point that when a patient is accompanied by relatives, addressing the patient together with the recognized ultimate decision maker, who could be an eldest son or daughter, is key to communicating diagnosis and care plan. It also creates a communication strategy for the family during their stay. People from Latin American, Asian, Arab, and Native American populations tend to prefer that bad news be discussed with this decision maker, not with the patient.[4] This, in their minds, spares the patient unneccsary stress. Respecting this choice – and also being cognizant of local medicolegal directives regarding this stance – is important.

### Case study 33.4

Mr. Khaled Al Wantaniyah is a 78-year-old Emirati gentleman who is visiting Zurich and presents to the ED. When the patient is brought into the ED with complaints of chest pain, he is seen by Dr. Williams, who conducts the entire care process and discusses the care plan with the patient. The next morning, the patient's eldest son and family register a complaint with the hospital's committee because they are upset about not being made aware of what happened to their father and why he was admitted. Dr. Williams recalls that all of these family members were present in and out of the room in the ED.

An open communication style is often taught in healthcare trainings. This style encourages an almost egalitarian vetting of the medical problem by the patient with the physician to determine the best plan of care. However, this is not acceptable in many cultures. For instance, for many Latino, Arab, and Asian patients, especially older patients, the doctor is the authority figure in the relationship. The doctor is expected to provide strict directives to the patient as to what needs to be done for the condition. A non-directive approach may be viewed by the physician as participatory, while patients of these cultures may view such an approach as meaning that the problem is not serious enough for the doctor to recommend strict action.

Other useful generalizations regarding many Arab and Asian cultures is the preference to be treated by medical providers and intrepretors of the same sex, especially for female patients. Also, many cultures, such as Latinos, Arabs, and Asians, are not accustomed to and resist social worker interventions. In these populations, reliance on family, close friends, and other relatives is preferable to seeking support from a stranger.

The perception of what is effective treatment is also different for different cultures. Using the 4C approach mentioned above is really important in such scenarios.

### Case study 33.5

Mr. Waheed is a 27-year-old Saudi male who presented for sudden, unilateral, sharp back pain. He received oral NSAIDs, an evaluation was negative for renal colic, and the most likely diagnosis was musculoskeletal pain. The nursing notes documented that the patient reported a decrease in his pain scale. Mr. Waheed was given oral NSAIDs to take home and counseled about back care. Upon discharge he complained that the emergency doctor "did not do anything for him." When the situation was explored further, the doctor realized that many patients, especially Arabs and Asians, prefer medical treatment in the ED that involves getting injections – the more intrusive the better – rather than pills and medical counseling.

She realized that the 4C approach upon initial history taking and then clarifying the plan and efficacy of IV, IM, or oral medications would have alleviated much of the stress of the situation.

Another important issue is that of the treatment of pain in the ED. The proper treatment of pain improves outcomes dramatically, but the assessment of the degree of pain is challenging in different ethnicities and cultures. Pain perception and its expression vary. Some cultures value expressiveness, and some value stoicism, in response to pain. Case study 33.6 illustrates the danger of stereotyping. Simply knowing a person's ethnicity is not an accurate prediction of pain response and how it should be managed. ED staff typically find it easier to take care of patients who are stoic and uncomplaining about their pain. They are labeled as "good" patients, while patients who are loud and verbalize their pain are termed "difficult." It is vital to be cognizant of these biases and determine the patient's true concern with a simple question. Another interesting caveat is that in some cultures, pain medication is viewed with suspicion (see Case study 33.7).

### Case study 33.6

Mrs. Guido was a 59-year-old Italian female who presented to the ED after sustaining a type III open left femoral fracture in a motor vehicle accident two hours earlier. She was stabilized with fracture reduction and immobilization by the trauma team. Parenteral opiates were begun using a PCA pump. Meanwhile, Mrs. O'Neill, an Irish woman, was also involved in the same accident and presented with a tibial fracture and shoulder dislocation. Once stabilized, she received a similar pain protocol. The Indian doctor and Jordanian nurse caring for the patient noted that Mrs. Guido constantly whimpered in pain, crying out in Italian frequently. Their comments to each other were that Italian women exaggerated her pain. Her vitals were checked and noted to be stable and, after speaking with the orthopedic team, her basal dose of morphine was adjusted upwards. Mrs. O'Neill was noted to be using her PCA regularly but refused any additional medications and did not call the nurse. As Mrs. Guido was being transferred to the surgical ward, it was noted that her left leg appeared pale and dusky. She was taken to the OR and found to have a near transection of her left femoral artery.

**Case study 33.7**

Mrs. Malik was a 78-year-old Pakistani female with lung cancer metastatic to the bone. She presented to the ED with excacerbation of her pain. Although she was on a hospice program, her family decided to bring her to the ED. It was determined that the family was not giving her morphine as prescribed because they did not want her to get "used to it." Explaining the rationale behind the pain medication, the nature of addiction and palliative care issues ameliorated the problem and the patient went back to her hospice care.

# Workforce diversity: the mosaic workplace

Staff shortages in many countries have led to cross-border staff recruitment. For instance, many nurses and assistants are recruited for North America from the Philippines and India. Physicians from countries where there is strife and limited opportunities for talent development and training relocate to more developed Western countries. These migratory patterns define the tapestry of healthcare providers and workforce diversity seen in healthcare facilities and EDs around the world. Such variety in ED workforce presents a blend of opportunity and challenge for employers. Mechanisms to recruit, manage, and retain staff are viewed by many human resource departments as beset with problems. Once an organizational decision is made to value and promote diversity among staff, the challenge lies in trying to manage this diversity through "systematic and planned commitment ... to recruit, train, reward, and promote a heterogeneous mix of employees."[7]

However ambitious the situation may appear, the necessity of supporting workforce diversity is important within the context of a patient population that reflects or matches the same diversity. The benefits of this approach include a workforce that:

- offers a broad pool of talent
- contributes different viewpoints and perspectives in concepts, initiatives, and decision making
- generates energy and creativity
- better represents and responds to our patients and our colleagues

However, in this environment staff–staff, staff–patient, and staff–administration issues arise that are derived from the diversity itself. It is worthwhile to review some of these scenarios and determine management strategies. Some cultures espouse rigid ideas about the role of the nurse. In many countries there is a visible, uneven hierarchy of the nurse–doctor, female–male relationship. In the countries of Asia, the Middle East, Africa, and the Far East, nurses are not considered part of the healthcare team. Nurses are perceived as helpers, not healthcare professionals, and their suggestions and advice are not taken seriously. Emergency physicians may need to explain the nurse's role to the patient. Additionally, in such cultures nurses with critical thinking skills are not valued, and this is not considered as a job success factor.[4] Nurses are marginalized to be order takers. However, it is a well-accepted fact that patient care and safety is enhanced and improved when nurses are integral and equal members of the team. Furthermore, they need to be able to confidently serve as the patient's advocate. Nurses should also be empowered to act as a patient advocate with confidence.

**Case study 33.8**

Jyoti, originally from India, was an ED nurse working in a US hospital. Jyoti was taking care of a severe asthmatic adult male. Dr. Abeke, a Nigerian and the current ED chief, ordered her to give the patient back-to-back nebulizer treatments. Jyoti noted that the patient was tachycardic with a heart rate of 178 after one treatment. She was afraid to question Dr. Abeke and noted that there was no order to adjust medications in this situation. She also did not feel comfortable advocating for the patient because she felt that she did not know how to open that conversation. Staff training to provide her with the confidence and verbal skills of query in a situation like this would have helped. Jyoti could then have approached Dr. Abeke, keeping in line with clearly demarcated and reciprocal ideas of authority, to present her dilemma, calmly asking for guidance in the current patient situation and what he might recommend if it worsened.

There is a wide variety of viewpoints on how to manage workforce diversity in healthcare settings. The most common are training sessions, subordinates' feedback, performance appraisals, and reward systems.[8] Despite the wide variety of choices, the ED's and the hospital's approach should maintain some common goals. These include fostering staff commitment to diversity, recruiting and empowering nursing staff champions, identifying and rewarding the value of differences.[9] Equally important are the operational changes and governance that empower staff with skill sets that foster effective communication and enhance patient safety. Specific strategies that have proven successful are increasing staff governance, mentorship, setting clear expectations, increasing communication, and increasing staff coaching and education.[10]

# References

1. McElroy JH. *American Beliefs: What Keeps a Big Country and a Diverse People United*. Chicago, IL: Ivan R. Dee, 1999.

2. McElroy A, Townsend PK. *Medical Anthropology in Ecological Perspective*, 2nd edn. Boulder, CO: Westview Press, 1989.

3. Saillant F, Genest S. *Medical Anthropology: Regional Perspectives and Shared Concerns*. Malden, MA: Wiley-Blackwell, 2006.

4. Galanti GA. *Caring for Patients from Different Cultures: Case Studies from American Hospitals*, 2nd edn. Philadelphia, PA: University of Pennsylvania Press, 1997

5. Banks JA, McGee Banks CA, Cortés CE, *et al. Democracy and Diversity: Principles and Concepts for Educating Citizens in a Global Age*. Seattle, WA: University of Washington, 2005.

6. Kim YH, Cohen D. Information, perspective, and judgments about the self in face and dignity cultures. *Personality and Social Psychology Bulletin* 2010; **36**: 537

7. Ivancevich JM, Gilbert JA. Diversity management: time for a new approach. *Public Personnel Management* 2000; **29** (1): 75–92.

8. Wallace PE, Ermer CM, Motshabi DN. Managing diversity: a senior management perspective. *Hospital and Health Services Administration* 1996; **41** (1): 91–104.

9. Spector RE. *Cultural Diversity in Health and Illness*, 6th edn. Upper Saddle River, NJ: Prentice-Hall, 2003.

10. McCullough-Zander K, ed. *Caring Across Cultures: the Provider's Guide to Cross-Cultural Health*, 2nd edn. Minneapolis, MN: Center for Cross-Cultural Health, 2000.

# Index

Printed in the United States
By Bookmasters